Food and Public Health

Food and Public Health

A Practical Introduction

Edited by
ALLISON KARPYN

Oxford University Press is a department of the University of Oxford. It furthers
the University's objective of excellence in research, scholarship, and education
by publishing worldwide. Oxford is a registered trade mark of Oxford University
Press in the UK and certain other countries.

Published in the United States of America by Oxford University Press
198 Madison Avenue, New York, NY 10016, United States of America.

© Oxford University Press 2018

Library of Congress Cataloging-in-Publication Data
Names: Karpyn, Allison, editor.
Title: Food and public health : a practical introduction / [edited by] Allison Karpyn.
Other titles: Food and public health (Karpyn)
Description: New York : Oxford University Press, [2018] |
Includes bibliographical references and index.
Identifiers: LCCN 2018006822 | ISBN 9780190626686 (pbk. : alk. paper)
Subjects: | MESH: Food Industry | Diet | Health Policy | United States
Classification: LCC HD9000.6 | NLM WA 695 | DDC 338.1/9—dc23
LC record available at https://lccn.loc.gov/2018006822

9 8 7 6 5 4 3 2 1

Printed by Sheridan Books, Inc., United States of America

Contents

Preface   vii

Acknowledgments   xi

Contributors   xiii

1. The History of Food and Public Health   1
   Emily Contois and Anastasia Day

2. History and Development of the 2015–2020 Dietary Guidelines
   for Americans   31
   Alice H. Lichtenstein and Allison Karpyn

3. Behavioral Design as an Emerging Theory for Dietary
   Behavior Change   47
   NCCOR Behavioral Design Working Group

4. Health Disparities: Race, Ethnicity, Gender, and Class   83
   Alison G.M. Brown and Sara C. Folta

5. Healthy Food Marketing   125
   Allison Karpyn

6. Policy Efforts Supporting Healthy Diets for Adults and Children   141
   *Courtney A. Parks, Eric E. Calloway, Teresa M. Smith,
   and Amy L. Yaroch*

7. Food Insecurity and Public Health   171
   Molly Knowles, Joanna Simmons, and Mariana Chilton

8. Obesogenic Environments and Public Health Mitigation Strategies   209
   Allison Karpyn

9. Food Controversies: The Healthy Pulse of a Democracy?   225
F. Bailey Norwood

10. The Obesity Pandemic and Food Insecurity in Developing
Countries: A Case Study from the Caribbean   255
Kristen Lowitt, Katherine Gray-Donald, Gordon M. Hickey,
Arlette Saint Ville, Isabella Francis-Granderson,
Chandra A. Madramootoo, and Leroy E. Phillip

11. Intersections of Food and Culture: Case Studies of Sugar and Meat
from Australia, Japan, Thailand, and Nigeria   281
Wakako Takeda, Cathy Banwell, Kelebogile T. Setiloane,
and Melissa K. Melby

12. From Soil to Stomach: Agritourism and Public Health   317
Erecia Hepburn and Allison Karpyn

Appendix: Answers to Quiz Questions   345
About the Editor   349
Index   351

Preface

Dietary issues, food policy, and obesity have received significant attention in the past 10 years while at the very same time public health programs have expanded dramatically. Each year, more than 26,000 students are enrolled in public health programs, creating a need for an introductory, comprehensive text on the topic of Food and Public Health. Our goal was to create a teacher-friendly textbook for students in public health or nutrition, though it also may be appropriate for seminars in other disciplines. Chapters are designed to stimulate discussion and create a platform for classroom activities and in-depth writing or research assignments.

In alignment with best practices in public health, the text focuses heavily on how facets of our food systems, cultures, and the policies that guide them inform diets in the United States and around the world.

Chapter 1 provides an introduction to the food system nested within the context of the history of food and public health. From food production to processing to consumption we provide a review of how the World Wars, urbanization, and modernization of the U.S. food system have shaped food safety, price, and availability. Authors also consider the role that consumer culture has had on our dietary habits, including the value placed on cookbooks, home economics, advertising, and a host of food media, from magazines and radio to blogs and social media. Finally, authors reflect on the history of the National School Lunch Program and use it as an example of how food production, processing, consumption, and policy converge.

Building on the brief discussion in Chapter 1, Chapter 2 provides a deep dive into the evolution of the dietary guidelines for Americans with a focus on changes over the past 40 years. Often with controversy, the evolution from Dietary Goals in 1977 to the 2015 Dietary Guidelines for Americans reflects a shift to recognizing the importance of the whole diet and how a variety of eating patterns can support good nutrition. Topics include concrete reporting on recommendations as well as a discussion of controversies borne by industry, lobbying groups, and government mandates.

In Chapter 3, authors review the core theories of health behavior for dietary change, while advancing new ideas about how the interaction between the individual and his/her environment creates our experience. Drawing from environmental psychology and behavioral design, authors integrate our newest understandings of human behavior within the context of the built and designed environments in which we live, work, play, and grow.

Chapter 4 provides an in-depth discussion of the ways in which food and health disparities have materialized. The chapter offers new perspectives on the importance of how disparities interact with race and class.

In Chapter 5, we discuss food marketing. The chapter summarizes the newer ways in which online marketing is taking shape via services like YouTube, which have unveiled a flurry of unregulated activities intended to influence youth perceptions of packaged foods. Organized in two parts, we begin with a review of recent efforts to curb unhealthy marketing to kids and then proceed to discuss current efforts to apply marketing strategies for health promotion. Topics include strategies to address healthy food purchases in the supermarket and in the school cafeteria.

Policy efforts that support healthy diets for adults and children are the focus of Chapter 6. Authors emphasize how policy-level action can result in impactful strategies to improve dietary behaviors and strengthen food environments. Policy levers such as taxation and regulation of businesses are discussed as important examples of the ways in which individual behavior change can be impacted by state and local policy. Authors review specific legislation, including the Healthy Hunger Free Kids (GMOs).

Food insecurity, the lack of access to enough food for an active and healthy life, is the cornerstone of Chapter 7. With a strong emphasis on the importance of a human rights approach to food, authors call for better food policy that more effectively recognizes the systemic structural inequalities that drive disparities in food insecurity, including discrimination against people of color, LGBTQ people, immigrants, people with disabilities, and women.

Chapter 8 provides an overview of the ways in which obesogenic environments can shape our food decisions. By looking at a variety of food environments and health policies intended to foster better nutrition, the chapter provides a succinct and informative overview of the building blocks of our modern nutrition environments.

From fights over access to food to debates about GMOs, food controversies abound. Chapter 9 explores how controversies persist due to insufficient facts to resolve them. It further sheds light on how a single controversy can actually be a proxy war over much bigger issues, and brings into our awareness ways we confuse specific policies with social movements. As readers we are led to re-think how and what shapes our opinions of food and to think more critically about the role of science in decision-making.

The last three chapters consider global challenges in food and public health. Beginning with a review of the obesity pandemic and food insecurity in developing countries, Chapter 10 reviews global trends in obesity and reflects on the impacts that a worldwide agri-food system is having. Public health professionals are called to recognize how global shifts have perpetuated and in many cases accelerated a "double burden of malnutrition." The chapter concludes with an overview of food security and obesity challenges facing the Caribbean Community (CARICOM) and profiles a "farm to fork" school feeding project in the island nation of St. Kitts-Nevis that was designed to reduce obesity and improve food security among children.

Chapter 11 considers the ways in which food and culture intersect by examining four case studies based in Thailand, Australia, Japan, and Nigeria. Around the world, culture influences food preferences and at the same time foods often are used to convey cultural values—such as convenience and modernity, urban lifestyle, hospitality, socialization, and moral education for children. Together these factors have implications for public health interventions and policies yet collectively require a locally nuanced understanding of culture.

We finish the text with Chapter 12 which focuses on agritourism, a novel but expanding approach to creating jobs and supporting small farms. Such efforts breathe new life into our global understanding of the connections between health and agriculture, all while supporting economic development for the worlds' most vulnerable populations.

In order to facilitate classroom discussions and teacher assessments of reading, the book begins each chapter with a bulleted synopsis of its key features. Further, at the end of each chapter, discussion and quiz questions are provided. Last, we have emphasized real-world examples and brought many global issues and strategies to the forefront. Although grounded more in U.S. policy than international, the text is intended to provide an understanding of food in public health which steps beyond the U.S. landscape into issues facing residents of nations across the globe.

Acknowledgments

To my beautiful and hilarious girls Lauren and Anna, I am particularly appreciative for your love and encouragement. My journey through this work was a result of many long nights and days, and I appreciate your support even though it required time away from you. And to my parents who have always supported me, I can't thank you enough for your always open arms in times of need.

Hillary O'Conner, thank you for your careful comments, dedication, and care for me and my family throughout the final stages of this book. Luci, your incredible heart and can-do, just get-it-done spirit has been a source of strength for me, and I cannot thank you enough. Andrea, Carrie, Liz, Fernando, Sarah, Jeanne, Leazona, David, and Shaun, thank you, too, for providing me inspiration an outlet to vent, new perspectives, a quick morning run, cup of coffee or cocktail, hug, wise word, or laugh.

I also would like to thank my University of Delaware family, including Henry May and Bahira Trask. Without your leadership, flexibility, and encouragement, this book would not have been possible. Tara and Layne, I know that in my long days and nights you kept the Center for Research in Education and Social Policy and all our research organized and moving forward, and I want to express my gratitude. Nicole Filion, your early support and incredible efficiency made working through the early phases of this book a breeze. Thank you.

Karen Glanz, I am deeply appreciative of your mentorship throughout the years. Your friendship, leadership, and downright brilliance have inspired me to believe I can make a difference in the world of food and public health.

And finally, to one of the best organizations on the planet, The Food Trust. Yael, John, and so many others, you have been a constant source of knowledge and inspiration and have given me the courage and environment to dive deep into the world of food and public health—but taught me to do so with care. Your support and advice have meant the world to me.

And to anyone I should have mentioned but neglected, please forgive me!

Contributors

Cathy Banwell, PhD
Associate Professor
National Centre for Epidemiology
  and Population Health
Research School of
  Population Health
Australian National University
Canberra
Australia

Alison G.M. Brown, PhD, MS
Post-Doctoral Fellow
Tufts Clinical and Translational
  Science Institute
Tufts Medical Center
Boston, Massachusetts

Eric E. Calloway, PhD, RD
Research Scientist
Gretchen Swanson Center for
  Nutrition
Omaha, Nebraska

Mariana Chilton, PhD, MPH
Professor
Department of Health Management
  and Policy
Drexel University
Dornsife School of Public Health
Philadelphia, Pennsylvania

Emily Contois, MA, MLA, MPH
PhD Candidate
American Studies
Brown University
Providence, Rhode Island

Anastasia Day, MA
Hagley Scholar and PhD Candidate,
  History
University of Delaware
Newark, Delaware

Sara C. Folta, PhD
Associate Professor
Nutrition
Friedman School of Nutrition
  Science and Policy
Tufts University
Boston, Massachusetts

Isabella Francis-Granderson, PhD
Department of Agricultural
  Economics and Extension
The University of the West Indies
St. Augustine, Trinidad and Tobago

Katherine Gray-Donald, PhD
Associate Professor (Retired)
School of Dietetics and Human
    Nutrition
McGill University
Ste-Anne-de-Bellevue, Quebec
Canada

Erecia Hepburn, PhD
Assistant Professor
Department of Biology
School of Chemistry and
    Environmental Life Sciences
University of the Bahamas
Nassau
The Bahamas

Gordon M. Hickey, PhD
Associate Professor
Department of Natural Resource
    Sciences
McGill University
Ste-Anne-de-Bellevue, Quebec
Canada

Molly Knowles, MPH
Research Manager
Department of Health Management
    and Policy
Drexel University
Dornsife School of Public Health
Philadelphia, Pennsylvania

Alice H. Lichtenstein, DSc
Gershoff Professor of Nutrition
    Science and Policy
Director and Senior Scientist,
    Cardiovascular Nutrition
    Laboratory
Tufts University
Boston, Massachusetts

Kristen Lowitt, PhD
Post-Doctoral Fellow
Department of Natural Resource
    Sciences
McGill University
Ste-Anne-de-Bellevue, Quebec
Canada

**Chandra A. Madramootoo,
PhD, P. Eng**
James McGill Professor
Bioresource Engineering
    Department
Faculty of Agricultural and
    Environmental Sciences
McGill University
Ste. Anne de Bellevue, Quebec
Canada

Melissa K. Melby, PhD
Associate Professor
Department of Anthropology
College of Health Sciences
University of Delaware
Newark, Delaware

F. Bailey Norwood, PhD
Professor
Department of Agricultural
    Economics
Oklahoma State University
Stillwater, Oklahoma

Leroy E. Phillip, PhD
Associate Professor (Retired)
Department of Animal Science
McGill University
Ste-Anne-de-Bellevue, Quebec
Canada

Courtney A. Parks, PhD
Senior Research Scientist
Gretchen Swanson Center for
   Nutrition
Omaha, Nebraska

Kelebogile T. Setiloane, PhD
Associate Professor
Department of Behavioral Health &
   Nutrition
University of Delaware
Newark, Delaware

Joanna Simmons
Member
Witnesses to Hunger
Penns Grove, New Jersey

Teresa M. Smith, PhD
Research Scientist
Gretchen Swanson Center for
   Nutrition
Omaha, Nebraska

Wakako Takeda, PhD
Lecturer
Institute for Population and Social
   Research
Mahidol University
Salaya, Nakhon Pathom
Thailand

Arlette Saint Ville, PhD
Department of Natural Resource
   Sciences
McGill University
Ste-Anne-de-Bellevue, Quebec
Canada

Amy L. Yaroch, PhD
Executive Director
Gretchen Swanson Center for
   Nutrition
Omaha, Nebraska

The History of Food and Public Health

Emily Contois and Anastasia Day

Chapter Highlights

- What should we eat to be healthy, and who decides?
- How does food make its way from farm to plate—and beyond?
- Are we what we eat?

This chapter considers questions like these as it focuses on four significant aspects of food and public health in the United States that have shifted over the last century. These transitions have profoundly shaped today's food system, food culture, and the health of the American people. First, the chapter addresses agricultural production. Urbanization, modernization, mechanization, and corporatization reconfigured food production, as did historical events such as the World Wars, the Dust Bowl, the Green Revolution, and the organic food movement. Secondly, the chapter tells the story of how our food system was industrialized. Innovations in transportation, preservation, retail, and packaging fostered a globalized food system that provided both opportunities and challenges for promoting food safety, nutrition, food access, and health. Third, the chapter chronicles the evolution of federal dietary guidelines and how they have navigated the relationship between scientific research, the food industry, consumer desires, and public health goals. Lastly, the chapter explores how the consumer culture has served as a complement and an antagonist to government dietary advice. Cookbooks, home economics, modern advertising, magazines, radio, television, celebrity chefs, blogs, and social media have all shaped what and how Americans eat.

Overall, these histories of agricultural production, the industrialization of food, dietary advice, and the consumer culture inform how today's students of food and public health understand the past, consider today's public health problems and solutions, and envision the future of food and public health.

Food Production: Agriculture And Gardens

At the dawn of the 20th century, the United States was a nation of farmers: just over 40% of Americans cultivated 37% of the land.[1] Sharecropping, a practice where farmers rented land in return for a share of the crops they raised on it, dominated huge swathes of the country, especially in the South where African Americans farmed plantations previously run on slave labor. By the dawn of the 21st century, farmers constituted 1% of the population cultivating 40% of the land.[2] Machines and migrant workers have replaced sharecropping as a system for procuring agricultural labor. This century-long transformation in agriculture forms the first link in the story of the nation's food supply, nutrition levels, and dietary habits.[3] Understanding the history of American nutritional policy begins with examining the supply and availability of various food crops.

War Reveals a "Backward" Agriculture

During World War I, American farmers grew as much food as possible to feed not only the domestic population, but also U.S. allies around the globe. Off the farm, a movement for citizens to produce their own wartime food captured the public imagination. Unlike in the subsequent war, however, the National War Garden Commission boasted a mere 5 million gardens.[4] At war's end, American farmers found themselves with too much product and falling demand; wartime loans to invest in more land and tools could not be repaid from the sales of their produce. Foreclosures swept the rural parts of the nation, seeming proof of farmers' inability to adapt to the modern era.[5]

In the 1920s, it became a national priority to help the so-called backward farmers of the nation avoid similar agricultural economic crises in the future. Agricultural modernizers in the United States Department of Agriculture (USDA) looked to industry and private business as models, endorsing standardization, mass production, elimination of skilled labor, and scientific methodology. Farmers were urged to adopt new technologies, including many that had been developed for the war.[6]

War had birthed an industry using the Haber process to fix nitrogen, creating ammonia. In the interwar period, this invention fostered a boom in synthetic fertilizer production and use.[7] Simultaneously, self-powered farming machinery made its debut. Henry Ford's Fordson tractor in 1917 marked the introduction of an internal-combustion engine to farming, followed shortly by threshers, combines, and pickers. The 1920s and 1930s also brought advances in plant biotechnology. USDA scientists created the first commercial hybrid seeds in the 1920s, leading to crops boasting greater yields, more standard fruit, and resistance to disease.[8]

Disaster Breeds a New Political Economy

The 1930s brought both the Great Depression and the Dust Bowl. The latter ravaged the southern plains of the United States, blowing away millions of cubic feet of topsoil in dust storms dense enough to block out the sun. Old World food crops such as wheat and potatoes, though staples of what Euro-Americans considered healthy diets, failed to hold the soil in place as drought-resistant indigenous grasses had for centuries previous. Industrial cultivation techniques like the plow, combined with annual crops instead of perennial flora, failed to replenish soil fertility while exposing bare topsoil to the wind every year. The result was colossal dust storms.[9]

Sharecropping peaked at the start of this decade; for example, in Tennessee sharecroppers worked one-third of all farms in the state.[10] Sharecroppers and homesteaders in the Dust Bowl states migrated westward in huge numbers, many going to work as hired labor on the still-flourishing fruit and vegetable farms of California. Black sharecroppers of the South, large numbers of whom had been moving northward since World War I in a movement known as the Great Migration, left for cities in the North. Many sharecroppers, however, white and black alike, found themselves too poor to finance the journey; stuck in place in a time of poverty and crises, sharecroppers organized into labor unions throughout the 1930s, culminating in the 1939 Missouri Sharecroppers Roadside Demonstration where over a thousand (mostly African American) sharecroppers camped out on major highways to protest mass evictions.[11]

In response to the twin crises of economy and agriculture, President Franklin Delano Roosevelt launched the New Deal, one plank of which was the "ever-normal granary." According to this plan, new federal entities, like the Agricultural Adjustment Administration (AAA) and the Commodity Credit Corporation (CCC), would buy surplus agricultural commodities when prices were low and sell when prices were high. This market manipulation would theoretically stabilize both consumer costs and farmer incomes.[12] This program was limited, however, to commodity crops such as wheat, soybeans, rice, and corn, as well as meat and dairy products. The American government would continue to aid farmers using production control, marketing aid, price-supporting loans, and direct income payments for the rest of the century. From this point on, ideas about what was healthy for Americans to eat would include considerations of what was economically healthy for the American farmer—represented by highly partisan farm lobby groups—under federal subsidy regimes.[13]

Conventional Agriculture Grows Victory

By 1941 more than a third of gross farm income came from payment for participation in federal agricultural programs.[14] That year's Lend-Lease Act shipped millions of dollars of agricultural products overseas as the United States joined World War II. With this outlet for surplus and the impetus of war, national food production increased 30% over prewar rates despite little expansion of crop land, a shortage of labor, and rationing of gas, machinery, and fertilizers.[15] A home food-production movement flourished in tandem; in 1943, "Victory Gardens" produced 42% of the fresh produce Americans consumed that year.[16] Government propaganda suggested homegrown vegetables might contain more nutritional value than store-bought, keeping Americans strong for the fight against the Axis (see Figure 1.1). Where farms might once have cultivated fields with a multitude of plant species, farmers shifted more toward commodity crops grown over many acres, or monoculture farming. American citizens then grew the varied fruits and vegetables necessary for healthy diets. The United States emerged as a postwar superpower due in no small part to its prodigious food production; Europe's farmland was one of the many victims of war.[17]

In the postwar era, subsidies continued to grow: By 1960 the CCC spent $7.7 billion dollars on agricultural products.[18] Fueled by this artificial market incentive, farmers increased production through new technologies. When fewer youth returned to farms than left them during the war (either for jobs or military service), farmers continued substituting machines for human labor. They sprayed a new generation of organophosphate pesticides, as well as chlorinated hydrocarbons such as DDT, developed for the recent war. Farmers

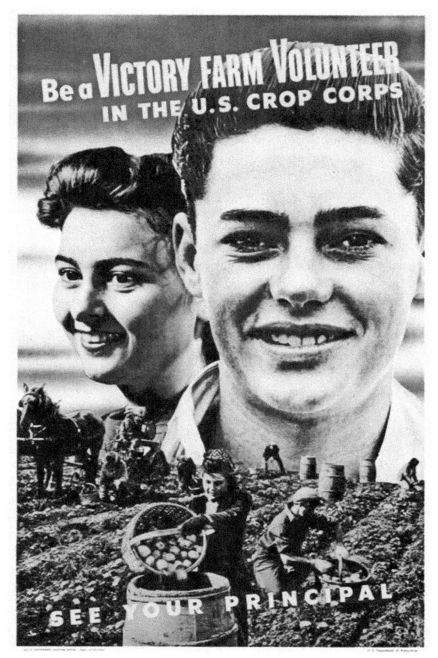

FIGURE 1.1 This 1943 poster worked to recruit youth to be victory gardeners and farmers.
http://www.idaillinois.org/cdm/ref/collection/isl5/id/38

also applied synthetic fertilizers to their fields, installed new automated feeding systems, and supplemented livestock feed with hormones and antibiotics. All these inputs increased overhead and operating costs, as well as risks to consumer health.[19] The financial pressures hit labor the hardest: Between mechanization and migration to cities, sharecropping was effectively eliminated in the 1940s and 1950s. To replace the labor of sharecroppers in jobs that couldn't be mechanized, farmers increasingly turned to immigrant and migrant labor that would work for little money. This had begun with the *Bracero* Program in 1942, where Mexican workers came to work on farms in the United States during the labor shortage of World War II, but the program reached its height only after the war was over. By the time the program ended in 1964, over 5 million Mexican workers had been brought to the United States as agricultural laborers.[20]

Despite the cheaper cost of labor, with higher total capital requirements came the collapse of family-operated farms with smaller acreage and the consolidation of U.S. agribusiness. In Iowa, for example, farmers almost halved in number from 1945 to 1970; yet the state still nearly doubled agricultural output while marginally decreasing acreage.[21] The national corporate agricultural interests profited from large-scale production of the same commodity crops that had been subsidized since the New Deal: as a result, American diets shrank in diversity while scientists developed more non-food uses for crops such as soy and corn to keep prices high.

Agricultural Critiques and Contested Futures

In this same postwar period of growth and consolidation, critiques of industrial agriculture based in environmental and health concerns flourished. Attacks on industrial farming entered mainstream American thought through figures such as J. I. Rodale, an organic farming advocate, and Rachel Carson, author of the 1962 bestseller *Silent Spring*.[22] Exposés of noxious algae blooms from fertilizer run-off, water tables tainted with pesticides, and cancer in the bodies of agricultural workers sent some people scurrying back to the land.[23] Most Americans, however, continued to leave agriculture to a shrinking number of farmers as land prices rose, threatened by suburban sprawl. A few of these Americans chose the middle ground of patronizing a growing selection of vegetarian, whole-grain, "natural," and organic foods at the grocery store.[24]

This tension continues in the 21st century. New technologies continue to fuel the productivity, profitability, and controversy of "conventional" agriculture, most prominent among these being genetically modified organisms (GMOs). Although GMOs have the potential to increase the nutritional value of foods, as in "Golden Rice" containing beta-carotene, some organic advocates maintain that organic foods have higher nutritional values.[25] New scholarship also illustrates the dangers of conventional agriculture for the environment, for agricultural labor, and for local economies, as well as for the planet through its relationship to climate change.[26] Farmers are now businessmen, while the agricultural laborers in fields are often abused and underpaid minorities: the USDA National Agricultural Worker survey found that 70% of farm workers in 2010 were born in Mexico, two-thirds spoke little or no English, and half were unauthorized immigrants. On the other hand, the organic agriculture industry has now industrialized, corporatized, and consolidated. Holdovers from the 1960s including local food movements, urban agriculture, and Community-Supported-Agriculture endeavors represent alternatives to both "Conventional Agriculture" and "Big Organic" for 21st-century consumers.

Commodification and Processing: The Industrialization of Food

Throughout the 20th century, the vast majority of Americans have not received their food directly from farms complete with dirt, blemishes, and a lack of preservation or packaging. However, the ways of processing food on its way from farm to table have changed radically from 1900 to the present day. Food processing developed in tandem with the industrial commodification of food, spurred by technological advances as well as social changes and values like convenience. At the same time, nutrition has been central to national discussions about processed foods, even if only through sanitation or purity concerns.

Regulation and Standardization

In 1906, Upton Sinclair published *The Jungle*: a best-selling exposé of the dangerous and unsanitary conditions in Chicago meatpacking plants (see Figure 1.2). Before the year was out, Congress passed the Pure Food and Drug Act, which required listing active ingredients on all food products, inspecting said products, and creating a bureau that in 1930 would be renamed the Food and Drug Administration, or FDA. In so doing, the Act promoted consumer faith in packaged foods, now with guaranteed federal oversight.

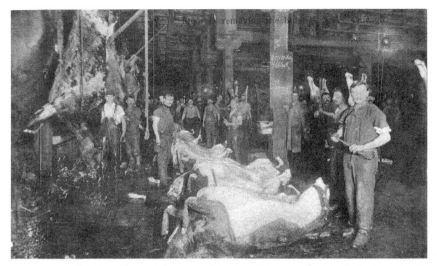

FIGURE 1.2 *The Jungle* revealed meatpacking conditions such as those depicted in this photograph in Chicago in the early 20th century.

https://en.wikipedia.org/wiki/File:Floorers_removing_the_hides_USY_Chicago_(front).tiff

This inadvertently pushed many local and non-industrial food processors out of business unless they wished to confine their activities within state lines.[27] The act also formalized the first stage of American food commodification: food became a fungible commodity. Rather than flour from Farmer Brown's southern field, for instance, consumers now bought flour made of wheat from many farms mixed into a homogenous product and sorted into grades according to government standards.[28]

Trust in Brands for Purity

Purity was a touchstone issue in the early 20th century.[29] As the chains linking food from farm to plate grew longer, consumers knew less about the food they purchased. Ignorance sparked fear and rumors, such as a rumor of bakers mixing plaster and sawdust into their bread flour. It was in this era that consumers learned to expect standard, unvarying, and trustworthy food products from national brands boasting reliable quality. In the 1910s and 1920s, the first national chain grocery retailers emerged, both fostering and pandering to these fears and beliefs.[30] This marks the second stage of food commodification: homogenous and standardized food products differentiated by brand name and distinct packaging.[31]

World War I accelerated this process. Stupendous growth in rail transportation capabilities nationalized food systems as never before. Cattle raised in Texas, then butchered and packed in the Midwest, were sold at delicatessen counters in neatly wrapped selections of rib or sirloin bearing the same brand trademark across the country.[32] Canned vegetables, soups, and other pre-cooked foods, previously considered unpalatable at best, were shipped to soldiers; only these heavily processed foods would keep through changes in temperature, humidity, time, and travel overseas.

Inventing New Foodstuffs

The final stage of American food commodification was technological, creating new products out of familiar foodstuffs. Through President Franklin Roosevelt's New Deal, government economic aid helped farmers remain on the land even though they continued to produce price-depressing surpluses of cotton, wheat, dairy products, and meat. This fueled research into how to reinvent these commodities, incorporating them into products new and old. Government scientists also worked with their industry counterparts to advance the science and use of synthetic flavorings, colorings, "enriching" vitamins, and other food additives. Jell-O represents the culmination of these trends. While aspics made from bone broth dated back centuries, the 1930s brought a craze for congealed foods made with powdered gelatin. Jell-O was industrially produced, synthetically flavored, and artificially colored. It was also made from surplus agricultural products: the bones and connective tissues of butchered animals discarded by meatpackers.[33] Thus, by the end of the Great Depression, once-simple agricultural crops had been homogenized, branded, and technologically reinvented: all three steps of the industrial commodification and processing of food were complete.

Processing for War

With the U.S. entry into the Second World War, the government became the nation's largest buyer of foodstuffs, with big implications for processors and distributors.[34] Food destined for soldiers and allies overseas needed to be stable for travel as in the First World War, but also to conserve materials scarce in the current war. New industrial drying technologies allowed powdered products such as dehydrated eggs to travel the world with little space and weight. The government ordered frozen foods en masse, which saved tin used for canned foods. Canned food sales also grew. For instance, Spam, a canned spiced ham product invented in 1937, was initially a regional curiosity; then the U.S. Army purchased 150 million pounds of it.[35] By war's end, Spam was a global product.

Food distribution also changed domestically in ways that favored processors. Under the War Food Administration, government attempts to coordinate a national food supply favored large chains and supermarkets that could afford staff to navigate red tape. Many independent, local, and ethnic grocers went out of business. Large corporate grocers were more likely to buy processed foods in bulk from other large food processors. With all these changes, per capita processed food production increased from 1940 to 1945 almost as much as it had over 1910–1940.[36]

TV Dinners Galore

Americans happily abandoned many wartime products (such as dried eggs) in the immediate postwar years. Nonetheless, they were more open to processed foods. Companies with colossal investments in food processing facilities took advantage of this nonchalance, leading to a renaissance of prepared and processed foods in the 1950s and 1960s. Middle-class mothers were more amenable to the ease and speed of prepared foods. Working in increasing numbers, women found their time was better spent on the clock than slaving away at the stovetop. Cake mixes provided married women a way to take pride in "home-baked" desserts for their families with a minimum of effort.[37]

Just as the world wars prompted advances in food processing, the Cold War space race fueled innovation. The 1959 introduction of Tang, a nutritionally lacking but tasty simulacrum of orange juice, was a failing product until the National Aeronautics and Space Administration (NASA) supplied astronaut John Glenn with some to drink in space in 1962, after which it became a national craze. Eating like astronauts was a more appealing pitch than eating like a soldier in a foxhole. As a result, processed foods of all types incorporated space explorations into their marketing in this decade.

It was not until the 1970s that Americans embraced frozen foods, in part because of lack of home freezers, undesirable textures upon reheating, and distrust of unfamiliar products.[38] Selling new products, such as frozen TV dinners, necessitated extended investment in marketing and promotions until consumers gave the product a chance. This need for capital contributed to the centralization of the food processing industry in the late 20th century.[39]

Backlash Against Processing and Health Concerns

Radicals of the 1960s critiqued processed American foodways. The counter-cuisine movement called prepared foods "plastic" and "unnatural," as well as nutritionally lacking. They proposed that Americans reconnect with their food through home preparation: baking sourdough whole wheat bread from scratch instead of buying white flour Wonderbread from national grocery chains, for example. Part of this movement was anti-corporate with calls for transparency in the food system. Counterculture concerns also were linked to fears that over-processing was stripping the nutritional content from the American diet.[40] These concerns went mainstream with diet cultures of the 1980s and 1990s; crazes such as the Atkins Diet and Sugar Busters Diet inevitably blamed processed foods for weight gain and poor health. This strain of distrust continues into the 21st century. Municipalities debate soda taxes in the name of public health, even as processed foods remain the backbone of the American diet.[41]

Dietary Guidelines: Nutrition Science, Food Policy, and the American Diet

Addressing minimally and ultra-processed foods alike, dietary guidelines first came about in the late-19th century.[42]

The First Food Guidelines, 1890s–1930s

The first U.S. food guidelines resulted from research conducted by Wilbur O. Atwater. Commonly referred to as "the father of American nutrition," he was the first director of the Office of Experiment Stations at the USDA.[43] Using cutting-edge technology like calorimeters, Atwater researched food composition, identifying the amount of energy (number of calories) contained in macronutrients—carbohydrate, fat, and protein. He also calculated the number of calories required for healthy sustenance, warning of the dangers of inadequate energy intake, as well as "the evils of overeating." Atwater published his findings in 1894 in the USDA's *Farmer's Bulletin*.[44] Although vitamins and specific minerals had yet to be isolated, his research formed the foundation of human nutrition science in the United States, as well as the content of the first published food guides.

In 1916, home economist Caroline Hunt published the first USDA food guide, *Food for Young Children*.[45] Recognizing—as maternal and child health initiatives do today—the importance of child nutrition, the guide instructed mothers on what and how much to feed children between the ages of three and six years. The guide promoted milk as one of the most important foods for children and included five food groups: milk and meat, bread and cereals, butter and wholesome fats, produce, and sweets. Aiming to sustain child health with foods that children would like, Hunt's guide urged mothers to "carefully prepare" and "attractively serve" foods. For example, the recipe for "Floating Island" is made with hearty ingredients such as eggs and milk, but is "decorated with small bits of jelly" to appeal to children visually and add a touch of sweetness. With Atwater's daughter, Helen Woodard Atwater, Hunt published *How to Select Foods* in 1917, which presented these food groups for both child and adult consumption.[46]

Early food guides presented the most recent scientific findings to specialists and to the public, including vitamin discoveries in the 1910s, 1920s, and 1930s. These scientific advancements are why some call the 20th century "The Golden Age of Nutrition Science."[47] Indeed, vitamin discoveries reoriented the science, earned 17 Nobel Prizes, and incited "vitamania" among the public, who were thrilled by the field's newfound abilities to address micronutrient deficiencies.[48]

Food guides also responded to the realities of American life. For example, during the economic hardship of the Depression, USDA head food economist, Hazel Stiebeling, developed food plans designed to meet nutrient needs at four incremental cost levels, depending upon a family's income.[49]

Foundation Diets to Eat Enough: 1940s to 1960s

In the 1940s, the USDA drafted the nation's first official government food guidelines. To ensure a well-nourished armed services and a productive citizenry, the Food and Nutrition Board of the National Academy of Sciences released in 1941 the first set of Recommended Dietary Allowances (RDAs). The RDAs sought to establish recommended intakes for calories and nine essential nutrients: protein, iron, calcium, vitamins A and D, thiamin, riboflavin, niacin, and ascorbic acid (vitamin C).[50] Based on the RDAs, the USDA published the "Basic Seven" food guide (see Figure 1.3). It was released as the *National Wartime Nutrition Guide* in 1943 to assist citizens to eat well even when certain goods were rationed or scarce. After the end of the war, the USDA revised the Basic Seven resource and published it as *The National Food Guide*.[51]

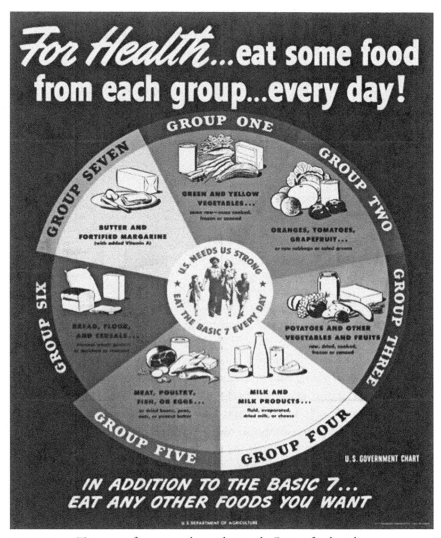

FIGURE 1.3 This poster from around 1945 depicts the Basic 7 food guide.
Records of the Office of Government Reports, RG 44; https://www.flickr.com/photos/usnation-alarchives/5589176479/in/album-72157626120220831/.

In 1956, *Food for Fitness–A Daily Food Guide*, popularly known as the "Basic Four," replaced the Basic Seven.[52] This guide recommended a minimum number of daily servings from four food groups: "some milk for everyone" (ranging from two to four or more servings depending upon one's age), two or more servings from the meat group, and four or more servings from both the fruits and vegetables group and the bread and cereal group. Outlasting all food guides, the Basic Four guided nutritional thought and policy for two decades.

Like previous guides, the Basic Four was a "foundation diet," encouraging consumption of enough nutritious foods to promote good health, while still liberally allowing for additional foods. For example, the Basic Seven endorsed, "In addition to the basic 7, eat any other foods you want," and the Basic Four concluded by stating, "Plus other foods as needed to complete meals and to provide additional food energy and other food values." These guides promoted nutrition messages about whole foods—"Eat green and yellow vegetables"—rather than quantified nutrient intakes, such as "Consume less than 300 mg per day of dietary cholesterol."

Nutrient-Based Food Guidelines to Combat Chronic Disease, 1970s to Present

Published in February 1977, the *Dietary Goals for the United States* reoriented the emphasis of dietary guidelines, as public health initiatives shifted focus from infectious diseases to chronic conditions. Unlike previous guidelines, which promoted consuming an adequate diet and enough food, new guidelines promoted avoiding excessive intake of the nutrients that appeared to be linked to chronic disease risk and body weight. Developed by the Senate Select Committee on Nutrition and Human Needs, the Dietary Goals set quantitative goals for the consumption of protein, carbohydrate, fat, fatty acids, cholesterol, sugars, and sodium. To communicate these recommendations to the public, the Committee published the *Hassle-Free Daily Food Guide* in 1979, which added an additional group of foods with low nutrient density to avoid—fat, sweets, and alcohol.[53] A yellow caution sign marked this group in the guide, marking a shift in how the government framed food consumption to the public and the connections between food, health, weight, and disease.

Emphasizing efforts to curb excessive consumption and focusing on specific nutrients, the USDA first published the *Dietary Guidelines for Americans* in 1980.[54] Every five years since then, the Dietary Guidelines Advisory Committee—a group composed of nutrition experts from both within and outside of government—has reviewed and revised the guidelines in light of published research, a review process mandated by federal law since 1990. The guidelines have wide-ranging effects, as they guide nutrition education, programs, and policies such as school food programs, Supplemental Nutritional Assistance Program (SNAP), and Women, Infants, and Children (WIC) program, to name but a few. The guidelines also influence the broader food industry.

Food Guides And Nutrition Education

The USDA has repeatedly endeavored to communicate the Dietary Guidelines to the American public. The USDA and American Red Cross developed "A Pattern for Daily Food Choices" in 1984, designed as a food wheel, much like the Basic Seven in appearance. It remained a little known resource, however. In comparison, the Food Guide Pyramid, published in 1992, was widely disseminated as the USDA's key nutrition education tool. Designed to promote dietary variety, proportionality, and moderation, the pyramid listed a specific number of recommended daily servings from each food group. At the peak of the pyramid, consumers were advised to use fats, oils, and sweets sparingly.[55]

In 2005, the MyPyramid Food Guidance System—which depicted a pyramid with multiple, vertical, colored segments of varying widths—replaced the Food Guide Pyramid, but experts and consumers alike found its conceptual graphic vague and confusing.[56] In 2011, the USDA moved away from the pyramid design altogether and launched MyPlate, which illustrated the proportions of the food groups on an individual dinner plate.[57]

Critiques of the Dietary Guidelines

Since their first publication in 1980, the Dietary Guidelines have incited criticism. Such critiques question the conflicting evidence that links food consumption and disease risk, as well as other matters, such as the guidelines' limited inclusion of ethnic and regional variation in diet and how a nutrient-focused approach to diet may do more harm than good.

Some critics of the USDA food guides have been particularly vocal. For example, Marion Nestle's *Food Politics: How the Food Industry Influences Nutrition and Health*, first published in 2002, claimed that the food industry's lobbying power influences the dietary guidelines and accompanying nutrition education resources.[58] Furthermore, in response to the USDA's tools, the Harvard School of Public Health issued its own Healthy Eating Pyramid and Healthy Eating Plate. These experts assert that their tools more accurately represent research on the connections between diet and health—namely, that the USDA tools promoted more dairy than necessary, did not limit red and processed meat consumption enough, and did not distinguish between whole and refined grains.[59]

Furthermore, the burgeoning field of critical nutrition studies examines, critiques, and, in some cases, rejects the primary role of nutrition science in food and eating.[60] Critical nutrition scholars endorse destabilizing nutrition's hierarchical position within food knowledge production. Such a move creates space to consider and emphasize additional aspects that affect diet and health, such as food production quality, degree of processing, food marketing, heritage, tradition, culture, identities, gastronomy, taste, and pleasure.

Consumer Culture: Cookbooks to Blogs Influence Food and Public Health

Although dietary guidelines are an important source of food and nutrition information, a 2011 survey done by the American Dietetic Association (now the Academy of Nutrition and Dietetics) found that people more often turn to television, magazines, and the Internet for dietary guidance than to registered dieticians, physicians, or the USDA's Dietary Guidelines.[61] Such a finding demonstrates the significant influence of media and popular culture—what can be called broadly the consumer culture—upon food and public health. Emerging in the early 20th century, the consumer culture includes aspects of food and nutrition such as cookbooks, home economics texts, advertisements, magazines, and radio. These sources have expanded across the course of the 20th century and into the 21st century with film, and television, as well as various digital and social media platforms.

Cookbooks and Home Economics

From the first cookbook published on U.S. soil featuring North American ingredients—Amelia Simmon's *American Cookery* in 1796 (see Figure 1.4)— early cookbooks instructed housewives and servants on what and how to eat, as well as how to manage a home, attend to cleanliness and sanitation, and treat common illnesses. Beyond mere instructional manuals, however, cookbooks and the recipes they contain also provide rich historical evidence for researchers to assess variables such as technological change, the average reader's cooking skill and embodied knowledge, the extent of mass-market consumption patterns, and class-based cultural aspirations.

Some cookbooks in the 19th century and in the early decades of the 20th were written by female domestic scientists, later called home economists. These food and nutrition professionals occupied a complicated space at the

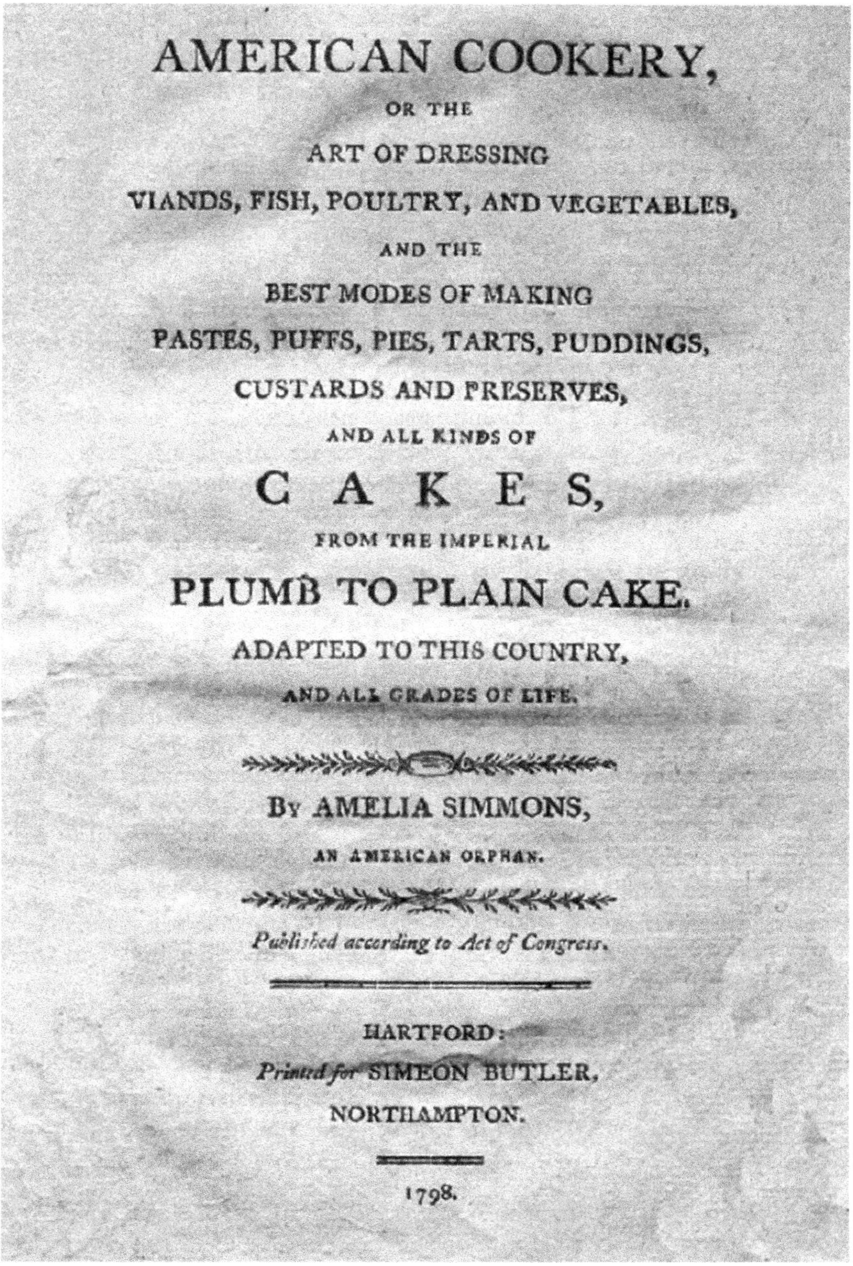

AMERICAN COOKERY,

OR THE

ART OF DRESSING

VIANDS, FISH, POULTRY, AND VEGETABLES,

AND THE

BEST MODES OF MAKING

PASTES, PUFFS, PIES, TARTS, PUDDINGS,

CUSTARDS AND PRESERVES,

AND ALL KINDS OF

CAKES,

FROM THE IMPERIAL

PLUMB TO PLAIN CAKE.

ADAPTED TO THIS COUNTRY,

AND ALL GRADES OF LIFE.

By AMELIA SIMMONS,

AN AMERICAN ORPHAN.

Published according to Act of Congress.

HARTFORD:

Printed for SIMEON BUTLER,

NORTHAMPTON.

1798.

FIGURE I.4 In 1796, Amelia Simmon's *American Cookery* was the first cookbook to be published on U.S. soil and feature North American ingredients.

http://digital.lib.msu.edu/projects/cookbooks/html/books/book_01.cfm

intersection of nutrition science discovery, modern agricultural production, and the ever-expanding consumer culture.[62] Focused on all aspects of domestic life, these women also brought the scientific findings of researchers like Wilbur O. Atwater to life in everyday kitchens.[63] They developed and disseminated nutrition education resources that emphasized rationalized consumption—through the foods one purchased and ate and how one engaged with the increasing menu of available mass-produced goods and media forms. It cannot be ignored, however, that domestic scientists promoted messages that moralized food. They also often targeted new immigrants and the urban poor, strongly encouraging dietary assimilation, which groups resisted. Home economists' messages influenced middle class culture through guidebooks, manuals, newspaper columns, magazine content, demonstrations, and exhibits. They shaped how generations of Americans thought about consumption, food, nutrition, and health, even if they did not fully alter consumption habits.

Modern Advertising

The marketing industry as known today first emerged in the early 20th century and has since extended its reach in the effort to establish consumer brand loyalty and to further market penetration. Just as cookbooks are more than instructional manuals, however, advertisements provide more than just product summaries. Although rooted in the capitalist desire for profit, advertisements, then and now, both shaped and reflected society as they constructed aspirational worlds of consumption and potential identities. Food advertising, in particular, communicated ideas about what and how one should eat, who one could become, and what life could be like.[64]

Beyond food makers and marketers, public health has also directly adopted marketing strategies, aiming to persuade the public to change behaviors and to make healthy choices. For example, Progressive Era reformers developed anti-tuberculosis campaigns in the 1910s and 1920s using modern marketing tactics. One also can see the mark of modern marketing in the propaganda posters distributed during World War I and World War II. These materials promoted efforts such as planting Victory Gardens, reducing food waste, and specific campaigns like Meatless Mondays and Wheatless Wednesdays, some of which have been revived today.[65] Contemporary "social marketing" interventions similarly harness these strategies to promote a healthy diet, among other lifestyle behaviors.[66]

Food Media: Magazines, Radio, Television, the Internet, and Social Media

Over the course of the 20th century, mass media also has spread messages about food that have shaped the nation's public health. Magazines were America's first mass medium and the *Ladies' Home Journal*, which began publication in 1883, was the first magazine to reach a circulation of one million subscribers.[67] Although not solely a food magazine, its content included domestic advice, recipes, and considerable food-related advertising. Magazines specifically dedicated to food emerged in the 20th century with periodicals like *Gourmet* in 1941, *Bon Appétit* in 1956, and *Food & Wine* in 1978. During these years, the publication of cookbooks also exploded. In a *New York Times* article in 1961, "Food: Cookbook Boom," June Owen wrote that more cookbooks were to be published that year than ever before, a trend that would only pick up speed in the years and decades to come.[68]

Over radio waves during the Depression and through the following decade, listeners (mostly women) also received a mix of cooking instruction, advice, and advertising with endorsements from figures like Betty Crocker and the USDA's Aunt Sammy, who both began broadcasting nationally in 1926.[69] These formats transitioned with the rise of television. Early forays into food television in the 1940s and 1950s included dozens of regional shows, as well as programs featuring iconic food figures, such as James Beard's short-lived *I Love to Eat* in 1946 and Dione Lucas's *The Dione Lucas Show,* which began airing locally on WCBS in New York in 1947. Although she had predecessors like Lucas, Julia Child and her television show, *The French Chef,* which began broadcasting on public television in Boston, Massachusetts in 1963, served as a watershed moment in the history of cooking on television.[70] Julia Child was considered America's first celebrity chef.

In our contemporary context, the food and eating aspects of the consumer culture have further infiltrated everyday life. Launched in 1993, the Food Network brought uninterrupted hours of cooking television—and mediated access to chefs, who have shifted within the public eye from blue collar cooks to venerated artisans and celebrities—onto screens for the first time.[71] The Internet also revolutionized the flow of food and nutrition information with websites dedicated to recipes, restaurant reviews, and other food news. Today's home cooks likely refer to online recipes, such as on blogs, at least as often as they turn to cookbooks. The *Merriam-Webster's Collegiate Dictionary* dates the term blog to 1999, and there are now tens of thousands of food blogs online.[72] Featuring recipes, stylized preparation, plating, photography, and personal narratives, blogs serve up entertainment and leisure alongside recipes, food facts, dietary advice, and an aspirational lifestyle.[73] In the 21st century, social media platforms such as Facebook, Twitter, and Instagram provide the means for users to both consume and produce food media that often overflow with "food porn" images.

Shaping American food and health, the consumer culture has brought and continues to bring ingredients, food products, recipes, and techniques into American homes. It has been made clear that food, more than strictly sustenance, also means entertainment, lifestyle, and identity.

Example In Practice: School Lunches

In the 21st century, school meal programs work to address food insecurity and promote national public health. And yet, school lunch programs often fail to provide the highest quality nutrition to students. They offer only limited employment opportunities for food workers and rarely provide adequate incomes for farmers. The root of many of these problems lies in the National School Lunch Program's (NSLP) insufficient funding and historical ties to agricultural subsidies. Understanding why such a relatively uncontroversial program struggles to achieve its goals necessitates an understanding of the roots of school meals in the Great Depression.[74]

Prior to the 1930s, various municipal and volunteer programs provided meals for students at schools, but these were few and far between. These programs primarily targeted immigrant populations, hoping to teach children American values through nutritionally sound American lunches. With the onset of the Great Depression, however, large numbers of hungry children spurred demands for state and federal funding to help provide lunches at schools. Under Roosevelt's New Deal, surplus agricultural commodities purchased by the Commodity Credit Corporation (CCC) were distributed to schools for lunch programs through the Works Progress Administration, which also employed out-of-work Americans to prepare and serve the lunches.

With the onset of the Second World War, the government was more interested in sending agricultural commodities to allies overseas than to school lunchrooms. More children needed lunches, however, because their mothers were working and unable to pack them lunches. With the dismantling of many New Deal programs in 1942, the War Food Administration temporarily ran the school lunch program, often fueled by Victory Gardens as much as agricultural surplus. At war's end, the 1946 National School Lunch Act established the modern NSLP. The ostensible reason for the act was promoting nutrition and public health in the aftermath of record numbers of youth turned away by draft boards for medical reasons.

On the federal level, however, the NSLP was administered not by the Office of Education but by the Department of Agriculture. Throughout the early years of the program, the NSLP benefited farmers more than it served the children of the nation. School lunches were organized around the commodities that farmers needed to sell as much or more than around nutritional guidelines. Few meals were free for needy children, and the majority of American children did not enjoy school lunches.[75] This prompted activism and changes in the administration of the NSLP, culminating in the 1966 Child Nutrition Act, which affirmed that the goals of the program were to be child-centered, not farmer-centered: a poverty-fighting program rather than an agricultural subsidy.

Still, the program was a financial disaster. As fast food chains took over American dining in the 1970s, they also encroached on school lunch programs. Privatized dining services were able to keep costs low enough to provide free meals to significant numbers of children for the first time in the program's history. The nutritional standards of these meals, however, continued to fall throughout the late 20th century.

In 2010, Congress passed the Healthy, Hunger-Free Kids Act, championed by First Lady Michelle Obama. While school lunch administrators boasted in the 1940s of their effectiveness in terms of pounds gained by underweight children, the 2010 act sought to fight both malnutrition and obesity. New and more stringent nutritional mandates now would guide school lunch meals.[76] To achieve the lofty goals of spreading nutrition, health, and vitality to America's youth, policymakers navigated the picky palates of children, local class politics, national budgets, the farm lobby, the large food processors, and the politics of welfare in the United States. History is crucial to understanding how and why each of these interests expects to be served by the school lunch program.

Discussion Questions and Activities
Activity: Investigate Your Food

Every meal you eat has a long journey from the soil to your stomach. On a single dinner plate there are often ingredients coming from multiple states, countries, and even continents. These foodstuffs may have traveled by multiple modes of transportation, as well as multiple stages of processing such as preservation, cooking, enrichment, and packing. Choose a single food product or food item you ate within the last week and try to tell the story of where it came from, what happened to it, and how it got to your plate. You may be surprised at how little or how much you are able to know about your food!

For this project, keep these questions in mind:

- Is your food identifiable as something from a farm? Or it is a processed commodity?
- Do you know what type of plant it grows on, animal it comes from (including breed!), or what ingredients it contains, without checking the ingredient list?
- How much or how little are you able to learn about your food simply from reading the packaging? (If it has any!)
- Who are the people at every step of your food's life story? Who grew it, harvested it, packaged it, distributed it, sold it?
- How easy is it to answer these questions? Why?
- Have the answers to these questions changed your feelings about your food item or your likelihood to eat it again in the future? Why or why not?

Activity: Reading and Analyzing Cookbooks

Too often dismissed as instructional manuals offering nothing but recipes, cookbooks are fascinating historical sources that can teach us much about food and public health during various time periods. For this activity, read and analyze a historic cookbook.

If you do have access to a library or archive with such texts, find one that interests you in an online archive, such as Feeding America: The Historic American Cookbook Project through Michigan State University (http://digital.lib.msu.edu/projects/cookbooks/) or the Internet Archive's collection of cookbooks and home economics texts (https://archive.org/details/cbk).

Consider the following questions as you read through the cookbook you have selected:

- What type of cookbook is it, or what is its main theme?
- Who is the author of this cookbook? What do we know about him/her/them?
- When and where was this cookbook published? What about that time period and place might be relevant?
- Who is the intended readership for this cookbook?

- Is it intended for a novice or an experienced cook? For a housewife or for servants? Is the readership male, female, or both?
- What ingredients, forms of measurement, technology, equipment, utensils, and techniques are called for in the recipes?
- How do these details relate to the historical context?
- What might they also tell us about the assumed cooking ability and class status of the cookbook's readership?
- How does the cookbook address nutrition, health, or disease?
- What does this cookbook tell us about how society at the time of publication conceived of categories of identity such as gender, race, ethnicity, class, religion, and/or region?

Quiz Questions

1. Which of the following is not a reason why farmers are now only 1% of the American population?
   a. Motorized farming machinery
   b. Suburban sprawl
   c. Farm boys sent to war rarely returned to the farm
   d. War gardens proved Americans could grow all of their own food
   e. Hybrid seeds, pesticides, herbicides, and other technologies to increase production
2. What did the ever-normal granary seek to do?
   a. Modernize agriculture through business models
   b. Promote home gardening for your family's food supply
   c. Stabilize farmer incomes and consumer food prices
   d. Conserve soil blown away in the Dust Bowl
   e. Standardize agricultural products
3. Which of the following were effects of the Pure Food and Drug Act?
   a. Inspection of food processing plants.
   b. Homogenous and standardized food products.
   c. Active ingredient lists on all foods
   d. Many small processors going out of business
   e. All of the above
4. What are the three stages of food commodification?
   a. Pure food, war food, space food
   b. Fungibility, branding, technological reinvention
   c. Pure Food and Drug Act, War Food Administration, countercuisine critiques

    d. Local farmers, factory processors, national corporations

    e. None of the above

5. Which of the following wartime foods achieved popularity through war?

    a. Spam

    b. Dried eggs

    c. Frozen vegetables

    d. Cake mixes

    e. Jell-O

6. Which of the following is false about the *Dietary Guidelines for Americans*?

    a. They were first published in 1980.

    b. They are updated every five years by an expert committee.

    c. They exert widespread influence upon public health nutrition programming and policies, such as school food, SNAP, and WIC.

    d. They have been critiqued by some scholars and nutrition experts.

    e. None of the above.

7. In what ways did government dietary advice change after approximately 1970?

    a. It became more focused upon whole foods, rather than specific nutrients.

    b. It primarily endorsed a foundation diet, liberally promoting the consumption of enough energy and nutrients to be healthy.

    c. It represented a shift in disease prevention strategy, away from a focus upon infectious diseases and toward a focus on chronic conditions believed to be diet-related.

    d. It focused more on social issues than scientific discoveries.

    e. None of the above.

8. Which of the following is NOT a food guide published at some point by the United States government?

    a. The Basic 10

    b. *Food for Fitness—A Daily Food Guide*, also known as the Basic Four

    c. The Food Guide Pyramid

    d. MyPyramid

    e. MyPlate

9. Which of the following is true about advertising?

    a. Modern advertising first emerged in the early 20th century.

    b. World War I and World War II food campaigns employed marketing techniques.

    c.   In addition to promoting products, advertising shapes and reflects society.

    d.   Public health campaigns have employed advertising strategies for nearly a century.

    e.   All of the above.

10. Which of the following is true about the history of food media?

    a.   The first magazine dedicated solely to the coverage of food and beverage was published in the 1890s.

    b.   Cooking shows had not appeared on television before the founding of the Food Network in 1993.

    c.   Taking off in the 2000s, food blogs and social media platforms have provided users the opportunity not only to consume food media, but also to produce it themselves.

    d.   (a) and (b) above.

    e.   None of the above.

References

1. *Historical Statistics of the United States—Colonial Times to 1970*. Part 1. Bicentennial edition. Washington, DC: Government Printing Office; 1975.
2. U.S. Census Bureau, Statistical Abstract of the United States. 129th Edition, Section 17. Agriculture; 2010. https://www.census.gov/library/publications/2009/compendia/statab/129ed/agriculture.html. Accessed May 2017.
3. Hurt DR. *Problems of Plenty: The American Farmer in the Twentieth Century*. Chicago, IL: Ivan R. Dee; 2003.
4. Pack CL. *War Gardens Victorious*. Philadelphia, PA: J. B. Lippincott; 1919; USDA National Agricultural Statistics Services. 1910 Census: General Report and Analysis.
5. Alston LJ. Farm foreclosures in the United States during the interwar period. *J Econ Hist*. 1983; (43)4: 885–903.
6. Fitzgerald D. *Every Farm a Factory: The Industrial Ideal in American Agriculture*. New Haven, CT: Yale University Press; 2010.
7. Johnson T. Nitrogen nation: the legacy of World War I and the politics of chemical agriculture in the United States, 1916–1933 (essay). *Ag Hist*. 2016; (90)2: 209–229.
8. Kloppenburg JR. *First the Seed: The Political Economy of Plant Biotechnology, 1492–2000*. Madison: University of Wisconsin Press; 2004.
9. Worster D. *Dust Bowl: The Southern Plains in the 1930s*. New York, NY: Oxford University Press; 1979.
10. McKenzie RT. Sharecropping. In: West C, ed. *The Tennessee Encyclopedia of History and Culture*. Knoxville: University of Tennessee Press; 2009. http://tennesseeencyclopedia.net/entry.php?rec=1193. Accessed May 2017.

11. Honey MK. *Sharecropper's Troubadour: John L. Handcox, the Southern Tenant Farmers' Union, and the African American Song Tradition.* New York, NY: Palgrave McMillan; 2013.

12. Phillips ST. *This Land, This Nation.* New York, NY: Cambridge University Press; 2007.

13. Hurt DR. *Problems of Plenty: The American Farmer in the Twentieth Century.* Chicago, IL: Ivan R. Dee; 2003.

14. Hurt DR. *Problems of Plenty: The American Farmer in the Twentieth Century.* Chicago, IL: Ivan R. Dee; 2003.

15. Backer K. *World War II and the Triumph of Industrialized Food.* Ph.D. dissertation, The University of Wisconsin—Madison; 2012.

16. *Manual For Company-Employee Gardens.* National Victory Garden Institute. New York, NY: The Institute; 1944.

17. Collingham L. *The Taste of War: World War II and the Battle for Food.* New York, NY: Penguin Press; 2012.

18. Hurt DR. *Problems of Plenty: The American Farmer in the Twentieth Century.* Chicago, IL: Ivan R. Dee; 2003.

19. Langston N. *Toxic Bodies: Hormone Disruptors and the Legacy of DES.* New Haven, CT: Yale University Press; 2010.

20. Ngai MM. *Impossible Subjects: Illegal Aliens and the Making of Modern America.* Princeton, NJ: Princeton University Press; 2004.

21. Anderson JL. *Industrializing the Corn Belt: Agriculture, Technology, and Environment, 1945–1972.* DeKalb, IL: Northern Illinois University Press; 2008.

22. Case AN. *Looking for Organic America: J. I. Rodale, The Rodale Press, and the Popular Culture of Environmentalism in the Postwar United States.* Ph.D. dissertation, The University of Wisconsin—Madison, 2012; Lytle, MH. *The Gentle Subversive: Rachel Carson, Silent Spring, and the Rise of the Environmental Movement.* New York, NY: Oxford University Press; 2007.

23. Beeman RS, Pritchard JA. *A Green and Permanent Land: Ecology and Agriculture in the Twentieth Century.* Lawrence, KS: University Press of Kansas; 2001.

24. Belasco WJ. *Appetite for Change: How the Counterculture Took on the Food Industry.* 2nd edition. Ithaca, NY: Cornell University Press; 2006.

25. Jenkins M. *Food Fight: GMOs and the Future of the American Diet.* New York, NY: Penguin Random House; 2017.

26. Industrial Agriculture. Union of Concerned Scientists; 2017. http://www.ucsusa.org/our-work/food-agriculture/our-failing-food-system/industrial-agriculture. Accessed June 2017; Chiotti QP, Johnston T. Extending the boundaries of climate change research: A discussion on agriculture. *J Rural Studies, Rural Conflict Change.* 1995; (11)3: 335–350; David P. *Organic and Conventional Farming Systems: Environmental and Economic Issues.* Ithaca, NY: Department of Entomology & Section of Ecology and Systematics, New York State College of Agriculture and Life Sciences, Cornell University; 2005.

27. Young JH. *Pure Food: Securing the Federal Food and Drugs Act of 1906*. Princeton, NJ: Princeton University Press; 1989.

28. Cronon W. *Nature's Metropolis: Chicago and the Great West*. New York, NY: W.W. Norton; 1991.

29. Smith-Howard K. *Pure and Modern Milk: An Environmental History Since 1900*. Cambridge, UK: Oxford University Press; 2014.

30. Deutsch T. *Building a Housewife's Paradise: Gender, Politics, and American Grocery Stores in the Twentieth Century*. Chapel Hill, NC: University of North Carolina Press; 2010.

31. Strasser S. *Satisfaction Guaranteed: The Making of the American Mass Market*. New York, NY: Pantheon Books; 1989.

32. Horowitz R. *Putting Meat on the American Table: Taste, Technology, Transformation*. Baltimore, MD: Johns Hopkins University Press; 2006.

33. Horowitz R. The great Jell-O controversy. In: *Kosher USA*. New York, NY: Columbia University Press; 2016.

34. Backer K. *World War II and the Triumph of Industrialized Food*. Ph.D. dissertation, The University of Wisconsin—Madison; 2012.

35. Smith A. *The Oxford Companion to American Food and Drink*. London, UK: Oxford University Press; 2007.

36. Backer K. *World War II and the Triumph of Industrialized Food*. Ph.D. dissertation, The University of Wisconsin—Madison; 2012.

37. Shapiro L. *Something from the Oven: Reinventing Dinner in 1950s America*. New York, NY: Viking; 2004.

38. Petrick GM. *The Arbiters of Taste: Producers, Consumers and the Industrialization of Taste in America, 1900–1960*. Ph.D. dissertation, University of Delaware; 2006.

39. Hamilton S. *Trucking Country: The Road to America's Wal-Mart Economy*. Princeton, NJ: Princeton University Press; 2008.

40. Belasco WJ. *Appetite for Change: How the Counterculture Took on the Food Industry*. 2nd edition. Ithaca, NY: Cornell University Press; 2006.

41. Nestle M. *Soda Politics: Taking on Big Soda (and Winning)*. Oxford, UK: Oxford University Press; 2015.

42. Welsh S, Davis C, Shaw A. A brief history of food guides in the United States. *Nutr Today*. 1992; November/December: 6–11.

43. Carpenter K. The life and times of W. O. Atwater (1844–1907). *J Nutr*. 1994; 124: 1707S–1714S.

44. Atwater W.O. Food: Nutritive value and cost. *Farmer's B*. 1894; 23: 1–30.

45. Hunt C. L. Food for young children. *Farmer's B*. 1916; 717: 1–20.

46. Hunt C.L. and Atwater H. How to select foods. *Farmer's B*. 1917; 808: 1–14.

47. Carpenter KJ. A short history of nutritional science: Part 3 (1912-1944). *J of Nutr*. 2003; 133: 3023–3032.

48. Apple R. *Vitamania: Vitamins in American Culture*. New Brunswick, NJ: Rutgers University Press; 1986.

49. Stiebeling H. Food budgets for nutrition and production programs. United States Department of Agriculture miscellaneous publication 183; 1933.

50. Davis C, Saltos E. Dietary recommendations and how they have changed over time. In: Frazao E, ed. *America's Eating Habits: Changes and Consequences*. Agriculture Information Bulletin No. (AIB-750); 1999: 33–50.

51. Davis C, Saltos E. Dietary recommendations and how they have changed over time. In: Frazao E, ed. *America's Eating Habits: Changes and Consequences*. Agriculture Information Bulletin No. (AIB-750); 1999: 33–50.

52. Mudry J. *Measured Meals: Nutrition in America*. Albany, NY: State University of New York Press; 2010.

53. Davis C, Saltos E. Dietary recommendations and how they have changed over time. In: Frazao E, ed. *America's Eating Habits: Changes and Consequences*. Agriculture Information Bulletin No. (AIB-750); 1999: 33–50.

54. Welsh S, Davis C, Shaw A. Development of the food guide pyramid. *Nutr Today*. 1992; November/December: 12–23.

55. Fargnoli J, Mantzoros CS. Food guide pyramids and the 2005 MyPyramid. In: Mantzoros CS, ed. *Nutrition and Metabolism: Underlying Mechanism and Clinical Consequences*. New York, NY: Humana Press; 2009: 195–207.

56. Fargnoli J, Mantzoros CS. Food guide pyramids and the 2005 MyPyramid. In: Mantzoros CS, ed. *Nutrition and Metabolism: Underlying Mechanism and Clinical Consequences*. New York, NY: Humana Press; 2009: 195–207.

57. Levine E, Abbatangelo-Gray J, Mobley, AR, McLaughlin GR, Herzog J. Evaluating MyPlate: An expanded framework using traditional and nontraditional metrics for assessing health communication campaigns. *J Nutr Educ Behav*. 2012; 44(4): S2–S12.

58. Nestle M. *Food Politics: How the Food Industry Influences Nutrition and Health*. Tenth Anniversary Edition. Berkeley, CA: University of California Press; 2013.

59. Harvard T.H. Chan School of Public Health. Healthy eating plate & healthy eating pyramid. *Nut Source*. 2011. https://www.hsph.harvard.edu/nutritionsource/healthy-eating-plate/.

60. Biltekoff C. Critical nutrition studies. In: Pilcher J, ed. *The Oxford Handbook of Food History*. New York, NY: Oxford University Press; 2012.

61. Nutrition and you: Trends 2011. Academy of Nutrition and Dietetics. http://www.eatrightpro.org/resources/media/trends-and-reviews/trends-survey. Accessed May 2017.

62. Goldstein C. *Creating Consumers: Home Economists in Twentieth Century America*. Chapel Hill, NC: University of North Carolina Press; 2012.

63. Shapiro L. *Perfection Salad: Women and Cooking at the Turn of the Century*. New York, NY: Farrar Straus and Giroux; 1986.

64. Parkin K. *Food is Love. Advertising and Gender Roles in Modern America*. Philadelphia, PA: University of Pennsylvania Press; 2007.

65. Bentley A. *Eating for Victory: Food Rationing and the Politics of Domesticity*. Champaign, IL: University of Illinois Press; 1998.

66. Kotler P, Roberto EL. *Social Marketing: Strategies for Changing Public Behavior.* New York, NY: Free Press; 1989; Grier S, Bryant C. Social marketing in public health. *Annu Rev Public Health.* 2005; 26: 319–39.

67. Scanlon J. *Inarticulate Longings. The Ladies' Home Journal, Gender, and the Promises of Consumer Culture.* New York, NY: Routledge; 1995.

68. Owen J. Food: cookbook boom. *New York Times.* October 23, 1961:32.

69. Collins K. *Watching What We Eat: The Evolution of Television Cooking Shows.* New York, NY: Bloomsbury Academic; 2010.

70. Shapiro L. *Julia Child: A Life.* New York, NY: Penguin Books; 2007.

71. Collins K. *Watching What We Eat: The Evolution of Television Cooking Shows.* New York, NY: Bloomsbury Academic; 2010; Ketchum C. The essence of cooking shows: How the Food Network constructs consumer fantasies." *J Com Inquiry* 2005; 29: 217–34.

72. Blog. http://www.merriam-webster.com/dictionary/blog. Accessed 12 May 2016.

73. Contois E. Healthy food blogs: Creating new nutrition knowledge at the crossroads of science, foodie lifestyle, and gender identities. *Yearbook of Women's Hist* 2016; 36: 129–145.

74. Levine S. *School Lunch Politics: The Surprising History of America's Favorite Welfare Program.* Princeton, NJ: Princeton University Press; 2008; Poppendieck, J. *Free For All: Fixing School Food in America.* Berkeley, CA: University of California Press; 2010.

75. Levine S. *School Lunch Politics: The Surprising History of America's Favorite Welfare Program.* Princeton, NJ: Princeton University Press; 2008.

76. Steisel S, Wengrovius E. "Healthy, hunger-free kids act of 2010 (P.L. 111-296) summary" National Conference of State Legislatures; 2011. http://www.ncsl.org/research/human-services/healthy-hunger-free-kids-act-of-2010-summary.aspx. Accessed May 2017.

2
_____

History and Development of the 2015–2020 Dietary Guidelines for Americans

Alice H. Lichtenstein and Allison Karpyn

Chapter Highlights

- Emergence of the Dietary Guidelines for Americans (DGAs) from controversy surrounding Dietary Goals
- Review of changes and recommendations presented in DGAs from 1980, 1985, 1990, 1995, 2000, 2005, 2010, and 2015
- Raise challenges in justifying changes in DGAs over time to the lay public

Though often with controversy, the Dietary Guidelines for Americans (DGAs) stands as the foundational document defining the federal government's nutrition policies. The reach of the guidelines is profound, influencing all federal educational outreach and guidelines for food assistance programs. Together the U.S. Department of Health and Human Services (HHS) and the U.S. Department of Agriculture (USDA) jointly publish revised recommendations every five years as mandated by Congress. Recommendations aim to "promote health, prevent chronic disease and help people reach and maintain a healthy weight."[1]

Each edition of the DGAs has evolved to address the most pressing public health and dietary concerns in an effort to support the nutrition needs of all Americans aged two years and older. That said, by 2020 it is expected that the dietary guidelines will be expanded to include specific guidance for infants and toddlers from birth to 24 months as well as for pregnant women.

In this chapter we provide a review of the DGA from their initial release in 1980 to the current 2015 edition.

Evolution of Dietary Guidelines for Americans, 1980 to 2015

The U.S. government has been issuing food and nutrition guidance since the late 1800s.

The forerunner to the Dietary Guidelines as we know them today did not appear, however, until 1977 when the Dietary Goals for Americans were released.[2] The goals recommended that Americans:

(1) increase carbohydrate intake to 55% to 60% of calories,
(2) decrease dietary fat intake to no more than 30% of calories, with a reduction in intake of saturated fat, and approximately equivalent distributions among saturated, polyunsaturated, and monounsaturated fats
(3) decrease cholesterol intake to 300 mg per day,
(4) decrease sugar intake to 15% of calories, and
(5) decrease salt intake to 3 g per day.

The concerns raised by both industry groups and the scientific community about these goals gave birth to what we now know as the DGAs, first issued in 1980.[3,4]

1980 Dietary Guidelines for Americans

In response to controversy associated with the development of the Dietary Goals for Americans, scientists at the USDA and at the Department of Health, Education and Welfare (later named HHS), with input from outside experts, formulated what has become the first edition of the DGAs.[5] The two departments released a brochure titled *Nutrition and Your Health: DGAs*. The guidelines were composed of seven principles of a healthful diet (Figure 2.1). These principles were based primarily on the 1979 Surgeon General's Report on Health Promotion and Disease Prevention, which described how, although "Americans Today are Healthier Than Ever," further improvements will be achieved only through the promotion of efforts to prevent disease and sustain health. It argued that a "reordering of health priorities" would be necessary.

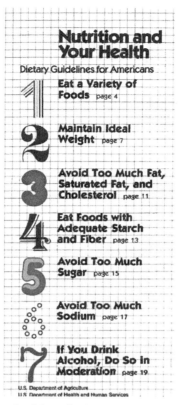

FIGURE 2.1 1980 Dietary Guidelines for Americans.

In addition to a thorough review of the current state of disease in America, the Surgeon General referenced and drew upon work from the Government of Canada, citing *A New Perspective on the Health of Canadians.*[6] In the 1979 U.S. report, Assistant Secretary for Health and Surgeon General Julius Richmond suggested that the Canadian framework for disease prevention, which emphasized investment across four elements including the importance of addressing key behavioral factors or unhealthy lifestyles. The report further advocated that more serious attention be given to the key diet related causes of disease and called for a stronger approach to health and improved quality of life for the American people. The emphasis represented a shift from more traditional discussions of diet, which largely focused on ingredients such as vitamins, minerals, and food additives to a broader preventative approach focused on lifestyle factors, such as diet and its effect on disease.[7]

As with the Dietary Goals, the 1980 DGAs generated a considerable amount of controversy from multiple sectors, including consumers, commodity and food industry groups, and nutrition scientists. Among the issues of concern were that the recommendations were premature without adequate scientific grounding on the connections between diet and health. The head of the American Medical Association's Council on Food and Nutrition at the time, for example, expressed concern, saying the guidelines seemed to "imply that all people must eat in the same way and would benefit from a reduction in fat or sugar or salt. The whole population should not be treated as if it were at risk of falling prey to diet-related diseases." Furthering the controversy were recommendations to limit cholesterol intake, which yielded vociferous rebuke from the National Livestock and Meat Board with statements such as, "There's tremendous potential for harm if the Government promotes highly controversial material on nutrition . . .the American public, as the Surgeon General says, is not in danger of extinction from poor eating."[8]

In response to this controversy in 1983 Congress directed the USDA and HHS to convene an advisory committee (Dietary Guidelines Advisory Committee [DGAC]) to revise future editions of the DGA. The specific mandate was that this committee be composed of scientific experts outside the federal government.

1985 Dietary Guidelines for Americans

In general, the second edition of the DGA (1985 DGA) was similar to the 1980 DGA.[9] Minor wording changes were made to some of the guidelines (Figure 2.2). Issues related to prevention of chronic disease were introduced, presumably in response to the growing overweight and obesity epidemic.

Two years after the 1985 DGA were issued, the House Committee on Appropriations directed the USDA and HHS to establish a Dietary Guidelines Advisory Group on a periodic basis. The intent was to task this group of scientists with reviewing the scientific data relevant to nutritional guidance and making recommendations to the Secretaries of USDA and HHS for updating the DGA.

Concurrent with this activity to ensure a periodic review and potential update of the DGA in 1990, the National Nutrition Monitoring and Related Research Act (Section 301 of Public Law 101-445, 7 USC 5341, Title III) was passed by the U.S. Congress. The law gave the responsibility for the DGA jointly to the Secretaries of USDA and HHS. It directed them to issue, at least every five years, a report titled *DGAs*, and mandated that the publication contain

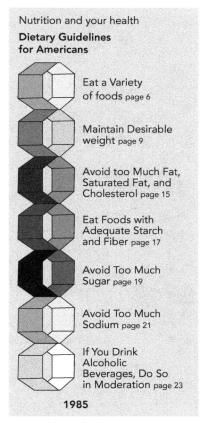

FIGURE 2.2 1985 Dietary Guidelines for Americans.

nutritional and dietary information for the general public, based on the preponderance of scientific and medical knowledge at the time of publication. It was further specified that the role of the committee was to advise the Secretaries of HHS and USDA, and it noted that the two Departments had the right to review and amend the text prior to publication. Importantly, it instructed that all federal policies and publications addressing issues related to nutrient and dietary guidance for the general public be consistent with the DGA.

1990 Dietary Guidelines for Americans

During the period when the legislation was developed, a scientific advisory committee had been convened by the Secretaries of HHS and USDA. This committee issued the third edition of the DGA (Figure 2.3).[10] For the most part the 1990 DGA recommendations were similar to 1985 DGA. The major

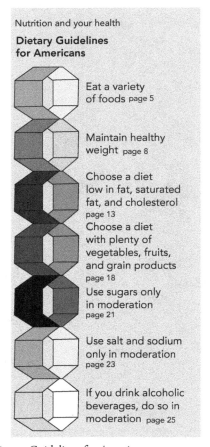

Nutrition and your health

**Dietary Guidelines
for Americans**

Eat a variety
of foods page 5

Maintain healthy
weight page 8

Choose a diet
low in fat, saturated
fat, and cholesterol
page 13

Choose a diet
with plenty of
vegetables, fruits,
and grain products
page 18

Use sugars only
in moderation
page 21

Use salt and sodium
only in moderation
page 23

If you drink alcoholic
beverages, do so in
moderation page 25

FIGURE 2.3 1990 Dietary Guidelines for Americans.

change was to reword the guidelines from negative (avoid) to positive (choose). The shift in wording from negative to positive was supplemented with text indicating that the DGA could be achieved by eating a variety of foods and eating those foods in moderation, rather than dietary restriction. It was emphasized that food could be both enjoyable and healthful. The 1990 DGA was the first to suggest quantitative goals for fat and saturated fat. Importantly and sometimes overlooked, it was clearly stated that these quantitative goals should be evaluated over several days, rather than a single meal or food.

1995 Dietary Guidelines for Americans

Whereas the 1980, 1985, and 1990 DGA editions were issued voluntarily by HHS and USDA, new regulations issued in 1990 by Congress in the

National Nutrition Monitoring and Related Research Act, mandated issuance of the 1995 DGA edition (Figure 2.4).[11] Changes included final shifts from negative to positive wording, and the inclusion of information linking the DGA to the Food Guide Pyramid and Nutrition Facts label. The importance of regular physical activity was added to the guideline for maintaining a healthy body weight.

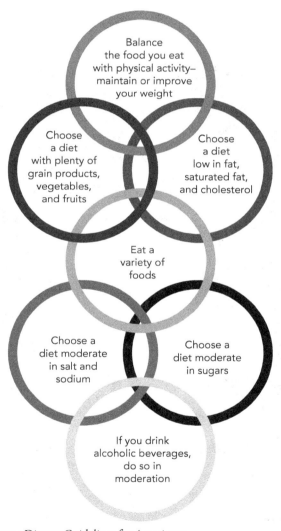

FIGURE 2.4 1995 Dietary Guidelines for Americans.

2000 Dietary Guidelines for Americans

Although the process used to develop the 2000 DGA was similar to that used for the 1995 DGA, significant changes were made to the guidelines themselves (Figure 2.5).[12] For the first time the number of guidelines was expanded from the original 7 to 10. Physical activity was separated from body weight, to recognize that there are health benefits of regular physical activity that are independent of energy balance. During the rewording of the DGA over the years, grains shared the same guideline as fruits and vegetables, encouraging consumption. Because the American public was consuming adequate amounts of grains but not fruits and vegetables, these food groups were separated into

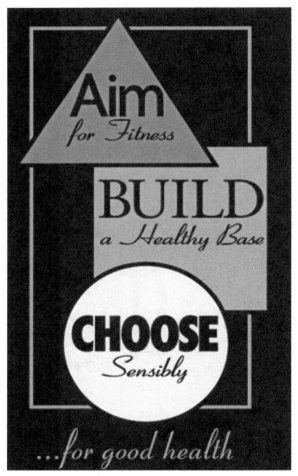

FIGURE 2.5 Dietary Guidelines for Americans.

two, fruits and vegetables, and grains. Furthermore, emphasis was placed on advising the American public to choose at least 50% of their grains as whole grains. Lastly, a guideline on safe food handling was added.

2005 Dietary Guidelines for Americans

The 2005 Dietary Guidelines Advisory Committee (DGAC) adopted a more formalized, systematic approach to review the literature than used previously, defining questions using the PICO (population, intervention, comparator, outcome) approach.[13] When using the DGAC report to formulate the dietary guidelines, the Departments shifted the focus of the DGA document from the general public to policymakers, healthcare professionals, nutritionists, and nutrition educators (Figure 2.6). The 2005 DGA included nine major dietary guideline messages that resulted in 41 Key Recommendations, of which 23 were for the general public and 18 were for specific population groups. A companion brochure, *Finding Your Way to a Healthier You,*[14] was issued for the general public.

2010 Dietary Guidelines for Americans

In 2008 the USDA established the Nutrition Evidence Library (NEL). One of the NEL's functions was to support the DGAC in identifying and reviewing the scientific literature in preparation for writing their report. The overarching theme of 2010 DGA was maintaining energy balance over time to achieve and sustain a healthy body weight, and consuming nutrient-dense foods and beverages (Figure 2.7).[15] The 2010 DGA included 23 key recommendations for the general population and six key recommendations for specific populations. This version of the guidelines introduced the concept of healthy eating patterns.

2015 Dietary Guidelines for Americans

The 2015 DGA used a similar approach to the 2010 DGAC to reviewing the literature. Reflecting the DGAC recommendations, the overarching theme of the 2015 DGA is to focus on the whole diet, emphasizing that a wide variety of eating patterns can result in a healthy diet (Figure 2.8).[16] The 2015 DGA includes five guidelines accompanied by key recommendations focused on describing elements of healthy eating patterns.

This latest round of dietary guidelines emphasizes the importance of lifelong healthy eating patterns coupled with limiting caloric intake to avoid

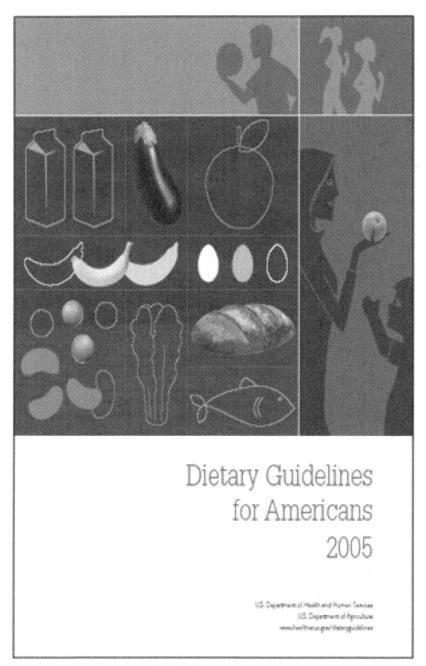

Dietary Guidelines
for Americans
2005

U.S. Department of Health and Human Services
U.S. Department of Agriculture
www.healthierus.gov/dietaryguidelines

FIGURE 2.6 2005 Dietary Guidelines for Americans.

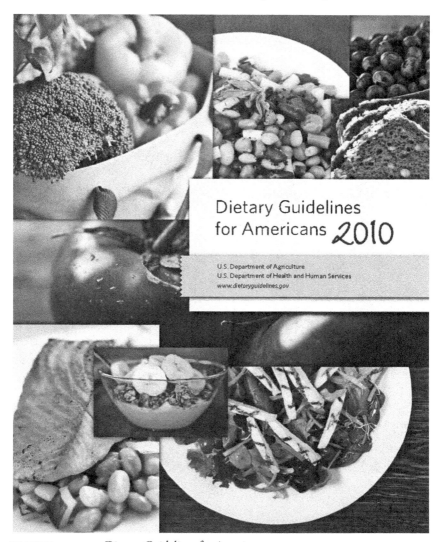

Dietary Guidelines
for Americans 2010

U.S. Department of Agriculture
U.S. Department of Health and Human Services
www.dietaryguidelines.gov

FIGURE 2.7 2010 Dietary Guidelines for Americans.

excess weight gain with advancing years. The guidelines further emphasize the importance of chronic disease risk reduction by consuming diets rich in vegetables, fruits, whole grains, low or non-fat dairy, seafood, legumes, and nuts; moderate in alcohol (among adults); lower in red and processed meat; and low in sugar sweetened foods and drinks, and refined grains.

New guidelines bode well for coffee lovers and indicate that moderate consumption of coffee is consistent with a healthy eating pattern.

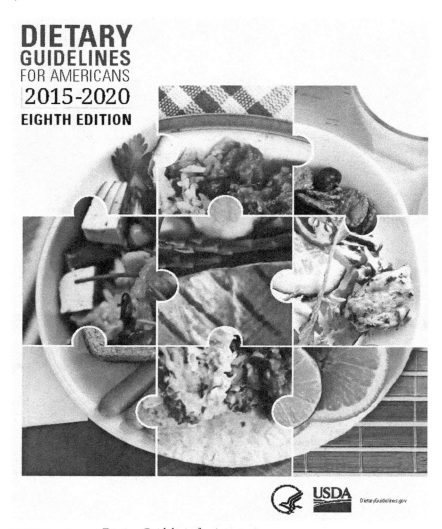

FIGURE 2.8 2015 Dietary Guidelines for Americans.

The same is not true, however, for products made from refined flour, including breads, cakes, and pastries. The 2015 DGA bring forward the recommendation initially made in the 2000 DGA that at least half of the grains we choose be whole grains and encourage limiting consumption of refined grains.

Red meat and processed meat continues to create controversy when it comes to dietary guidelines and recommendations. The DGAC report recommended reducing red and processed meat intake. This wording was modified in the DGA document to advice that a variety of protein-rich foods be incorporated into healthy eating patterns, including plant-based protein-rich foods. Finally, added sugars were perhaps the hardest hit in the 2015 guidelines with clear recommendations to limit added sugars to less than 10% of daily calories. Such recommendations are aligned with current efforts to limit sugar-sweetened beverage consumption and incorporate added sugar on the Nutrition Facts Panel label.

Conclusions and Reflections

The evolution of the DGA demonstrates progress toward clearer and more specific recommendations but also illuminates several important underlying themes of controversy, which we will likely continue to face. Concerns for mixed messages, inadequate nutrition science, and a relatively limited understanding of which diets are best for whom, consistently pepper concerns across the decades.[17,18]

One underlying cause may be the realities faced by the USDA's original role as an advocate for growers. Serving the dual role of industry advocate and dietary guideline author has created challenges when it comes to balancing the needs of the American diet with agricultural policy. Almost 30 years ago, a telling 1989 *New York Times* article takes the position that the USDA creates "mixed messages on nutrition" and emphasizes the apparent contradiction between the dietary guidelines and the fact that the position of the agency is one which could not suggest any foods are "bad" or "good." Quoting from a memo of the time, "essentially any food can be combined with other foods in numerous ways in diet that conform to the dietary guidelines principles of variety, moderation and balance." Spokesperson for the USDA's health and nutrition information service was also quoted saying, "if you start giving rules and regulations, it's too dictatorial."[19]

These issues continue to surface. It is difficult to explain to the general public why the focus has shifted from the total amount of fat in the diet to the type of fat in the diet, or why the emphasis is on dietary patterns rather than individual nutrients without going into the details of all the studies evaluated by the DGAC. We need to find better ways to educate the public as new information emerges that causes the scientific community to step back, revaluate all the available information in its totality, and determine whether the evidence is strong enough to change recommendations. That is certainly what happened in the area of dietary fat and we are just now understanding the challenges of communicating why the change is appropriate.

This acknowledgment that science evolves over time served as the basis for the mandate to review and potentially adjust the DGA every five years. As new guidelines for young children emerge and science for the whole population expands, it will be eye-opening to see the extent to which these common themes continue to guide our dietary guidelines.

Quiz Questions

1. The aim of the dietary guidelines for Americans is to:
   a. Help people reach and maintain a healthy weight
   b. Promote health
   c. Prevent chronic disease
   d. B and C above
   e. All of the above
2. The dietary guidelines for Americans were initially released in 1970. True or false?
3. What federal agency initially released the dietary guidelines for Americans?
   a. DHHS
   b. CDC
   c. NIH
   d. USDA
   e. A and D above
4. In 1990 major change was made to the dietary guidelines, which recommended:
   a. Eating foods in moderation rather than restricting your diet
   b. Avoiding foods high in carbohydrates
   c. Reaching mealtime goals for saturated fat
   d. Achieving new quantitative recommendations for sodium
5. The 1995 dietary guidelines were the first to be issued as a mandate from Congress. True or false?
6. Despite common belief, the dietary guidelines for Americans the food guide pyramid, and the nutrition facts label are not formally linked. True or false?
7. In 1995 the dietary guidelines for Americans included physical activity guidelines. True or false?
8. The NEL serves to:
   a. Collect data from households about dietary intake
   b. Monitor compliance with the dietary guidelines for Americans

    c. Report to Congress on the progress of the dietary guidelines for Americans' recommendations

    d. Identify and review scientific literature

    e. A and C above

9. The 2015 dietary guidelines for Americans includes five guidelines and key recommendations. Guidelines emphasize:

    a. A diet rich in fruits and vegetables

    b. Limiting food insecurity

    c. Lean meats containing little or no saturated fat

    d. A and C above

    e. All of the above

10. Current guidelines include coffee as part of a healthy eating pattern. True or false?

Discussion Questions

- What do you think should be in the 2020 DGA?
- On what scientific evidence do you base your recommendations?
- To what extent have the DGAs changed since 1980 and to what extent have they remained the same?
- How do programs such as SNAP and WIC support or detract from the recommendations provided in the DGAs?

References

1. U.S. Department of Health and Human Services and U.S. Department of Agriculture. 2015–2020 Dietary Guidelines for Americans, 8th Edition December 2015 .

2. Dietary Goals for Americans. https://health.gov/dietaryguidelines/dga2005/report/HTML/G5_History.htm 1977.

3. Schneeman BO. Evolution of dietary guidelines. *J Am Diet Assoc* 2003;103:S5–S9.

4. Watts ML, Hager MH, Toner CD, Weber JA. The art of translating nutritional science into dietary guidance: history and evolution of the Dietary Guidelines for Americans. *Nutrition Reviews* 2011;69:404–412.

5. Dietary Guidelines for Americans. https://health.gov/dietaryguidelines/1980.asp 1980.

6. Labelle H. A new perspective on the health of Canadians. *AARN News Lett* 1976;32:1–5.

7. Brody JE. U.S. Acts to Reshape Diets of Americans. *New York Times* (1923–Current file) 1980 02/05/1980 Feb 05;Sect. 1.

8. King SS. U.S. to Publish Diet Guides for Consumers. *New York Times* (1923–Current file) 1979 10/10/1979 Oct 10;Sect. 1.

9. Dietary Guidelines for Americans. https://health.gov/dietaryguidelines/1985.asp 1985.

10. Dietary Guidelines for Americans. https://health.gov/dietaryguidelines/1990.asp 1990.

11. Dietary Guidelines for Americans. https://health.gov/dietaryguidelines/1995.asp 1995.

12. Dietary Guidelines for Americans. https://health.gov/dietaryguidelines/2000.asp 2000.

13. Dietary Guidelines for Americans. https://health.gov/dietaryguidelines/dga2005/ document/ 2005.

14. U.S. Department of Health and Human Services USDoA. Finding your way to a healthier you: Based on the Dietary Guidelines for America. Washington DC: U.S. Independent Agencies and Commissions; 2005:12.

15. Dietary Guidelines for Americans. https://health.gov/dietaryguidelines/2010/ 2010.

16. Dietary Guidelines for Americans. https://health.gov/dietaryguidelines/2015/ 2015.

17. Brody JE. What's New in the Dietary Guidelines. *New York Times* January 18, 2016.

18. Brody JE. We Are What We Eat, But Only Some of Us. *New York Times* (1923– Current file) 1980 02/10/1980 Feb 10;Sect. 1.

19. Burros M. Eating Well: From the USDA Mixed Messages on Nutrition. *New York Times* (1923–Current file) 1989 06/14/1989 Jun 14;Sect. 1.

3

Behavioral Design as an Emerging Theory for Dietary Behavior Change

NCCOR Behavioral Design Working Group

Chapter Highlights

- Further integrate and explain how theories of behavior and design, and relevant fields of application (e.g., nutrition, physical activity) intersect to form a more comprehensive understanding of how theory and practice connect
- Focus on enabling the development of behavioral design applications to the built and natural environments

Introduction

"The taste of the apple . . . lies in the contact of the fruit with the palate, not in the fruit itself; in a similar way . . . poetry lies in the meeting of poem and reader, not in the lines of symbols printed on the pages of a book. What is essential is the aesthetic act, the thrill, the almost physical emotion that comes with each reading."—J.L. Borges

What humans "do" is a complex interplay of our intrapersonal and external experience. This interplay of relationships changes over time not only as we move through our individual stages of development, but also as human society and culture evolve. Group norms and behaviors (culture), as well as the physical and informational world (society), exist in reciprocity with the intrapersonal (physical and psychological) to form, adapt, and condition human experience.

Recognizing these complexly interwoven ideas at varying levels, such as through socio-ecologic, behavioral change, and systems models, public health efforts to improve healthy eating and active living attempt to include individual and environmental approaches via multilevel—intrapersonal, interpersonal, organizational, community, and policy—interventions.[1,2,3,4,5,6,7,8,9,10,11,12]

The ability to construct and efficiently apply these approaches is facilitated by increasing the awareness of how individual (agent) and environmental (exposure) qualities intertwine to create our experience. Recognizing the necessary complexity, note that agent and exposure are also plural, as in group agency or a multifaceted exposure.

As a science to practice framework, behavioral design facilitates our understanding and the ability to influence how the agency-exposure interaction produces experiences. Behavioral design, in turn, can incentivize the design and building process to maintain health as a proximate performance outcome.

The past few decades have seen increasing work in science, philosophy, art, and their sub-domains to refine and resolve the intricate connectivity that we call experience and its connection to the agent-exposure interface. Efforts include increasingly realistic behavioral and cognitive models that focus on what humans do and can do in lieu of a history of cultural expectation and idealism.[13]

The behavioral sciences and economics, choice architecture, and numerous commercial endeavors (e.g., marketing, architecture, and design), often working in conjunction with emerging technologies, have examined and applied these concepts to influence individuals and groups toward particular physical actions or psychological mind states.[14,15]

In this chapter, we work to further integrate and explain how theories of behavior and design, and relevant fields of application (e.g., nutrition, physical activity) intersect to form a more comprehensive understanding of how theory and practice connect. The chapter has a specific focus on enabling the development of behavioral design applications to the built and natural environments.

Many factors influence the use and effectiveness of behavioral design to alter feelings, perceptions, choices, actions, and behaviors relative to lifestyle factors that, in turn, influence health outcomes. This effort focuses on applying these concepts to the areas of healthy eating and active living for children and their families in the context of the built environment and community (Figure 3.1). This chapter is informed by 2015–2016 National

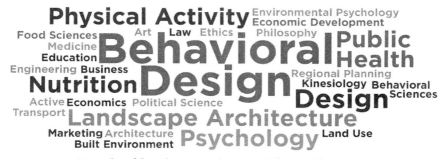

FIGURE 3.1   Examples of disciplines contributing to behavioral design.

Collaborative on Childhood Obesity Research (NCCOR) meetings re-lated to deriving and applying behavioral design principles to foster active living and healthy eating.

Gathering these concepts under a single rubric of behavioral design can facilitate systemic and systematic considerations and approaches for developing and applying strategies. Beginning with the most basic relationship that defines experience, agent, and exposure, behavioral design provides needed context and resolution (details on specific issues) to guide and inform the development and application of public health strategies (Figure 3.2).

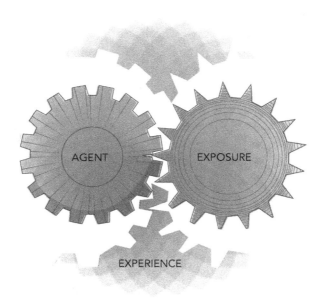

FIGURE 3.2   Experience as the integration of our agency with exposure.

The Roots of Behavioral Design

Behavioral design's maturation requires drawing from the base domains of human experience to explore, contextualize, and guide our understanding of the relationship between our actions and the natural and built environment.[16,17] The importance of a domain-level approach should not be underestimated, because this approach goes beyond systems or even ecologic approaches and, if done with care, enforces considerations from the different ways we think and act. The fields of psychology, environmental psychology, behavioral economics, and public health have all had a strong influence on emergence and development of behavioral design.

Behavioral design is not a new endeavor, though the past century has greatly enriched our empirical understanding of human behavior and cognition and the application of this understanding to personal, community, and commercial design and layout. The technology, trade, and tricks of behavioral design extend to prehistory. The way we organize and lay out communities, design structures or buildings, use information posturing to sell material goods or ideas, and entertain are all richly poignant aspects of our history and archaeological record.[18,19] Infiltrating the primary historic currency of artistic intuition, advances in empirical evidence of environmental design's influence on behavior has led to design and designers being major actors in industry and architecture. The increased recognition of the role of design in influencing human action builds on previous efforts to organize and design tools, buildings, and communities with intent or an artistic inclination. As the scope of design increases and its impact becomes increasingly robust via scientific research, this trend may accelerate.

Current common uses of design are numerous; some examples include using layout, placement, lighting, color, and signage to influence purchasing decisions of food and other consumer goods; the interface and physical design of electronic goods; laying out forms or websites for enrollment programs (e.g., insurance, retirement, job applications); and designing buildings, parks, playgrounds, and communities.[39]

Businesses, architecture firms, community planners, and governments have taken note, applying these strategies to increase sales, improve the human experience, save money, increase safety, and benefit public health and well-being. For example, governments including the United States, Canada, United Kingdom, the Netherlands, Germany, France, Denmark, Singapore, and Australia have created behavioral insight teams in recent years.[20,21,22,23,24] General public-sector approaches tend to focus on organizing the decision environment such that the easy and default options maximize the public good.

Environmental Psychology and Behavioral Design

The environmental psychology field began in the 1960s, emerging from the work of social psychologists who recognized that the physical environment played a role in social phenomenon such as cooperation and competition, and from the work of cognitive scientists interested in how environment affected cognitive processes.[25] A third impetus for the formation of the environmental psychology field was concern regarding environmental degradation[26] and a desire to understand and promote ecological or "pro-environment" behavior. Thus traditionally, environmental psychologists have focused on:

(1) Factors that encourage people to engage in ecological behaviors such as recycling and using public transportation[27]
(2) Understanding how the environment affects function, behavior, or well-being. For example, environmental psychologists interested in how the environment affects humans explore topics such as environmental stressors including noise and crowding.[28] In recent years, the environmental psychology empirical findings and theoretical frameworks increasingly have been leveraged to affect public health.

In the past two decades, the public health field has recognized the limitations of education-only intervention strategies aimed at individuals, and instead, has embraced multilevel, broad-brush interventions that employ environment and/or policy to promote healthy behaviors.[29,30] With this paradigm shift has come greater connection between public health and environmental psychology[31] and an opportunity to leverage environmental psychology concepts and theories to promote healthy eating and active living. A few core environmental psychology concepts and theories of potential relevance to behavioral design will be highlighted here.

Lessons from Sustainable Behavior

It may be possible to leverage lessons from strategies to promote pro-environmental behavior toward the promotion of active living. These lessons may be particularly appropriate when behaviors have dual positive outcomes: good for the environment and good for human health. For example, behaviors that save energy and increase human movement include using a clothesline rather than a gas or electric clothes dryer, taking the stairs instead of using an elevator, and using public transportation rather than driving a private vehicle.

Layout

Environmental psychologists have examined various aspects of the physical layout of interior spaces. Although limited published research has examined the implications of interior layout for healthy eating and active living, these topics are rife with opportunity, individually or collectively, for obesity prevention and control purposes. Environmental psychology researchers have discovered that the configuration of seating arrangements profoundly influences social interaction. *Sociopetal* arrangements, characterized by moveable seating that can be configured for face-to-face interaction at comfortable interpersonal distances, promote social interaction. *Sociofugal* arrangements, which discourage social interaction, are typically inflexible shoulder-to-shoulder seating in rows, such as in a train station or church. Space syntax theory provides tools to examine the effects of spatial configuration on human behavior.[32] Among the concepts from space syntax is *architectural depth,* which refers to the number of spaces one must pass through to reach a given room. Research suggests that in crowded residential settings, architectural depth allows people greater control over social interaction and thereby dampens the impact of crowding on social withdrawal and psychological distress.[33] Another aspect of layout is *floorplan openness.* An open floorplan is one with few walls and is visually permeable, while a closed floorplan has walls and doors. Recent research suggests that due to the greater visibility and convenience of food access, an open kitchen–dining room floorplan in the home environment (compared to a closed floorplan) directly affects the number of food trips made to the kitchen and indirectly affected the amount of food consumed.[34] Focusing mainly on convenience, behavioral economists have begun to examine the impact of some aspects of layout on children's dietary intake within a school lunchroom.[35]

Affordance

One of the key concepts in the field of environmental psychology is **affordance.** An affordance is a characteristic of the environment that signals how an object or environmental feature can be used.[36] By providing the user of a space with clues, an affordance can foster certain behaviors. Flat surfaces afford sitting, while knobs afford turning, for example. Affordances can, therefore, nudge building occupants. The notion of affordance can be contrasted with *environmental determinism*, which suggests that environments *cause* behavior.[122]

Behavior Setting

In the 1940s, Roger Barker proposed the notion of ***behavior settings*** as the unit of analysis to examine small-scale social systems within their natural, ecological context. Behavior settings can be examined in terms of the number of people and the number of roles they contain. A setting that is ***overstaffed*** (or "overmanned") has fewer roles than people, while a setting that is "***understaffed***" has more roles than people, leading, according to staff theory, to people feeling more needed and obligated to fill a role. The ratio of roles to occupants has implications for the social dynamics of the environment and the activities completed. Understaffed environments tend to encourage people to work harder on more diverse tasks.

Human Behavior: Reflective and Automatic Systems

Despite the evolution of public health models, a traditional and dominant model of human behavior is that of the deliberative, intentional, and rational actor. This human behavior model posits that decisions and behaviors are the result of a reflective process where individuals consciously analyze information and make decisions based solely on their preferences. Many health behavior theories come from this model, including the Health Belief Model,[37] the Theory of Reasoned Action,[38] and the Theory of Planned Behavior.[39] Public health researchers and practitioners have developed multiple interventions based on the rational actor model. Many interventions based on the tenants of the rational actor model use information and incentives to achieve behavior change. These interventions, however, have had limited effectiveness.[40] According to the rational actor model, actors' intentions would directly lead to their behaviors. Empirical research on the relationship between intentions and behaviors, however, shows that intentions are weakly correlated with behaviors[41] and that intentions account for little of the variance in behavior change.[42]

Much of the advancement in our understanding of human behavior comes from a shift from the rational actor model to the dual-system model of cognition.[66] The dual-system model posits human cognition as taking place via two parallel systems—a reflective system and an automatic system. The reflective system is deliberative and slow; it is associated with rational, rule-based thought and requires conscious effort and control. The automatic system, in contrast, is uncontrolled and fast; it operates at an unconscious level that requires no noticeable effort and is characterized by automatic, associated thought. The automatic system is responsive to external stimuli and, as such, is heavily influenced by context and environment.

Thinking Automatically

As mentioned above, much of human behavior is influenced by automatic thought processes. If human decisions were based solely through the reflective system, humans would attend to and account for all available information and make deliberate rational decisions based on that information and their preferences. Human decisions, however, do not solely operate through the reflective system but rather are influenced by the automatic system. As such, humans have certain automatic and unconscious biases that influence their decisions and behaviors. One of the biases is known as the status quo bias, which is the human bias to select status quo options when making a decision. This bias leads to the large effects of defaults on behaviors. Experiments show that manipulating default options leads to behavior changes including organ donation, financial decisions, and health care utilization.[100] Another bias in human decision-making is that we tend to make decisions based not on the universe of information available, but rather on what is current and proximal.[43]

Human decisions then tend to be influenced by stimuli that are most salient in a given context and environment. Salient stimuli tend to be simple, novel, and accessible.[73] Previous research showed that changing the salience of healthy foods in a physical microenvironment led to positive eating behaviors.[44] A third bias is that priming, or the unconscious exposure to stimuli, influences our decisions and behaviors. In the realm of eating behavior, much of priming takes place via advertisements in physical microenvironments. These advertisements tend to be for food with low nutritional value. It is possible, however, for priming to take place via mechanisms other than advertising and to be used toward the end of promoting healthy eating. Furthermore, priming may be used in physical microenvironments to promote physical activity. Lastly, human decisions and behaviors are biased by affect, that is, the experience of feeling or emotion. In addition to making cognitive evaluations when making a decision, individuals also make unconscious and automatic affective evaluations. These affective evaluations influence behavior in that individuals are more likely to engage in behaviors and select options that they associate with positive affect, and they are less likely to engage in behavior and select options that they associate with negative affect.

Knowing this, physical microenvironments involved in eating and physical activity can be manipulated such that healthy eating and physical activity are associated with positive affect.

One key factor that influences automatic thought, particularly around eating behavior, is the sensory stimuli found in a particular environment. Much research has shown that sensory stimulation regarding food can later influence behaviors. For example, both the sight[45] and smell[46] of food can affect food choice and eating behavior. This relationship, in part, is due to the fact that individuals make automatic associations between sight and smell with taste and satiating properties. Many restaurants and grocery stores manipulate their environments to take advantage of the fact that individuals think automatically through the use of visuals and smells associated with delicious foods.[47]

Thinking Socially

In addition to thinking automatically, people also think socially. Just as thinking automatically results in people being influenced by the effects of defaults, salience, priming, and affect, thinking socially results in people being influenced by the effects of norms and ego. Traditional rational actor models assume that humans are selfish and inward looking. More recent research, however, shows that humans are very attuned to their social environments, and that these social environments influence their decisions and behaviors. Social norms are one way in which social environments influence decisions and behaviors. People are more likely to engage in behaviors and to make decisions that they perceive to be normative. As it pertains to physical microenvironments where eating behaviors and physical activity take place, interventions can make healthy eating and physical activity appear normative. Ego is another aspect of thinking socially that influences behaviors and decisions. People fundamentally want to view themselves positively, and they automatically and unconsciously compare themselves with others. As a result, people are more likely to engage in behaviors that are in line with their positive self-image and that are associated with higher status. Similar to how physical microenvironments can be designed to present healthy eating and physical activity as normative, they can also present these behaviors as socially desirable and positive.

Thinking with Mental Models

Beyond thinking automatically and socially, individuals also think with mental models.[48] According to the World Bank (2015), "mental models include categories, concepts, identities, prototypes, stereotypes, causal narratives, and worldviews." Mental models heavily influence individuals' decisions and behaviors. Affect is one avenue through which mental models may operate. Individuals may have mental models about healthy eating and physical activity that directly relate to affect. For example, children may have mental models that healthy food is disgusting, and that physical activity is boring. Changing mental models to associate more positive affect with healthy behaviors may increase the likelihood that children engage in these behaviors. One aspect of mental models is the power to influence how individuals perceive environments. Mental models can change what individuals attend to in an environment. As such, mental models can affect the salience of certain aspects of an environment. It is possible, at least theoretically, that activating a healthy mental model may make certain aspects of an environment associated with healthy behaviors more salient to individuals. Mental models also operate through identities. We already have discussed how ego can influence behaviors and decisions. A key part of ego is identity, which is one of our strongest mental models. Individuals often make decisions and engage in behaviors because they are consistent with their identity. Knowing that individuals think with mental models, and specifically through identities, we know that we can facilitate healthy behaviors through activation of certain identities.

Making Decisions: Experience, Environment, and Exposure

> "There are significant challenges and no doubt inherent error in any attempt to dissect experience into agent-exposure, observer-observed, subject-object, or human-environment."—William James

As William James and others have pointed out, we do not experience separate conditions of agent and exposure but rather a singular synthetic experience. Nevertheless, our experience is not passive in its emergence. Indeed, our experiences are an artificial reciprocity informed, molded, and driven by the behavioral (agent) and design (exposure) aspects. Behavioral design represents an experiential control locus, achieved by altering and aligning aspects of agent and exposure. Experience, that is, agent-exposure immediacy, is of course also mediated, reinforced, moderated, and guided by numerous informational aspects, which are critical aspects of behavioral design. Other than this brief recognition of its importance, however, we only address the use of information as a medium for factual education. Internal exposure is discussed in the psychology section (i.e., mindsets, mental models, and developmental stages) and external exposure is discussed in the section on the physical (natural and built) and informational environments. Figure 3.3 portrays a working descriptive geography of experience and roughly pictorializes the foundations of behavioral design.

Recognizing the reciprocal nature of "agent and exposure" is foundational to developing an understanding of behavioral design. At a low resolution, this might be referred to as feedback loops, but more specifically it includes those items left as time passes, such as conditioning, resilience, expectation, repeated

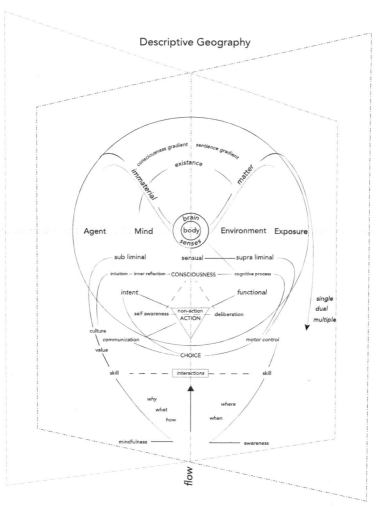

FIGURE 3.3 Descriptive geography of experience, foundations of behavioral design.

behaviors, and normality. Regardless of our desires, these effects are decisive in our relationship with the world. This conceptual perspective recognizes "experience" as the central and iterative influence on the momentum of our lives; this momentum contains and modifies our whole being including our biologically dictated but changing propensities such as our developmental stage and our physical or psychological assets or limitations.

With this momentum, our actions lie on a continuum from the planned, informed, or highly intentional (aware) to the unaware, reactive, or default (referred to as mindless, fast thinking, or automatic).[13] Decision-making, suggestive of intent, tends toward the "aware" side of this continuum (i.e., slow thinking). At least semantically, it might be argued that a choice made without awareness is still a decision, but in general what is referred to as a decision trends on the aware side. This does not imply that decisions are well informed and balanced or effectively consider alternatives (so called "rational" decisions), instead that decision-making advances are based on available information and overall context (so called bounded rationality).[13]

Physical and informational exposure enables, guides, encourages, requires, informs (or the reverse of these), while agents react in accordance with their abilities and desires (physical attributes, information processing, goals, ambitions, routines, etc.). Contributing to this reciprocity are the less-aware parts of experience, in general the experiential load, which is conditioned, reactive, instinctual, and subliminal. Further, cognitive load, ego depletion, tiredness, and other trying or will power–depleting experiences may influence the balance of experience between agent and exposure.[49,50] Thus, both actions and decisions are closely intertwined with exposure and can support or detract from health behaviors (i.e., our actions or decisions related to eating or physical activity).

Providing specifics in a few areas can be illustrative, however, as in many areas of human behavior, isolated single behavioral design activities within the larger context may negate or complement their effects. This caution is warranted as popular descriptions of this work may overstate possible outcomes. Therefore, the potential impacts of single exposure issues may be small; however, the cumulative aspect of the total behavioral design environment and the cumulative effect over time can be significant. Pragmatically, it is also critical to consider the degree to which behavioral design interventions address the inherent behavioral milieu or are modified by individual variables (age, gender, culture, etc.).

On the physical side, the environment can affect how much effort is required for any specific action. In the case of eating behaviors, for example, environmental factors may be the distance to a grocery store, the placement of items in a store, or the layout of items in a cafeteria or on a restaurant menu. The easy and default option environment, presented as related to physical distance, time needed, distance from the present, or overall required effort, creates gravitational centers of likelihood for particular outcomes. A person's previous exposure compounds these effects as time layers experience and creates routines, habits, and norms manifesting as ingrained eating practices or a certain level of physical activity. These personal routines can come from or become group routines, norms, or cultural practices.[51] The cognitive states and conative/affective states are closely bound (in our relationship) to exposure. Our limited mental energy and bandwidth to engage in conscious decision-making for frequent and repetitive behaviors, such as eating and moving, are taxed by emotional implications and our ability to process information.[52,53,54,55] Exposure may complement, enable, or retard cognitive capacity, affecting functionality, energy expenditure (for the same task), or awareness (of actions) and ultimately the quality of decisions when viewed retrospectively. Prior exposure and the way it is integrated, maintained, and influences emotions, is instrumental in how we manage time and may be predictive of our levels of intention, decisions, and actions. For example, our response to living with adversity and insecurity—such as threats, poverty, or social class—can be the development of a scarcity mindset, which leads to effects such as short-term decision-making that overvalues the present over the future.[100,101,102,56]

Physical exposure influences affective states such as emotion, feeling, and mood, as well as cognitive abilities such as focus.[57,58] For example, the soundscape can trigger post-traumatic stress disorder (PTSD) responses or alleviate them, increase aggressiveness in children or reduce it, and influence our ability to think clearly and focus.[105,59]

Cognitive, affective, and physical responses to sensory perception also influence higher brain functions of learning, memory, and creativity. To give one example, exposure to background noise and/or color (e.g., computer screen or wall paint) can cause stress or calming responses.[104,105,60,61] Another example is how enhancing the spaciousness of a room with a high ceiling may improve our ability to focus our efforts, thoughts, or actions.[62] These effects tend to be on a continuum and threshold dependent, with adverse sensual experiences leading to difficulties in decision-making, default option choice, and negative stress responses.[63]

To iterate, specifics types of exposures exerting negative or positive effects on health-related actions or behaviors have been demonstrated but largely with a focus on a limited number of variables (e.g., how sound influences concentration). The entirety of the "whole" exposure is less well studied, although commercial environments are specifically designed to modify sensory experiences to produce often unconscious actions, such as what foods to choose and how long to spend eating. This "whole" exposure is not simply about a single event, as in going to a restaurant, but a day, month, or years of events that modify or enforce single or recurrent actions.

The Built and Designed Environment

In the modern world, our exposure and thus experience are heavily influenced by the built world, which may or may not be intentionally designed to have specific behavioral outcomes. This lack of behavioral focus is, in part, the compromise in managing competing requirements but is also frequently simply a lack of awareness or interest in how the environments we construct actually affect people. Construction and design are driven by factors such as cost, time, tradition, or priorities, while also addressing the functional necessities, such as structural soundness, safety, durability, and aesthetics—based on a given price, time frame, and preferences. If behavioral outcomes are desired and attempted, limitations exist in knowledge and understanding of how design affects behavior, and in the standards and skills of designers, architects, and others on how to apply these theories to practice most effectively. Regardless of the quality and extent of the environment's design aspects, agentic response may vary as it is influenced or even dictated by inherent individual factors (such as development stage, gender, mindset, or difficulty of influencing a specific behavior) and competing and holistic influences.

Design considerations are relevant to health behaviors in most if not all settings, such as homes, buildings in general, schools, playgrounds and parks, community layout and content, transportation, and worksites. Many aspects of these settings are designed and have the ability to influence behavior, from seemingly small issues, such as the shapes of rooms, types of furniture, or paint color in buildings, to the broader scale issues of connectivity of streets and access to public transportation.[89,90]

Commercial, business, economic, and political influences all play a role in the built environment's design. Differing opportunities and costs are presented by whether an effort encompasses development/build or redevelopment/rebuild. The former represents expensive and long-term impacts; in such efforts, it is critical to include behavioral design consideration early in the process, although time may be limited for such considerations. Regarding the latter, which is more common and can be done at many levels from full renovations to minor updates, behavioral design components can be added based on available funds. In both cases, important parameters to consider are operational policies, such as tobacco cessation or food service policies, and contracts that do not require overt changes to physical structures. Such approaches may be particularly useful when funds are limited to enact physical changes.

Strategies to facilitate the integration of behavioral design into practice include legislative (e.g., zoning and land use regulations), business approaches (e.g., rating and certification systems), and their amalgam (e.g., community planning and requirements for certification).

The Food and Beverage Environment

Enabling effective thinking about the potential impact of behavioral design on food and eating patterns requires moving past basic assumptions that taste, price, and convenience are the sole or even primary drivers of dietary choice. "Food" in this section is inclusive of foods and beverages. Our relationship to food is intertwined with much of what it means to be human and stands as a starkly unique quality in the animal world. Food as nourishment and pleasure is physically and viscerally desired and needed. Fluid is essential to hydration. Collectively, food is the social and cultural currency where traditions pass, stories are told, deals are made, and relationships are formed and bonded.

Food is a primary activity of our species, in one way or another we spend much of our time, use most of our land, and a good deal of planetary resources to produce, process, prepare, transport, sell, buy, eat, and dispose of food. Food is omnipresent—everywhere and at all times—and thus our personal and commercial environments are rich in designed materials and structures that influence and often facilitate food and our relationship with food.

At the individual and family levels, food selection, preparation, and consumption are influenced by numerous factors. These include how food is made available in communities and how it is prepared, served, presented, priced, and marketed, as well as the myriad of personal, social, and cultural issues alluded to above. Overlaying virtually all aspects that connect us to food is the potential to influence our actions through physical and informational design. Probably because food is intricately and intimately related to the human psyche, connecting as physical necessity and visceral identity, using behavioral design to influence our actions related to food is common and traditional though increasing in sophistication in the modern commercial sector.

Commercial and academic research has explored and demonstrated—in structured experiments and real-life marketplace implementation—the ability to influence food choices with a myriad of approaches, including packaging, portion sizes, salience, health claims, labeling, design in general, visceral stimulants (e.g., sounds, smells), and cultural/social/normative approaches. Notably, people generally lack insight about the influence of these strategies on their personal dietary choices.[110]

Behavioral design strategies can support better food and beverage choices by informing, encouraging, enabling, and generally making the healthier choices easier, default, normative, and less expensive. Behavioral design also may be able to increase the transparency of how food environments may be driving choice, enabling people to recognize persuasive intention even if near awareness thresholds. As a result, behavioral design potentially brings more awareness to one's actions. Evidence-based behavioral design strategies include numerous approaches that can be roughly classified as ambience, functional design, labeling, presentation, sizing, pricing, priming, prompting, default, and normalization.[15] These strategies are widely employed to sell food but are not limited in their influence and play a general role in ways humans act and persuade.

Therefore, the concepts used in behavioral design traditionally have not been discrete, nor do they require intention or understanding of the concepts to be used (i.e., they are used to some degree inadvertently whenever we offer food). These and other strategies in our food environment produce a concerted exposure. The ideal combination and specifics of application depend on many issues, may vary by circumstances, and not be fully understood, thus limiting the provision of comprehensive and accessible guidance on application.

Ethics of Modifying Exposure

Influencing actions through design is generally seen as less ethically controversial than influencing action by limiting people's choices or by constraining their actions (e.g., bans on the use of *trans* fat or portion-control policies). Influencing actions through design is also generally seen as less ethically controversial than influencing action by financially disincentivizing certain actions—such as taxing sugar-sweetened beverages—which some view as regressive, and, thus, strike some people as unfair.[64] Influencing actions through design, however, is seen as *more* ethically controversial than influencing action by just providing information and education. A primary ethical concern is that using behavioral design to influence action is manipulative and is an ethically inappropriate way to exert control over people. As design expert Dan Lockton puts it: "All design influences our behavior, but as designers we don't always consciously consider the power this gives us to help people (and, sometimes, to manipulate them)."[65] Multiple ethicists have articulated the concern that nudges (one kind of behavioral design) can be manipulative.[66,67,68,69]

As a first response to these concerns about manipulation, it is important to note that design—through sounds, colors, smells, signs, and the physical layout of spaces—can slow people down, prompt them to engage in reflection, and put them into more reflective mind states. Thus, behavioral design is not always used to make our experience less reflective and deliberative. Another important response to concerns about manipulation is that the intention behind behavioral design can be made transparent, through the use of signs or design features that are overt.

But what about behavioral design that does not enhance reflection and reflective mind states, but instead influences behavior without prompting reflection about this behavior (e.g., prompting people to take the stairs rather than the elevator, but without prompting any reflection about that matter)? What about behavioral design that is not fully transparent to people who encounter it—or design that is transparent to us but nonetheless influences us emotionally and psychologically in ways that we cannot control? Should we worry that behavioral design could be manipulative?

Whether behavioral design *is* manipulative and *is* ethically problematic for those reasons are complex ethical questions. The case that behavioral design is manipulative might go roughly as follows: It is manipulation whenever someone's action is influenced by means other than rational persuasion or by means other than engaging her in reflection and deliberation. Behavioral design does not influence action by rationally persuading people to act in a certain way, nor does it influence action by engaging people in reflection and deliberation, but instead bypasses reflection and deliberation. Thus, behavioral design is manipulative. But this argument is based on an understanding of manipulation and rationality that many scholars would reject. There are countless examples of influence that do not engage people in reflection and deliberation, and are not rational persuasion, yet are not manipulative. Rather than understanding manipulation as influence that does not engage people in rational deliberation, a better understanding is this: Manipulation is influence that intentionally makes people fall short of various rational ideals and behavioral ideals. With this way of defining manipulation, designers' and policymakers' use of behavioral design is not inherently manipulative, but only manipulates us when it intentionally makes us fall short of rational ideals and behavioral ideals.[70,71] Thus, one could argue that using behavioral design to promote health is not manipulative because it aims to influence people to act in healthier ways, which better aligns people's behavior with their goals and values. Continuing this line of thought, one might argue that the use of behavioral design by many in the private sector is different. That is, many in the private sector are not using behavioral design to make a consumer behave in ways that better align with a consumer's goals and values, but rather most in the private sector are primarily aiming to produce behavior that is profitable for commercial interests.

This alternative understanding of manipulation makes sense in light of work on "bounded rationality." Behavior is not consistently produced by informed deliberation that culminates in a "rational" choice; this is a lesson of work on "bounded rationality."[72,73] And at baseline, many people are not behaving in ways that are "rational" or align with their goals and values.[137,74] Thus, the ethical standard by which we assess whether influence is manipulative should not be whether that influence encourages rational deliberation, but instead whether that influence encourages behavior that better aligns with people's goals and values. Furthermore, as Cass Sunstein has argued, reducing the number of choices that people make can enhance their autonomy: "If we had to make far more decisions, our autonomy would be compromised, because we would be unable to focus on what concerns us."[139]

Therefore, arguments can be made that behavioral design is not inherently manipulative—it can prompt reflective engagement with the world, and even when it doesn't, it can help align people's behavior with their goals and values. A further argument in favor of behavioral design is that it can enhance our ability to make good choices when it counts by reducing the number of choices we must actively make. Although these ethical defenses of behavioral design have merit, a note of caution is needed. It is not defensible to assume that healthier behavior *always* aligns with people's goals and values, so it is not defensible to assume that behavioral design for health *always* helps people align their behavior with their goals and values. Nor is it ethically defensible to assume that it always makes people better off. A theme in the ethics literature is that unhealthy behavior has benefits and healthy behavior has costs—for example, when people drink less soda, they might experience less pleasure or lose out on valuable social experiences.[75,76,77] Thus, the most ethically preferable behavioral design efforts are those that not only produce healthier behavior, but which also *make healthier behavior less costly and more rewarding* for individuals and groups. In this context, it may be useful to draw a distinction between uses of behavioral design that provide people with new opportunities or experiences, or make existing options better—for example, making walking paths and parks safer or more beautiful—and uses of behavioral design that do not. An example of the latter would be setting an option as the default to take advantage of the psychological propensity to stick with the default, but without making that option any better. Although the latter strategies may be ethically defensible in many cases, the former are generally ethically preferable, all other things equal.

Another way to defend behavioral design for health against the charge of manipulation is to concede that it may be manipulative. Nonetheless, the argument would go, this manipulation may be ethically acceptable when it makes enough individuals better off or provides sufficient benefit to the public.[134] This defense also allows us to distinguish behavioral design for health from much behavioral design in the private sector, which arguably does not primarily aim to make individuals better off or to benefit the public.

It is also important to distinguish behavioral design that has paternalistic aims—it aims to change individuals' behavior to improve *their own* health and well-being—and behavioral design that is not just paternalistic, but also aims to change individuals' behavior to protect or benefit others. Ethicists generally agree that it is harder to justify paternalism, especially if a society's shared political values include valuing extensive personal liberty and individual freedom, but easier to justify measures that benefit third parties or protect them from harm.[78,79,80,81] For example, tobacco control measures have been justified as protecting bystanders from the harms of secondhand smoke, not just as protecting smokers themselves.[72] That government has a responsibility to protect citizens' health from others' harmful behavior is an idea that has resonance even with those who think individuals should be free to harm themselves.[71,72,145,146] Similarly, the view that government and civil society have a responsibility to protect children's health and well-being may be accepted even by those who think that adults should be free to adopt unhealthy lifestyles.

The Physical Activity Environment

The relationship of behavioral design to the physical activity environment has similarities to that of its relationship to the food and beverage environment, but the interfaces may be more direct and immediate. Movement is inherent and feels good to many, and the built environment is largely where physical activity happens and has the potential to be shaped in ways that not only encourage but require physical activity. Unfortunately, the modern built environment has progressively made physical activity difficult, for both in-tentional and unintentional reasons. If environments are designed and con-structed with humans in mind, it may be supposed that we might achieve sufficient exercise simply by going through our usual daily routines. It is gen-erally presupposed that in the past the ambient level of physical activity re-quired by the demands of daily living may have been sufficient for a healthy lifestyle.[82] A variety of issues, however, have slowly eroded our physical ac-tivity levels in response to the demands of daily living.

As with food, physical activity is a continuous and cumulative habit, and thus small repetitive changes over long periods of time are sufficient to cre-ate notable outcomes (positive or negative). For example, many labor-saving devices reduce our physical activity. A few illustrative examples in homes in-clude dishwashers, garage door openers, and remote controls; other examples from our work or social environment include inactive transport, elevators, fewer jobs with manual labor, generally more automation and labor-saving devices, and, in general, increasing screen time from all devices.

Numerous aspects of the modern built environment impede activity. For example, walking, biking, and other active transport are difficult and dangerous in a car-centric environment; wide-ranging safety issues, real or perceived, reduce free and open outdoor play for children; and car-based transportation systems generally reduce physical activity. Adding to the gen-eral trend toward sedentary behavior, where movement only happens from couch to car and car to work, is the general decline of access to the beau-ties of the natural world. Improving access to sidewalks may improve activity, but we also need open engagement with natural areas and clean, safe, and appealing built environments to reduce the cognitive barriers. Recent place-making efforts have highlighted the need for places for these activities; one example that addresses this issue is the Project for Public Spaces, which is a nonprofit planning, design, and educational organization that is dedicated to helping people create and sustain public spaces that build stronger com-munities (See Application of Design Strategies to Food and Physical Activity Environments).

A relative consensus exists on recommendations for how built environments—such as schools, playgrounds/parks, communities, cities, and transport systems—can be designed to encourage and enable more active living. Reviews report a variety of successful approaches to increase activity that potentially may be facilitated and augmented by integrating behavioral design concepts. Behavioral and social approaches include social support within communities and worksites, physical education, classroom activities, after-school sports, and active transport in schools. Environmental and policy approaches include access to places for physical activity and informational activities, community and street-scale urban design, active transport policy and practices, and community-wide policies and planning.

Numerous groups have developed these strategies for recommendations; for example, the Centers for Disease Control and Prevention (CDC) recommended strategies, briefly summarized below, to create environments that encourage physical activity (https://www.cdc.gov/healthyplaces/healthtopics/physactivity.htm):

- Improve access to outdoor recreational facilities such as parks and green spaces.
- Build or enhance infrastructures such as sidewalks, paths, and trails to support walking and bicycling for transportation and recreation.
- Support locating schools within easy walking distance of residential areas.
- Improve access to public transportation.
- Support mixed-use development where people can live, work, play, and meet everyday shopping and lifestyle needs within a single neighborhood.
- Enhance personal and traffic safety in areas where people are or could be physically active.
- Participate in community coalitions or partnerships to address obesity.

Operationalizing these strategies from ideation and information campaigns to policies can benefit from including behavioral design. Incorporating behavioral design to facilitate physical activity efforts can systemize synthetic approaches to the whole environment.

Application of Design Strategies to Food and Physical Activity Environments

This section provides an overview of the research on the application of behavioral design strategies to foster active living and healthy eating among children, teenagers, and their families, along with the communities in which they live, learn, work, and play.

Although a detailed summary of the many behavioral design approaches and strategies is beyond the scope herein, we have attempted to capture aspects to consider when evaluating or intervening in the behavioral design process (Figure 3.4).

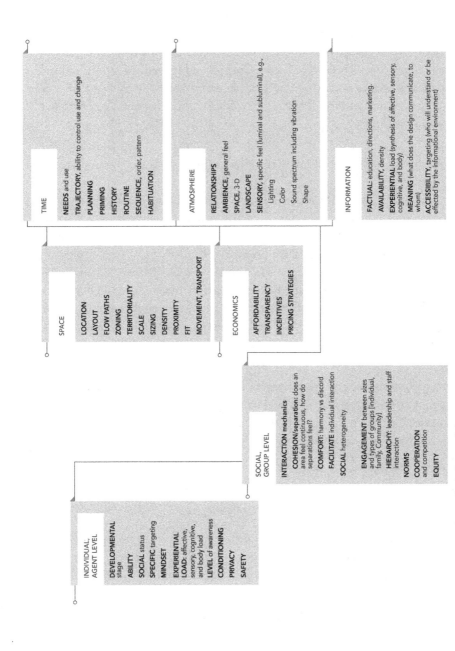

TIME

NEEDS and use
TRAJECTORY, ability to control use and change
PLANNING
PRIMING
HISTORY
ROUTINE
SEQUENCE, order, pattern
HABITUATION

ATMOSPHERE

RELATIONSHIPS
AMBIENCE, general feel
SPACE, 3-D
LANDSCAPE
SENSORY, specific feel (luminal and subluminal), e.g.,
Lighting
Color
Sound spectrum including vibration
Shape

INFORMATION

FACTUAL: education, directions, marketing.
AVAILABILITY, density
EXPERIENTIAL load (synthesis of affective, sensory, cognitive, and body)
MEANING (what does the design communicate, to whom)
ACCESSIBILITY, targeting (who will understand or be effected by the informational environment)

SPACE

LOCATION
LAYOUT
FLOW PATHS
ZONING
TERRITORIALITY
SCALE
SIZING
DENSITY
PROXIMITY
FIT
MOVEMENT, TRANSPORT

ECONOMICS

AFFORDABILITY
TRANSPARENCY
INCENTIVES
PRICING STRATEGIES

SOCIAL, GROUP LEVEL

INTERACTION mechanics
COHESION/separation: does an area feel continuous, how do separations feel?
COMFORT: harmony vs discord
FACILITATE individual interaction
SOCIAL heterogeneity

ENGAGEMENT between sizes and types of groups (individual, family, Community)
HIERARCHY: leadership and staff interaction
NORMS
COOPERATION and competition
EQUITY

INDIVIDUAL, AGENT LEVEL

DEVELOPMENTAL stage
ABILITY
SOCIAL status
SPECIFIC targeting
MINDSET
EXPERIENTIAL LOAD: affective, sensory, cognitive, and body load
LEVEL of awareness
CONDITIONING
PRIVACY
SAFETY

FIGURE 3.4 Aspects to consider in the behavioral design process.

Healthy Eating

Although several sectors of society affect a child's eating and exercise behaviors, as well as health outcomes, research indicates that well-designed, well-implemented school programs can effectively promote physical activity, healthy eating, and reductions in television viewing time.[83] In the United States, almost all (more than 95%) children and adolescents are enrolled in school.[84] American students also attend school for more than 13 years of their lives and spend an average of 6.7 hours a day there during the school year. Research indicates the school's physical environment influences student behavior, attitudes, and academic achievement.[85] Studies have examined the role of seating position, classroom design, density, privacy, noise, the presence or absence of windows, and open space.

Several facets make up the school food environment, and a variety of factors influence the foods children are offered and, ultimately, eat at school.[86] Increasingly, researchers and practitioners are exploring the application of behavioral design principles to the school food environment,[87] especially within the USDA-sponsored National School Lunch Program in which more than 30 million students participate every school day.[88] The Pew Charitable Trust Kids' Safe and Healthful Foods Project assessed school kitchen equipment and infrastructure challenges across the United States and found that 88% of surveyed school districts needed at least one piece of kitchen equipment and 55% needed kitchen infrastructure changes such as electrical upgrades.[89]

A recent systematic review identified 102 studies reporting evidence regarding the influence of the school physical environment on healthy-eating outcomes.[90] Most of these studies (n = 71; 70%) were from the United States. Using a causal loop diagram, this review determined that architecture and design helped create supportive, healthy-eating school environments and positively affected healthy-eating outcomes. A range of influential physical factors emerged from the studies reviewed; specifically, serving style, water access, vending machines, on-site food production such as school gardens, and educational signage. The school physical environment review discussed how potential synergistic influences could potentially impact the role of physical space and design. In particular, the review noted how the adoption and use of healthy-eating programming and practices were critical, yet it acknowledged major implementation barriers such as competing priorities and inadequate resources.

To improve the schools' ability to adopt healthy nutrition curriculum and promote healthy eating using design principles, a recent National Collaborative on Childhood Obesity Research (NCCOR) sponsored tool was developed, known as Healthy Eating Design Guidelines for School Architecture.[91] Based on a pilot of this tool in a rural school district in Virginia, the guidelines helped remove physical barriers; nonetheless, unanticipated challenges emerged and school staff varied in their awareness and comfort with using the new healthy-eating features.[92] Often, the school-based interventions used multiple modifications to improve the intake of fruits and vegetables, while others used them to target low-fat milk and water. Some interventions simultaneously used behavioral design strategies to target improvements in physical activity. Several studies also rigorously evaluated specific strategies such as using attractive names for vegetables or serving sliced fruit. In conclusion, infrastructural changes are increasingly being explored in the school food environment, and they generally help promote healthy eating when complemented by nutrition education and promotion, along with changes in meal preparation practices and procurement strategies.

Efforts to promote healthy eating outside of the school food environment have examined a range of design strategies and have mainly targeted the following key eating settings: home, childcare centers, worksite, retail food outlets, and restaurants.[84] Special attention has generally been given to improving access to healthier foods and beverages among the most high-risk, underserved populations. To illustrate, an innovative social experiment conducted from 1994 to 1998 randomly assigned 4,498 women with children living in public housing in high-poverty, urban census tracts to one of three groups, namely to:

(1) receive housing vouchers, which were redeemable only if they moved to a low-poverty census tract and had counseling on moving;
(2) receive unrestricted, traditional vouchers, with no special counseling on moving;
(3) offered neither of these opportunities (control group).[93]

From 2008 through 2010, various health outcomes were examined among participants, and results found that the opportunity to move from a neighborhood with a high-level of poverty to one with a lower level of poverty was modestly associated with reductions in extreme obesity and type 2 diabetes. A recent randomized controlled trial with children aged 3 to 5 years participating in a home-based intervention tested the effects of a strategy that paired positive stimuli (i.e., stickers and cartoon packaging) with vegetables and presented them as a default snack; the study found significant effects on vegetable intake.[94] In childcare centers, interventions have not been as extensively explored as compared to the school food environment. Nevertheless, evidence is emerging that shows the promise of applying behavioral design principles in this developmentally important setting. For instance, a recent study found building a garden at a childcare center was positively associated with the attending preschoolers' intake of fruits and vegetables.[95] Although not a key sector for affecting healthy eating among children and adolescents, research in institutional food service settings has furthered or laid the foundation for the evidence base to inform the use of design strategies in school or childcare center food environments; specifically studies conducted in worksite,[96] military,[97] healthcare,[98] and university[99] settings.

Over the past decade, the application of design strategies to the retail food environment has been considered at the local, state, tribal, and national levels, particularly to address disparities in access to healthy foods[100] and with special attention on promoting healthy eating among participants in federal food and nutrition assistance programs.[101] Strategies have ranged from product labeling to point-of-purchase prompts, to zoning provisions supporting the development of community gardens and farmers' markets, to public–private partnerships incentivizing the building or renovating of grocery stores.[103,102] An in-store example used a randomized controlled trial to evaluate the effects of in-store marketing strategies to promote the purchase of specific healthier items in five product categories. The intervention resulted in significantly greater sales of the skim and 1% milk, water, and two of the three types of frozen meals, compared with the control store sales during the same time period.[44] On the other hand, a recent study evaluating the introduction of a government-subsidized supermarket into an underserved, urban neighborhood did not find any significant changes in household food availability or children's dietary intake.[103] Indeed, healthy-food store interventions have had mixed results on positively influencing eating behaviors and health outcomes.[104] A recent commentary recognized these mixed findings and acknowledged how addressing access is a critical ingredient, and went on to emphasize how initiatives to improve diet quality and, ultimately, health outcomes need to consider innovative approaches beyond just building a retail food outlet and must aim to build the infrastructure necessary within and around a retail food outlet to promote healthy eating.[105] Moreover, multidisciplinary evaluations are needed that examine the influence of these healthy retail interventions on increasing access to healthy foods and nutrition-related behaviors and health outcomes, as well as their impact on improving community and economic development.[106]

Recognizing that more Americans are eating food prepared away from the home,[107] behavioral design strategies have been applied to promote healthy eating in restaurants. A 2013 review examining the use of choice architecture on eating behavior reported that nutrition labeling at the point-of-purchase was associated with healthier food choices.[108] This review also identified other behavioral design strategies that are being used in self-service settings, such as manipulating the plate and payment options; however, the review determined the evidence base was too limited to understand how the strategies impact the selection and consumption of healthier food and beverage choices. Notwithstanding, studies conducted at this stage indicate how minor changes, such as varying the proximity of more and less healthier items or the serving utensils, can positively affect selection.[109] The majority of behavioral design-related research in restaurants centers on menu engineering.[110] Key menu positioning strategies include shifting attention and taste expectations toward healthier items by using descriptive words, placement, or formatting. Another approach is to increase the perception of value by, for example, deemphasizing attention on the price of the entrees and placing the price at the end of an item description. Even among children, a recent study found menu modifications are associated with healthier ordering patterns without removing choice or reducing revenue.[111] Much work remains to understand the full potential of menus (along with other facets of restaurants, including playgrounds) on promoting the selection and consumption of healthier foods and beverages.

Conclusions

Research and evaluation will play an instrumental role in determining which combination of strategies has the greatest potential to positively impact active living and healthy eating among youth. Case studies will be an invaluable learning tool, particularly ones detailing multidisciplinary approaches. Equally important, periodic reviews and meta-analyses may help identify the most promising strategies, relevant rigorous methodologic designs for addressing various types of questions, and future research needs and opportunities.

Quiz Questions

   1. Behavioral design primarily examines interactions between:
      a. Agents and environments
      b. Environments and exposures

    c.   Health and environments

    d.   agents and exposures

    e.   Both B and D above

2. Behavioral design offers a single rubric for the design and application of public health strategies. True or false?

3. Ecologic approaches are contained in behavioral design. True or false?

4. The concept of *affordance* differs *from environmental determinism* because it:

    a.   Suggests that environments cause behavior

    b.   Indicates behaviors determine environments

    c.   Suggests cost is critical to environmental change

    d.   Indicates the way spaces are arranged signals object use and fosters behavior

    e.   A and D above

5. Human decisions often are influenced by *stimuli* that are perceived as most salient in a given context and environment. True or false?

6. The following is an example of *priming*:

    a.   Putting salt out before a storm

    b.   Smell of fresh baked pizza in a grocery store

    c.   Reading a book about nutrition before going on a diet

    d.   Planning how to manage eating out before you leave the house

7. People are more likely to engage in behaviors that are in line with:

    a.   A positive self-image

    b.   A negative self-image

    c.   A higher status

    d.   A lower status

    e.   A and C above

8. Physical exposure influences affective states such as emotions, feelings, and moods. True or false?

9. Design considerations are primarily relevant in parks. True or false?

10. Which of the following is *not* a strategy to integrate behavioral design into practice:

    a.   Zoning regulations

    b.   Certification systems for businesses

    c.   Cooperative agreements with churches

    d.   Community planning requirements

    e.   Land use regulations

Acknowledgments

NCCOR Behavioral Design Working Group Members

Joel Kimmons, Ph.D.*
David Berrigan, Ph.D., M.P.H.
Michael Burke, Ph.D., M.P.H.
Deirdra Chester, Ph.D., R.D.
Rachel Fisher, M.S., M.P.H., R.D.
Sheila Fleischhacker, Ph.D., J.D.
Nadine Budd, Ph.D.

Rachel Ballard, M.D., M.P.H.*
Laura Kettel-Khan, Ph.D., M.I.M.
Elizabeth Rahavi, R.D.
Jesus Soares, Sc.M., Sc.D.
Matthew Trujillo, Ph.D.
Kathleen Watson, Ph.D.

External Contributors and Participants of 2015–2016 Behavioral Design Meetings

Lydia Ashton, Ph.D.
Anne Barnhill, Ph.D.
Jamie Chriqui, Ph.D., M.H.S.
Samuel Dennis, Jr., Ph.D.
Matthew Finn, R.A.
Terry Huang, Ph.D., M.P.H.

Katie Janson
Robin Moore, Honorary ASLA
Matthew Trowbridge, M.D.
Francine Welty, MD, Ph.D.
Nancy M. Wells, Ph.D.
Mark Wentzel, M.A.

NCCOR Coordinating Center, FHI 360

Elaine Arkin
Jordan Broderick, M.A.
LaVerne Canady, M.P.A.
Mari Nicholson, M.H.S.
*NCCOR Working Group Co-Chairs

Todd Phillips, M.S.
Anne Rodgers
Amanda Samuels, M.S., M.P.H.
Namita Vaidya, M.P.H.

References

1. Bronfenbrenner U. Toward an experimental ecology of human development. American Psychologist. 1977; 32: 513–531.
2. Kersell MW, Milsum JH. A systems model of health behavior change. Behavioral Science. 1985; 30(3): 119–126.
3. McLeroy KR, et al. An ecological perspective on health promotion programs. Health Education Quarterly. 1988; 15(4): 351–377.

4. Cockrell Skinner A, Foster EM. Systems science and childhood obesity: a systematic review and new directions. J Obes. 2013; 2013: 129193

5. Vandenbroeck IP, Goossens J, Clemens M. Foresight tackling obesities: Future choices—building the obesity system map. Government Office for Science, UK Government's Foresight Programme. 2007; retrieved on January 13, 2016 from https://www.gov.uk/government/uploads/system/uploads/attachment_data/file/295154/07-1179-obesity-building-system-map.pdf.

6. Skinner BF. The behavior of organisms: an experimental analysis. Oxford, England: Appleton-Century; 1938.

7. Bandura A. Social foundations of thought and action. Englewood Cliffs, NJ: Prentice Hall; 1986.

8. Ajzen I. The theory of planned behavior. Organizational Behavior and Human Decision Processes. 1991; 50(2): 179–211.

9. Prochaska JO, Redding CA, Evers K. The transtheoretical model and stages of change. In Glanz K, Rimer BK, Lewis FM, editors. Health behavior and health education: theory, research, and practice. 3rd edition. San Francisco, CA: Jossey-Bass, Inc.; 2002.

10. Schwarzer R. Self-efficacy in the adoption and maintenance of health behaviors: theoretical approaches and a new model. In Schwarzer R, editor. Self-efficacy: thought control of action. Washington, DC: Hemisphere; 1992. p. 217–243.

11. Sallis J, Glanz K. Physical activity and food environments: solutions to the obesity epidemic. The Milbank Quarterly. 2009; 87(1): 123–154.

12. Stokols D. Translating social ecological theory into guidelines for community health promotion. Am J Health Promot. 1996; 10(4): 282–298.

13. Kahneman D. A perspective on judgment and choice: mapping bounded rationality. Am Psychol 2003; 58(9):697–720.

14. Arno A, Thomas S. The efficacy of nudge theory strategies in influencing adult dietary behaviour: a systematic review and meta-analysis. BMC Public Health. 2016; 16: 676.

15. Hollands GJ, Shemilt I, Marteau TM, et al. Altering micro-environments to change population health behaviour: towards an evidence base for choice architecture interventions. BMC Public Health. 2013; 13: 1218.

16. Datta S, Mullainathan S. Behavioral design: a new approach to development policy. CGD Policy Paper 016. Center for Global Development. Washington, DC. Available at: http://www.cgdev.org/content/publications/detail/1426679; 2012.

17. Alexander C. The phenomenon of life: the nature of order: an essay on the art of building and the nature of the universe. Berkeley: CES Publishing; 2003.

18. Alexander C. The timeless way of building. New York: Oxford University Press; 1979.

19. Kopec D. Environmental psychology for design. 2nd edition. Canada: Fairchild Books; 2012.

20. Exec. Order No. 13707, 3 C.F.R. 56365; 2015.

21. Dolan P, Hallsworth M, Halpern D, et al. Influencing behaviour: the mindspace way. J Econ Psychol. 2012 Feb; 33(1): 264–277.

22. The Behavioural Insights Team. Update Report 2015–16; 2016. Available at: http:// 38r8om2xjhhl25mw24492dir.wpengine.netdna-cdn.com/wp-content/uploads/ 2016/09/BIT_Update_Report_2015-16-.pdf .

23. Lourenço JS, Ciriolo E, Almeida SR, et al. Behavioural insights applied to policy: European Report 2016. EUR 27726 EN.

24. NSW Department of Premier and Cabinet—Behavioural Insights Unit. Understanding people, better outcomes; 2014. Available from http://bi.dpc.nsw. gov.au/library/ .

25. Wells NM, Evans, GW, Aldred Cheek KL. Environmental psychology. In Frumkin H, editor. Environmental health: from global to local. Hoboken (NJ): John Wiley & Sons; 2016.

26. Carson R. Silent spring. Boston: Houghton Mifflin; 1962.

27. De Young R. New ways to promote proenvironmental behavior: expanding and evaluating motives for environmentally responsible behavior. Journal of Social Issues. 2000; 56(3): 509–526.

28. Evans GW. Environmental stress. CUP Archive; 1984.

29. Sallis JF, Bauman A, Pratt M. Environmental and policy interventions to promote physical activity. American Journal of Public Health. 1998; 15(4): 379.

30. Story M, Kaphingst KM, Robinson-O'Brien R, et al. Creating healthy food and eating environments: policy and environmental approaches. Annu Rev Public Health. 2008; 29: 253–272.

31. Wells NM, Evans GW, Yang Y. Environments and health: planning decisions as public health decisions. Journal of Architectural and Planning Research. 2010; 27(2): 124–143.

32. Hillier B. Space is the machine: a configurational theory of architecture. London, UK: Space Syntax. 2007.

33. Evans GW, Lepore SJ, Schroeder A. The role of interior design elements in human responses to crowding. Journal of Personality and Social Psychology. 1996; 70(1): 41.

34. Rollings KR, Wells NM. Effects of residential kitchen floor plan openness on eating behaviors. Environment & Behavior; in press.

35. Hanks AS, Just DR, Smith LE, et al. Healthy convenience: nudging students toward healthier choices in the lunchroom. Journal of Public Health. 2012; fds003: 1–7.

36. Gifford R. Environmental psychology: principles and practice. 5th edition. Colville (WA): Optimal Books; 2014.

37. Becker MH. *The health belief model and personal health behavior*. Thorofare, NJ: Slack; 1974.

38. Ajzen I, Fishbein M. Understanding attitudes and predicting social behavior. Englewood Cliffs, NJ: Prentice-Hall;1980.

39. Ajzen I, Madden TJ. Prediction of goal-directed behavior: attitudes, intentions and perceived behavioral control. J Exp Soc Psychol. 1986 Sept; 22(5): 453–474.

40. World Health Organization (WHO). Behaviour change strategies and health: the role of health systems. WHO: Tbilisi, Georgia; 2008.

41. Sheeran P. Intention-behaviour relations: a conceptual and empirical review. Eur Rev Soc Psychol. 2002; 12: 1–36.

42. Webb T, Sheeran P. Does changing behavioral intentions engender behavior change? A meta-analysis of the experimental evidence. Psychol Bull. 2006 Mar; 132(2): 249–68.

43. Kahneman D, Thaler R. Anomalies: utility maximisation and experienced utility. J Econ Perspect. 2006; 20(1): 221–234.

44. Foster GD, Karypn A, Wojtanowski AC, et al. Placement and promotion of strategies to increase sales of healthier products in supermarkets in low-income, ethnically diverse neighborhoods: a randomized controlled trial. Am J Clin Nutr. 2014; 99: 1359–1368.

45. Wansink B. Environmental factors that increase the food intake and consumption volume of unknowing consumers. Annu Rev Nutr. 2004; 24: 455–479.

46. Ferriday D, Brunstrom JM. "I just can't help myself": effects of food-cue exposure in overweight and lean individuals. Int J Obes. 2011; 35(1): 142–149.

47. McCrickerd K, Forde CG. Sensory influences on food intake control: moving beyond palatability. Obes Rev. 2016; 17(1): 18–29.

48. World Bank. World development report 2015: mind, society, and behavior. Washington, DC: World Bank; 2015.

49. Baumeister RF, Bratslavsky E, Muraven M, et al. Ego depletion: is the active self a limited resource? J Pers Soc Psychol. 1998; 74(5): 1252–1265.

50. Weir, K. What you need to know about willpower: the psychological science of self-control. American Psychological Association; 2012. Available at: http://www.apa.org/helpcenter/willpower.pdf.

51. Project for Public Spaces. The case for healthy places: improving health outcomes through placemaking. Project for Public Spaces; 2016. Available at: https://www.pps.org/wp-content/uploads/2016/12/Healthy-Places-PPS.pdf.

52. Hagger MS, Wood C, Stiff C, et al. Ego depletion and the strength model of self-control: a meta-analysis. Psychol Bull. 2010; 136(4): 495–525.

53. Morsella E, Poehlman TA. The inevitable contrast: conscious vs. unconscious processes in action control. Front Psychol. 2013; 4: 590.

54. Muraven M, Baumeister RF. Self-regulation and depletion of limited resources: does self-control resemble a muscle? Psychol Bull. 2000; 126(2): 247–259.

55. Baumeister RF, Masicampo EJ, Vohs KD. Do conscious thoughts cause behavior? Annu Rev Psychol. 2011; 62: 331–361.

56. Shah AK, Shafir E, Mullainathan S. Scarcity frames value. Psychological Science. 2015; 26(4): 204–212.

57. Brown B, Rutherford P, Crawford P. The role of noise in clinical environments with particular reference to mental health care: a narrative review. Int J Nurs Stud. 2015; 52(9): 1514–1524.

58. Stansfeld SA, Matheson MP. Noise pollution: non-auditory effects on health. Br Med Bull. 2003; 68: 243–257.

59. Mehta R, Zhu R, Cheema A. Is noise always bad? Exploring the effects of ambient noise on creative cognition. Journal of Consumer Research. 2012; 39(4): 784–799.

60. Mehta R, Zhu RJ. Blue or red? Exploring the effect of color on cognitive task performances. Science. 2009; 323(5918): 1226–1229.

61. Genschow O, Reutner L, Wänke M. The color red reduces snack food and soft drink intake. Appetite. 2012; 58(2): 699–702.

62. Meyers-Levy J, Zhu R. The influence of ceiling height: the effect of priming on type of processing that people use. J Consum Res. 2007; 34(2): 174–186.

63. Cohen DA, Babey SH. Contextual influences on eating behaviors: heuristic processing and dietary choices. Obes Rev. 2012 May; 13(9): 766–779.

64. Barry CL, Niederdeppe J, Gollust SE. Taxes on sugar-sweetened beverages: results from a 2011 national public opinion survey. American Journal of Preventive Medicine. 2013; 44 (2): 158–163.

65. Lockton D. Introduction to the design with intent toolkit. Design with Intent; 2016. Accessed November 11. http://designwithintent.co.uk/introduction-to-the-design-with-intent-toolkit/ .

66. Conly S. Against autonomy: justifying coercive paternalism. Cambridge: Cambridge University Press; 2013. p. 29–32.

67. Waldron J. It's all for your own good. The New York Review of Books; 2014 Oct.

68. Sunstein CR. Making government logical. The New York Times. 2015 Sept 19. http://www.nytimes.com/2015/09/20/opinion/sunday/cass-sunstein-making-government-logicalhtml.html .

69. Eyal N. Nudging and benign manipulation for health. In Cohen IG, Fernandez Lynch H, editors. Nudging health: health law and behavioral economics. JHU Press; 2016. p. 83–96 .

70. Noggle R. Manipulative actions: a conceptual and moral analysis. American Philosophical Quarterly. 1996; 33(1): 43–55.

71. Barnhill A. What is manipulation? In Coons C, Weber M, editors. Manipulation: theory and practice. Oxford; New York: Oxford University Press; 2014. p. 51–72.

72. Thaler RH, Sunstein CR. Nudge: improving decisions about health, wealth, and happiness. New Haven: Yale University Press; 2008.

73. Kahneman D. Thinking, fast and slow. 1st edition. New York: Farrar, Straus and Giroux; 2011.

74. Sunstein CR. Why nudge?: the politics of libertarian paternalism. New Haven: Yale University Press; 2014.

75. Resnik D. Trans fat bans and human freedom. The American Journal of Bioethics. 2010; 10(3): 27–32.

76. Noe A. The value in sweet drinks. NPR.org; 2013. Accessed August 1. http://www. npr.org/blogs/13.7/2012/09/24/161277720/the-value-in-sweet-drinks .

77. Barnhill A, King KF, Kass N, Faden R. The value of unhealthy eating and the ethics of healthy eating policies. Kennedy Institute of Ethics Journal. 2014; 24(3): 187–217.

78. Feinberg J. Harm to self. New York: Oxford University Press; 1986.

79. Bayer R. The continuing tensions between individual rights and public health. Talking point on public health versus civil liberties. EMBO Reports; 2007; 8(12): 1099–1103.

80. Gostin LO, Gostin KG. A broader liberty: J.S. Mill, paternalism and the public's health. Public Health. 2009; 123(3): 214–221.

81. Verweij M. Infectious disease control. In Dawson A, editor. Public health ethics. Cambridge and New York: Cambridge University Press; 2011. p. 100–117.

82. Lieberman DE. Is exercise really medicine? An evolutionary perspective. Curr Sports Med Rep. 2015;14(4):313–319.

83. Wechsler H, McKenna ML, Lee SM, et al. The role of schools in preventing childhood obesity. The State Education Standard. 2004. Available at: http://www.cdc. gov/healthyyouth/physicalactivity/pdf/roleofschools_obesity.pdf.

84. Story M, Kaphingst KM, French S. The role of schools in obesity prevention. The Future of Children. 2006; 16(1): 109–142.

85. Weinstein, CS. The physical environment of the school: a review of the research. Rev Educational Res. 1979; 49(4): 577–610.

86. Johnson DB, Podrabsky M, Rocha A, et al. Effect of the healthy hunger-free kids act on the nutritional quality of meals selected by students and school lunch participation rates. JAMA Pediatr. 2016; 170(1): e153918.

87. Gorman N, Lackney JA, Rollings K, et al. Designer schools: the role of school space and architecture in obesity prevention. Obesity (Silver Spring). 2007; 15(11): 2521–2530.

88. Mancino L, Guthrie J. When nudging in the lunch line might be a good thing. USDA Economic Research Service. Amber Waves. 2009;7(1). Available at: http:// smarterlunchrooms.org/sites/default/files/mancino_guthrie_2009_when_nudging_in_the_lunchline_might_be_a_good_thing.pdf .

89. The Pew Charitable Trusts Kids' Safe and Healthful Foods Project. States need updated school kitchen equipment. Released March 26, 2014. Available at: http://www.pewtrusts.org/en/research-and-analysis/reports/2014/03/26/ states-need-updated-school-kitchen-equipment-b .

90. Frerichs L, Brittin J, Sorensen D, et al. Influence of school architecture and design on healthy eating: a review of the literature. Am J Public Health. 2015; 105(4): e46–e57.

91. Huang TT, Sorensen D, Davis S, et al. Healthy eating design guidelines for school architecture. Prev Chronic Dis. 2013; 10: E27.

92. Frerichs L, Brittin J, Intobubbe-Chmil L, et al. The role of school design in shaping healthy eating-related attitudes, practices, and behaviors among school staff. J Sch Health. 2016; 86(1): 11–22.

93. Ludwig J, Sanbonmatsu L, Gennetian L, et al. Neighborhoods, obesity, and diabetes—a randomized social experiment. N Engl J Med. 2011; 365(16): 1509–1519.

94. Cravener TL, Schlecher H, Loeb KL, et al. Feeding strategies derived from behavioral economics and psychology can increase vegetable intake in children as part of a home-based intervention: results of a pilot study. J Acad Nutr Diet. 2015; 115(11): 1798–1807.

95. Namenek Brouwer RJ, Neelon SE B. Watch me grow: a garden-based pilot intervention to increase vegetable and fruit intake in preschoolers. BMC Public Health. 2013; 13: 363.

96. Hipp JA, Reeds DN, Van Bakergem MA, et al. Review of measures of worksite environmental and policy supports for physical activity and healthy eating. Prev Chron Dis. 2015; 12: 140410.

97. Arsenault JE, Singleton MC, Funderburk LK. Use of the go-for-green nutrition labeling system in military dining facilities is associated with lower fat intake. J Acad Nutr Diet. 2014; 114: 1067–1071.

98. Thorndike AN, Riis J, Sonnenberg LM, et al. Traffic-light labels and choice architecture: promoting healthy food choices. Am J Prev Med. 2014; 46(2): 143–149.

99. Cioffi CE, Levitsky DA, Pacanowski CR, et al. A nudge in a healthy direction. The effect of nutrition labels on food purchasing behaviors in university dining facilities. Appetite. 2015; 92: 7–14.

100. Larson NI, Story MT, Nelson MC. Neighborhood environments: disparities in access to healthy foods in the U.S. Am J Prev Med. 2009; 36(1): 74–81.

101. Just DR, Mancino L, Wansink B. Could behavioral economics help improve diet quality for nutrition assistance program participants? US Department of Agriculture Economic Research Service; 2007 June; Economic Research Report Number 43. Available at: http://www.ers.usda.gov/media/196728/err43_1_.pdf.

102. Glanz K, Bader MDM, Iyer S. Retail grocery store marketing strategies and obesity: an integrative review. Am J Prev Med. 2012; 42(5): 503–512.

103. Elbel B, Moran A, Dixon LB, et al. Assessment of a government-subsidized supermarket in a high-need area on household food availability and children's dietary intakes. Public Health Nutr. 2015; 18(15): 2881–2890.

104. Williams J, Scarborough P, Matthews A, et al. A systematic review of the influence of the retail food environment around schools on obesity-related outcomes. Obes Rev. 2014; 15(5): 359–374.

105. Block JP, Subramanian SV. Moving beyond "food deserts": reorienting United States policies to reduce disparities in diet quality. PLoS Med. 2015; 12(12): e1001914.

106. Fleischhacker SE, Flournoy R, Moore LV. Meaningful, measurable, and manageable approaches to evaluating healthy food financing initiatives: an overview of resources and approaches. J Public Health Manag Pract. 2013; 19(6): 541–549.

107. Yen S, Lin B, Davis C. Consumer knowledge and meat consumption at home and away from home. Food Policy. 2008; 33(6): 631–639.

108. Skov LR, Lourenço S, Hansen GL, Mikkelsen BE, Schofield C. Choice architecture as a means to change eating behaviour in self-service settings: a systematic review. Obes Rev. 2013; 14(3): 187–196.

109. Rozin P, Scott S, Dingley M, et al. Nudge to nobesity I: minor changes in accessibility decrease food intake. Judgement Decision Making. 2011; 6(4): 323–332.

110. Wansink B, Love K. Slim by design: menu strategies for promoting high-margin, healthy foods. Int J Hospitality Management. 2014; 42: 137–143.

111. Anzman-Frasca S, Mueller MP, Sliwa S, et al. Changes in children's meal orders following healthy menu modifications at a regional US restaurant chain. Obesity. 2015; 23s: 1055–1062.

4

Health Disparities

RACE, ETHNICITY, GENDER, AND CLASS

Alison G.M. Brown and Sara C. Folta

Chapter Highlights

- Explore how race, ethnicity, gender, and socioeconomic status influence diet-related health outcomes, such as malnutrition, obesity, hypertension, diabetes, and cardiovascular and cerebrovascular disease, and the complexity of the underlying causes of these health disparities and inequities.
- Provide a foundational understanding of the terms and concepts as well as the historical nature of these disparities.
- Discuss the array of factors that contribute to health disparities, including the social determinants of health such as educational level, employment status, environmental factors, access and affordability of healthy food, neighborhood segregation, chronic stress, and access to health care.
- Given the growing number of immigrants in the United States and their important role in society, discuss the healthy immigrant hypothesis and the dietary acculturation process among various immigrant groups in the United States.
- Elaborate on global diet-related health disparities and the global and societal factors that perpetuate these differences in outcomes.

Consideration of Definitions
Health Disparities versus Health Inequities

Although the title of this chapter includes the term "Health Disparities," in considering definitions, it is important to note the differences between health disparities and health inequities. According to the Centers for Disease Control and Prevention, health disparities are defined as any difference in disease or health status between population groups in which disparities are measured in comparison to the most favorable group or segment of the population. Health inequities, however, include an element of unfairness and injustice, in which the disparity in disease rates is due to avoidable differences in social, economic, environmental, or health care resources. For example, there is a disparity in breast cancer rates between women and men that is unrelated to inequities; but the disparity in diabetes between Native Americans and whites is considered a health inequity because it has historical roots in discriminatory practices and policies in the United States. Many of the disparities in diet-related diseases that we will be highlighting in this chapter, in fact, pertain to underlying inequities.

When observing differences in diet-related diseases, it is important to consider the underlying factors that may contribute to these disparities. Is it solely due to individual practices and decision making around food choice? What environmental factors (such as the availability and affordability of healthy, nutritious food) influence food-related decisions? Are there current and/or historical social, economic, and political factors at play that shape these environmental characteristics?

Race and Ethnicity

Race and ethnicity are commonly used in public health and epidemiological literature to compare the prevalence and risk of certain diseases and health outcomes between different groups. However, the classification system by race, both in the United States and globally, is now widely considered a social construct; that is, there is *no meaningful biological basis* for the classification.[1] Rather, it is a classification system that developed largely to justify systems of oppression such as slavery in the Americas and thereafter evolved to continue to socially and economically divide populations.[2] Today, in health disparities research, the race variable is thought to measure a combination of some aspect of social class, culture, and genetics, serving, however, only as a rough proxy for each.[3,4] Converse to race, ethnicity is generally used to describe a more distinctive cultural tradition; there is, however, no clear consensus on a standardized definition of either race or ethnicity. These labels are, in fact, often used interchangeably.[3]

In 2010, the U.S. Office of Management and Budget classified individuals under four distinct racial categories (white, Black or African American, American Indian or Alaskan Native, or Native Hawaiian or another Pacific Islander) and one ethnic category (Hispanic or Latino and Not Hispanic or

Latino)[5]. A major limitation of this categorization structure is the breadth of these categories, which may prevent public health practitioners from being able to gauge health disparities accurately. For example, the African American/Black racial category includes African Americans whose families have been in the United States for many generations as well as immigrants from countries throughout Africa and the Caribbean, each with meaningful differences in culture and lifestyle patterns that influence food preferences and diet quality. Comparatively, the Census in England more accurately captures the heterogeneity within each larger racial category. To help address the diversity that exists within the broad categories used in the United States, the proposed 2020 U.S. Census questions, taking a lead from other countries such as the United Kingdom, will provide granular information. (See Figure 4.1 for comparison of 2010 census questions compared with the proposed 2020 questions and the U.K. census.)

Throughout this chapter, the above foundational understanding of race and ethnicity will be helpful as we discuss health disparities based on these constructs. As we will discuss later in the chapter, perceptions of racism and ethnocentrism are considered social determinants of health that relate to diet-related diseases such as hypertension and heart disease.

Gender

Sex and gender are also terms that often are used interchangeably despite their distinctly different meanings. Sex is descriptive of the anatomy of an individual's reproductive system and secondary sex characteristics (i.e., facial hair, increased muscle mass, deepening of voice in males and enlargement of breasts in females). Gender, on the other hand, is socially based according to one's internal awareness, identity, and/or sexual orientation. In terms of gender identity, an individual can therefore be female, male, transgender, non-binary, or gender nonconforming. Both sex-based and gender- and sexual-orientation based diet-related health disparities will be discussed in this chapter; the latter has received less attention from researchers and more work is necessary.

Diet-related Health Disparities by Race and Ethnicity in the United States
Hispanic/Latino

Hispanic/Latino is an ethnic group that includes individuals of Cuban, Mexican, Puerto Rican, South or Central American, or other Spanish culture

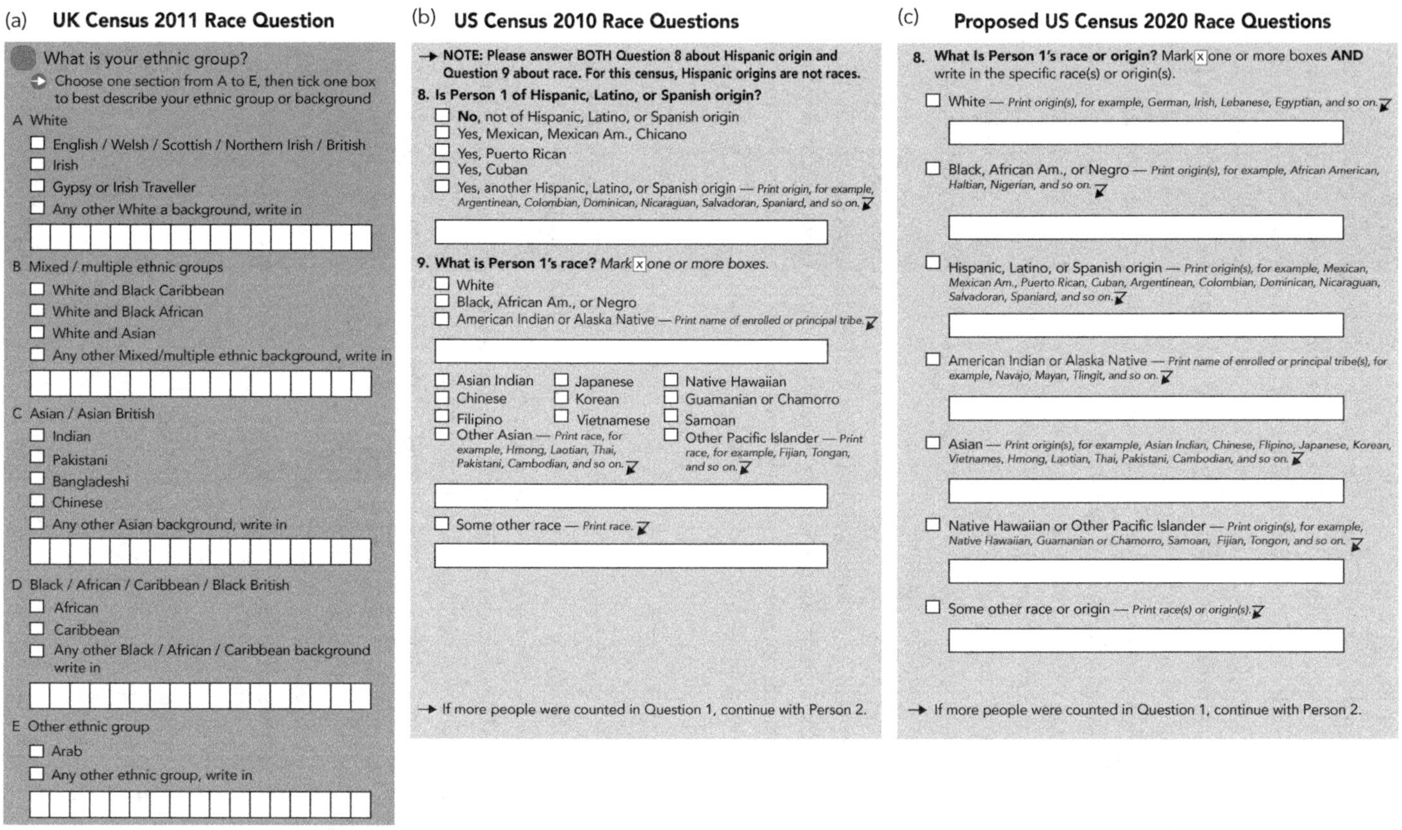

(a) UK Census 2011 Race Question

What is your ethnic group?

→ Choose one section from A to E, then tick one box
   to best describe your ethnic group or background

A White
☐ English / Welsh / Scottish / Northern Irish / British
☐ Irish
☐ Gypsy or Irish Traveller
☐ Any other White a background, write in
   [   ]

B Mixed / multiple ethnic groups
☐ White and Black Caribbean
☐ White and Black African
☐ White and Asian
☐ Any other Mixed/multiple ethnic background, write in
   [   ]

C Asian / Asian British
☐ Indian
☐ Pakistani
☐ Bangladeshi
☐ Chinese
☐ Any other Asian background, write in
   [   ]

D Black / African / Caribbean / Black British
☐ African
☐ Caribbean
☐ Any other Black / African / Caribbean background
   write in
   [   ]

E Other ethnic group
☐ Arab
☐ Any other ethnic group, write in
   [   ]

(b) US Census 2010 Race Questions

→ NOTE: Please answer BOTH Question 8 about Hispanic origin and
   Question 9 about race. For this census, Hispanic origins are not races.

8. Is Person 1 of Hispanic, Latino, or Spanish origin?
☐ No, not of Hispanic, Latino, or Spanish origin
☐ Yes, Mexican, Mexican Am., Chicano
☐ Yes, Puerto Rican
☐ Yes, Cuban
☐ Yes, another Hispanic, Latino, or Spanish origin — Print origin, for example,
   Argentinean, Colombian, Dominican, Nicaraguan, Salvadoran, Spaniard, and so on. ↘
   [   ]

9. What is Person 1's race? Mark ☒ one or more boxes.
☐ White
☐ Black, African Am., or Negro
☐ American Indian or Alaska Native — Print name of enrolled or principal tribe. ↘
   [   ]

☐ Asian Indian   ☐ Japanese   ☐ Native Hawaiian
☐ Chinese   ☐ Korean   ☐ Guamanian or Chamorro
☐ Filipino   ☐ Vietnamese   ☐ Samoan
☐ Other Asian — Print race, for   ☐ Other Pacific Islander — Print
   example, Hmong, Laotian, Thai,   race, for example, Fijian, Tongan,
   Pakistani, Cambodian, and so on. ↘   and so on. ↘
   [   ]   [   ]

☐ Some other race — Print race. ↘
   [   ]

→ If more people were counted in Question 1, continue with Person 2.

(c) Proposed US Census 2020 Race Questions

8. What is Person 1's race or origin? Mark ☒ one or more boxes AND
   write in the specific race(s) or origin(s).

☐ White — Print origin(s), for example, German, Irish, Lebanese, Egyptian, and so on. ↘
   [   ]

☐ Black, African Am., or Negro — Print origin(s), for example, African American,
   Haitian, Nigerian, and so on. ↘
   [   ]

☐ Hispanic, Latino, or Spanish origin — Print origin(s), for example, Mexican,
   Mexican Am., Puerto Rican, Cuban, Argentinean, Colombian, Dominican, Nicaraguan,
   Salvadoran, Spaniard, and so on. ↘
   [   ]

☐ American Indian or Alaska Native — Print name of enrolled or principal tribe(s), for
   example, Navajo, Mayan, Tlingit, and so on. ↘
   [   ]

☐ Asian — Print origin(s), for example, Asian Indian, Chinese, Filipino, Japanese, Korean,
   Vietnamese, Hmong, Laotian, Thai, Pakistani, Cambodian, and so on. ↘
   [   ]

☐ Native Hawaiian or Other Pacific Islander — Print origin(s), for example,
   Native Hawaiian, Guamanian or Chamorro, Samoan, Fijian, Tongan, and so on. ↘
   [   ]

☐ Some other race or origin — Print race(s) or origin(s) ↘
   [   ]

→ If more people were counted in Question 1, continue with Person 2.

FIGURE 4.1 Census captions in the United States and United Kingdom.

or origin, regardless of race. According to the 2015 U.S. Census estimates, 17.6% (56.5 million) of the population is Hispanic, making this the largest minority group in the United States.[6] Mexicans, Puerto Ricans, Central Americans, South Americans, and Cubans represent the largest percentages within this ethnic category. Although united through Spanish origins and language, within this ethnic group there is substantial heterogeneity in language dialects, cuisines, cultural preferences, and taste preferences, which may influence diet-related disease risk.

Based on the epidemiological data, Hispanics are more likely to be diagnosed with certain diet-related diseases and less likely to be diagnosed with others compared with non-Hispanic whites. For example, in the United States, Hispanics are almost twice as likely as non-Hispanic whites to be diagnosed with diabetes and also have higher rates of end-stage renal disease. Conversely, Hispanics are less likely to have coronary heart disease or to die from heart disease than non-Hispanic white adults (see Figure 4.2 for trends in death rate from cardiovascular disease by race). See additional statistics below.

In the United States:

- Hispanics are 1.2 times more likely to be obese than non-Hispanic whites.[6]
- Among Mexican American women, 77% are overweight or obese compared with 64% of non-Hispanic white women. [6]
- Hispanics are 30% less likely to die from heart disease than non-Hispanic whites.[6]
- Hispanics are 10% less likely to have coronary heart disease than non-Hispanic whites and Hispanic women are 30% more likely to have a stroke than non-Hispanic white women.[6]

Further disaggregation of the epidemiological data suggests poorer health outcomes among different subgroups within the Hispanic ethnic group. For example, Puerto Rican Americans have the highest hypertension-related death rate among Hispanic subgroups, while those of Cuban heritage have the lowest overall hypertension-related deaths.

Variations in disease are a result of a combination of factors including diet, the acculturation process and changes in diet after migrating, availability of culturally appropriate foods, and other social factors. Unlike other racial/ethnic groups, some Hispanic groups have shown better health outcomes than their white counterparts despite having lower educational attainment and being of lower socioeconomic status.[7] This phenomenon has been termed the "Latino/

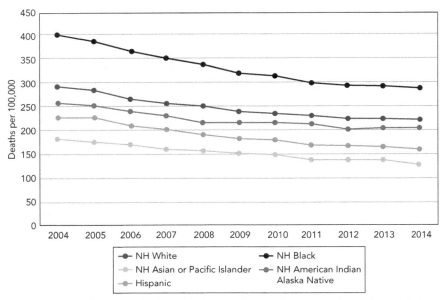

FIGURE 4.2 U.S. age-standardized death rates from cardiovascular disease by race/ethnicity, 2000 to 2014.

From: Benjamin, Emelia J., et al. "Heart disease and stroke statistics—2017 update: a report from the American Heart Association." Circulation 135.10 (2017): e146-e603.

Hispanic paradox."[8,9] One explanation includes the "healthy immigrant effect," which posits that those who immigrate are healthier than those who stay in the home country.[10-12] Others argue that the Latino/Hispanic paradox is mainly driven by health behaviors among less acculturated Hispanics and to a lesser extent among those of other generations who have acculturated to the Western diet and lifestyle behaviors.[13] The "salmon bias" is another theory that posits that the return of Hispanics to their home country for reasons of employment, retirement, or severe illness distorts Hispanic mortality rates in the United States, given that these deaths are not accounted for in the U.S. mortality reports.[14]

Black or African American

African Americans are the second largest minority group in the United States, making up 12.7% of the total population (or 40.7 million people) based on 2015 U.S. Census Bureau estimates.[15] Blacks/African Americans have some of the highest rates of diet-related diseases and conditions such as cardiovascular and cerebrovascular disease, diabetes, and hypertension, in comparison to other racial groups in the United States. For example, compared with their white counterparts,[1] Blacks are 40% more likely to be diagnosed with hypertension and 30% more likely to die from heart disease.[16-18] Other notable diet-related health inequities include:

- African American adults are 80% more likely than white adults to have been medically diagnosed with diabetes.[15]
- Non-Hispanic Blacks were 4.2 times more likely to be diagnosed with end stage renal disease compared with non-Hispanic whites.[15]
- African Americans are 1.5 times more likely to be obese than whites.[15]

There are also notable differences in disease rates by both race and gender:

- African American women are 60% more likely than non-Hispanic white women to have high blood pressure.[15]
- African American women were twice as likely to be obese than non-Hispanic white women.[15]
- African American men are twice as likely to have a stroke compared with adult non-Hispanic white men.[15]
- African American girls are 50% more likely to be overweight than non-Hispanic white girls.[15]

These higher rates of diet-related chronic diseases among Blacks are caused by a myriad of influences, including dietary and lifestyle factors, genetic predisposition to salt sensitivity, and physiological responses to chronic stress. Other upstream social determinants of health underpinning these disparities include inequities in the U.S. educational system, socioeconomic deprivation in Black communities, racial segregation, racially biased practices within the U.S. judicial system, and disproportionate advertisement of processed and fast foods to African Americans and other minority groups. These will be discussed in more detail later in the chapter.

American Indian and Alaskan Native

The American Indian/Alaskan Native racial category includes those having origins among any of the original peoples of North America, South America, and/or Central America and who maintain tribal affiliation or community

---

I. Counterparts are defined as a comparative group in which demographic factors such as socioeconomic status, sex, age, and level of educational attainment are controlled for.

attachment. Based on 2012 data, 2% of the total U.S. population (5.2 million) self-identified as American Indian and Alaska Native alone or American Indian and Alaska Native in combination with one or more other races.[19] In terms of geographic distribution, 22% of the American Indians and Alaska Natives live on reservations or other trust lands and 60% of American Indians and Alaska Natives live in metropolitan areas.[19]

Based on epidemiological data, American Indians and Alaska Natives are more likely than non-Hispanic whites to be diagnosed with diet-related diseases such as chronic liver disease, obesity, hypertension, stroke, diabetes, and end stage renal disease. Related to the high prevalence of chronic liver disease—the leading cause of death among this demographic—these high rates are thought to be associated with chronic alcoholism, obesity, and exposure to Hepatitis B and C viruses among this group.[19]

Specific data include:

- American Indian/Alaska Native adults are 2.5 times more likely to be diagnosed with chronic liver disease compared with non-Hispanic whites.[19]
- The mortality rate for American Indian/Alaska Natives is 2.3 times higher than for the white population.[19]
- American Indian/Alaska Native adults are 2.4 times more likely to be diagnosed with diabetes compared with white adults.[19]
- American Indians/Native Americans are 2.7 times more likely to be diagnosed with end stage renal disease than non-Hispanic whites.[19]
- American Indian/Alaska Native adults are 30% more likely than white adults to have high blood pressure.[19]
- American Indian or Alaska Native adults and adolescents are 50% more likely to be obese than non-Hispanic white counterparts.[19]
- American Indian/Alaska Native adolescents are 50% more likely than non-Hispanic whites to be overweight.[19]
- American Indians/Alaska Native adults are twice as likely to have a stroke as their white adult counterparts.[19]

Although genetic predisposition to these diseases may a play role, as evidenced by the Pima Indians case study, the above described health disparities and inequities are a result of environmental factors related to the access to healthy, traditional, and culturally appropriate foods, which ultimately have roots in historical and arguably unjust actions of American settlers in the late 1800s and early 1900s and unfair policies of the U.S. government (Box 4.1).

BOX 4.1

The Changing Diet and Environment of the Pima Indians: The Role of History in Creating Disparities

The Pima Indians of the Gila River Indian Community of Arizona have some of the highest rates of diabetes in the United States. A 2006 study found that 38% of U.S. Pima Indians had diabetes compared with only 6.9% of the Pima Indians living in Mexico, providing support for the role of diet, as well as behavioral and environmental factors in the development of type 2 diabetes. Although diet was not compared between the two groups, other studies have found that the composition of the U.S. Pima Indian diet has changed over the last century from a diet high in complex carbohydrate and high fiber foods to that of high-fat, high-sugar processed modern foods. This change in the Pima Indian diet parallels the increase in diabetes.

To fully understand these dietary shifts and the health of Pima Indians in the United States, the historical underpinnings must be considered. Native Americans who lived in an area that is now in northwestern Mexico and southern Arizona have lived in the valleys of the Gila and Salt rivers in what is now Arizona for over 2,000 years. Here, they practiced subsistence farming of crops such as wheat, maize, beans, and squash. They hunted and gathered foods from the desert such as saguaro cactus fruit, mesquite beans, cholla cactus buds, prickly pear fruit, wild berries, and wild greens. As the area became more settled by white Americans in the 1880s, the upstream waters of the Gila River were overtaken and diverted to the extent that farming in these desert regions was no longer possible for the Pima. They consequently became more reliant on trading posts and subsidized food from the United States government—much of it containing sugar and white flour.

Sources:
Schulz, Leslie O., et al. "Effects of traditional and western environments on prevalence of type 2 diabetes in Pima Indians in Mexico and the US." *Diabetes Care* 29.8 (2006): 1866–1871.
Boyce, Vicky L., and Boyd A. Swinburn. "The Traditional Pima Indian Diet: Composition and adaptation for use in a dietary intervention study." *Diabetes Care* 16.1 (1993): 369–371.
Narayan, KM Venkat. "Diabetes mellitus in Native Americans: The problem and its implications." *Population Research and Policy Review* 16.1-2 (1997): 169–192.

Asian

People having origins of the original people of the Far East, Southeast Asia, or the Indian subcontinent are included in the Asian racial category. Based on 2015 Census data, 17.3 million Asian Americans live in the United States, making up 5.4% of the nation's population.[20] Unlike other racial/ethnic groups, Asian Americans generally have better health outcomes than their white counterparts, with a few exceptions. For example, Asian adults are less likely than white adults to die from a stroke and have lower rates of being overweight or obese and of having hypertension. Specifically, Asian Americans are 20% less likely to die from diabetes compared with whites; however, they are 10% more likely to be diagnosed.[20] Asian Americans are also 50% less likely to die from heart disease than whites.[20] Conversely, Asians are at greater risk for end stage renal disease than whites.

There is considerable and noteworthy heterogeneity in diet-related diseases among the Asian American population. For example, Asian Indians have the highest prevalence of type 2 diabetes among the Asian subgroups. Also, compared to all Asian Americans, Filipino adults are 70% more likely to be obese. Meanwhile, 10% of Vietnamese and Korean adults are considered underweight.[20] The heterogeneity in diet-related disease outcomes among the Asian racial category underscores the importance of considering the diversity within the larger racial categories.

Native Hawaiian/Other Pacific Islander

This racial category includes any people who have origins among any of the original peoples of Hawaii, Guam, Samoa, or other Pacific Islands. According to the 2015 U.S. Census Bureau estimate, roughly 1.3 million Native Hawaiians/Pacific Islanders, alone or in combination with one of more races, reside within the United States.[21] This group represents about 0.4% of the U.S. population.[21]

In comparison to other racial/ethnic groups in the United States, Native Hawaiians/Pacific Islanders have higher rates of alcohol consumption and obesity. According to the Centers for Disease Control and Prevention (CDC), leading causes of death among Native Hawaiians/Pacific Islanders include cancer, heart disease, stroke, and diabetes. Based on national survey data, Native Hawaiians/Pacific Islanders are 2.4 times more likely to be diagnosed with diabetes in comparison with their white counterparts. Additionally, in 2014, Native Hawaiians/Pacific Islanders were 50% more likely to be obese than non-Hispanic whites.[21] In terms of coronary heart disease, 2012 data suggests that Native Hawaiians/Pacific Islanders were 70% more likely to be diagnosed with coronary heart disease than non-Hispanic whites.[21]

Immigrants and Health Disparities

Relevant to the concept of health disparities is the immigrant experience in the United States. According to the Migration Policy Institute, 13.5% of the U.S. population (more than 43.3 million people) are considered immigrants.[22] Between 2014 and 2015, the foreign-born population increased by 2.1%. According to the 2016 Current Population Survey (CPS), immigrants and their U.S.-born children now account for 27% of the overall U.S. population (84.3 million people).[22] With this increasing number of immigrants in the United States comes increased diversity in experiences and cultural backgrounds, as well as diet and lifestyle behaviors. Relevant to the immigrant experience is the acculturation process.

Acculturation is a process of cultural and psychological change resulting from intercultural contact and the extent to which ethnic minorities and immigrant groups participate in the dominant cultures' values, beliefs, assumptions, and practices.[23-26] Additional cultural domains include interpersonal relationships and language preferences. Originally described by psychologist John Berry, some researchers view acculturation as a combination of two different dimensions—adherence to the dominant culture and maintenance of original culture.[25] In this view, the acculturation process comprises four aspects: assimilation, separation, integration, and marginalization.[24-26] Other researchers argue that acculturation is unidimensional, ranging from immersion in the existing cultural context to immersion in the individual's culture of origin on either end of the spectrum.[27] Both viewpoints of the acculturation process have been difficult to operationalize, and a variety of proxy measures are used to estimate levels of acculturation. These proxy measures include immigration status, length of residence, nativity, and language, as well as more complex scales.[28]

In public health studies, acculturation has been used to explore the relationship between cultural change, changes in diet, and health outcomes. Although various conceptual models have been proposed to explain the general process of acculturation,[24] the Satia-Abouta model of dietary acculturation (Figure 4.3) specifically posits several key contributors to changes in diet among immigrant groups, including socioeconomic, demographic, and cultural factors.[29] These factors are thought to predict the process of change

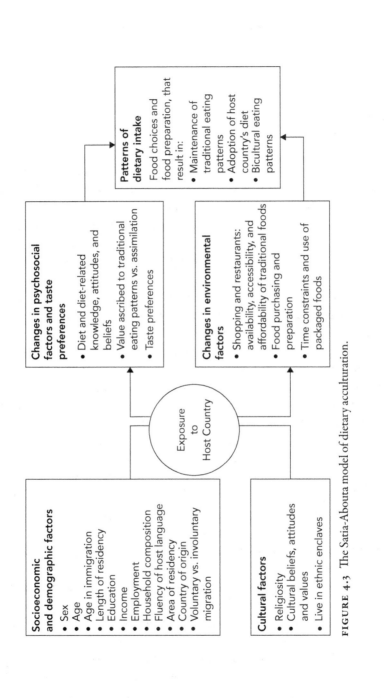

FIGURE 4.3 The Satia-Abouta model of dietary acculturation.

in psychosocial factors, such as attitudes and beliefs about food, taste preferences, and food availability and preparation.[29] This model is particularly relevant given the limited research among immigrants.[30-32] Most of the acculturation literature focuses on Hispanic and Asian groups, in which, albeit mixed, research shows an association between migration and acculturation and changes in disease risk, lifestyle behaviors, and dietary composition.[33-36] A study among Mexican Americans, for example, found that risk of cardiovascular disease was highest among U.S.-born, Spanish-speaking Mexicans and lower among foreign-born Mexicans.[34] Studies that examined dietary change among Hispanics overall have varied results—from an association between acculturation and fat avoidance among women to greater levels of acculturation and lower intakes of fiber and higher intakes of calorically dense foods.[37,38] A systematic review on this topic concluded that overall, less acculturated Hispanics consumed less sugar and sugar-sweetened beverages, and consumed more fruit, rice, and beans.[39] Many of these studies, however, used inconsistent measures of both acculturation (i.e., nativity vs. language preferences) and dietary intake.[39] Nevertheless, the importance of examining the level of acculturation among immigrants to assess diet-related disease risk is noteworthy.

Health Disparities and Cultural Influences

The cultural cuisines of various racial/ethnic groups in the United States may either help protect against or contribute to health disparities (Box 4.2). For the Hispanic ethnic group, diets vary depending on the country and region of ancestry, which may play a role in the heterogeneity in diet-related disease risk in this population. For example, while food from Mexico includes corn-based products, beans, and a variety of fruits and vegetables, the typical cuisine from Puerto Rico includes yellow rice, beans, roasted pork, and plantains. For African Americans, the traditional historically based diet includes fried foods, refined grains, yams, collard greens, processed meats, and few fruit. Meanwhile, Blacks who have migrated to the United States from different countries have cultural cuisines that vary throughout the African diaspora.[40-42] Based on the available flora and fauna in the countries of origin, many of these cultural diets comprise foods associated with lower chronic disease risk, such as fruit, vegetables, legumes, and seafood. For Asians, the typical cuisines of countries such as China, Korea, and Japan include a variety of green leafy vegetables and seafood, which are foods encouraged for a healthy diet. See Chapter 11 for an in-depth look at how culture influences food choice.

BOX 4.2

Cultural Niche Construction: Interrelationship among Genes, Culture, and Food Choice

Cultural niche construction is a term used to describe the process by which organisms or species modify their own genes through their activities and cultural behaviors, in what is known as gene-culture interactions. Culturally based behaviors, including those related to diet, can have a profound effect on human evolution, and anthropologists are investigating cultural practices that may modify current selection. It is quite possible that genes related to nutrient metabolism and digestion have been positively selected to provide an advantage in certain groups of people based on the available flora and fauna available in the region of settlement in the world. More research, however, is necessary to determine the nature of these gene-culture interactions that may have shaped the human genome and any possible role that genetics may play in creating the racial/ethnic-related health disparities that exist. For example, discordance between the nutrients of the Western Diet and genes may be worth further exploration.

Sources:
Laland, Kevin N., and Michael J. O'Brien. "Cultural niche construction: An introduction." *Biological Theory* 6.3 (2011): 191–202.
Laland, Kevin N., John Odling-Smee, and Sean Myles. "How culture shaped the human genome: bringing genetics and the human sciences together." *Nature reviews. Genetics* 11.2 (2010): 137.

Differences in perceptions of beauty, body image, and weight, as well as attitudes and behaviors related to eating also have a cultural basis, which might influence health disparities, particularly among women. Studies consistently show differences in body dissatisfaction by race/ethnicity.[43,44] For example, several studies show that African American women have lower levels of body dissatisfaction and disordered eating despite higher BMIs than white and Asian women.[44,45] Cultural values around body weight and attractiveness may, therefore, contribute to the acceptance of overweight/obesity among this demographic.

Health Disparities by Gender and Sexuality

There are reported disparities by gender of diet-related diseases such as cardiovascular disease, diabetes, and hypertension.[17,46] Although CVD is the leading cause of mortality for both men and women, there are significant differences in the prevalence, onset, and mortality from this disease. For example, the absolute number of women dying of CVD and stroke is higher than men, given the longer life expectancy of women.[17,46] However, the age adjusted mortality rates by CVD are higher among men; specifically, in 2007, the age-adjusted CVD death rate in men was 300 per 100,000 compared with 212 per 100,000 in women.[46] There are also differences in hypertension diagnosis by gender and age, in which women older than 65 years have a higher prevalence of hypertension as compared to men of the same age. Women and men, however, have similar prevalence of hypertension when not stratifying by age.

Also noteworthy are the racial/ethnic differences of CVD by gender. Black women have the highest prevalence of CVD and related risk factors among women 20 years or older. The prevalence of CVD is 47% among Black women compared with 34% among white women and 31% among Mexican American women. Black women also have the highest rate of hypertension in the United States, with 44% of Black women age 20 years or older diagnosed with the disease. Mortality caused by hypertension was 37.0 per 100,000 for Black women and 14.3 per 100,000 for white women.

With the notable exception of HIV/AIDS, limited public health research has explored the association between gender identity and sexual orientation and physical and mental health outcomes. As demonstrated in the PRIDE case study, disparities among the LGBT community are an issue that is gaining increased attention (Box 4.3). An early study found that despite higher socioeconomic status, 50- to 79-year-old lesbian and bisexual women had an increased prevalence of risk factors for cardiovascular disease

---

BOX 4.3

Exploring Health Disparities in the LGBT Community: The PRIDE Study

The first of its kind, the Population Research for Identity and Disparities for Equality (PRIDE) study, based at the University of California, San Francisco, is a longitudinal cohort study of people who identify as lesbian, gay, bisexual, transgender, queer, or another sexual or gender minority. The purpose of the study is to determine how sexual and/or gender identity influences physical and mental health through the lens of health disparities.

For information about the study, go here https://pridestudy.org/study

(obesity, smoking, and low fruit and vegetable intake) compared with heterosexual women.[47] A more recent study found disparities in cardiovascular disease biomarkers between young adult gay and bisexual compared with heterosexual men.[48]

Diet-Related Health Disparities and Socioeconomic Status

Numerous studies have explored the association between socioeconomic status and health, particularly diet-related diseases such as heart disease, hypertension, and diabetes. Although operationalization of socioeconomic status differs by study, generally, research conducted in the United States shows an inverse relationship between educational attainment and income and optimal health outcomes. A study based on data from the U.S. National Health Interview Survey of adults aged 25 years and older measured socioeconomic status by educational level and family income.[49] Even after controlling for age, gender, race/ethnicity, marital status, and body mass index (BMI), having less than a high school education was associated with a twofold higher odds of mortality from diabetes in comparison with study participants with a college degree or higher.[49] Similarly, being below the poverty level was also associated with a twofold higher mortality in comparison with families of higher income levels. Results are similar in studies conducted in Canada and the United Kingdom.[50,51]

Most studies have reported better diet quality and food purchasing behaviors in accordance with dietary guidelines among those of higher socioeconomic status compared with those of lower socioeconomic status.[52-56] A recent trend analysis of National Health and Nutrition Examination Survey (NHANES) data from 1999 to 2010, for example, revealed a positive association between both income and educational level with total diet quality (using the Alternative Health Eating Index–2010) and an increase in the disparity between low and high socioeconomic during the examined time period.[55]

Another relevant topic is the association between poverty, low socioeconomic status, and issues of hunger and ultimately malnutrition. In 2015 in the United States, 42 million people faced issues of hunger and lived in households that were considered food insecure, including 13 million children and 5.4 million seniors.[57] Of these households, 59% participated in at least one federal food assistance program, such as the Supplemental Nutrition Assistance program, the National School Lunch Program, or the Supplemental Nutrition

Program for Women, Infants, and Children.[57] Despite these safety-net programs, food insecurity and hunger are persistent concerns.

The global context also matters in the relationship between obesity and socioeconomic status. For example, research in the late 1980s found a consistent inverse relationship between obesity and socioeconomic status among women in developed countries.[58] Conversely, in developing societies, a strong direct relation was observed for women, men, and children, with a higher likelihood of obesity among persons in higher socioeconomic strata.[58] With globalization, however, this pattern is not as striking today, although the associations persist.[59]

Underlying Causes: Social Determinants of Health

Differences in disease outcomes are not solely based on individual-level behaviors and beliefs, but also are related to a variety of factors at broader levels that may serve to perpetuate health inequities. These factors can be considered as social determinants of health, or "the structural determinants and conditions in which people are born, grow, live, work and age."[60] Some of these factors include, but are not limited to, income, access to quality education and educational attainment, transportation access, neighborhood characteristics, and healthy food accessibility and affordability. As evidenced in the socioecological model, behaviors and the outcomes they may produce are a result of an interrelated combination of factors at multiple levels. Figure 4.4 and Table 4.1 depict a socioecological framework to explain race/ethnicity-based health inequities in the United States and illustrate how various forms of racism relate to each domain. These levels of influence and examples of each are listed here:

- *Individual*: Beliefs, behaviors, socioeconomic status
- *Interpersonal*: Race-based microaggressions, relationship with family and social networks
- *Community*: Inequitable distribution of resources, such as access to quality education, recreational spaces, grocery stores; race-based residential segregation
- *Organizational*: Hiring practices, sick leave policies, health insurance coverage
- *Policy*: Redlining, minimum wage laws, globalization contributing to unemployment

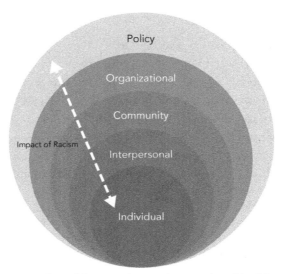

FIGURE 4.4 Socioecological framework to explain race-based health inequities in the United States.

Table 4.1 Socioecological Framework to Explain Race-Based Health
Inequities in the United States

Socioecological Domain	Forms of Racism	Examples
Policy	Institutionalized	• Redlining (historic) • Property tax-based public school funding • Minimum wage laws • Globalization and "exportation" of jobs
Organizational		• Decision of some companies within the food industry to disproportionately market unhealthy foods to Hispanic and Black youth • Human Resource policies within wage working industries (sick leave policies, health insurance, etc.)
Community		• Inequitable distribution of resources (access to quality education, grocery store access) • Racial/ethnic segregation
Interpersonal	Personally mediated	• Race/ethnic-based microaggressions (interpersonal or personally mediated racism)
Individual	Internalized	• Beliefs, attitudes ("can't do" mentality), self-perceptions, socioeconomic status (wealth gap), educational level

Historical Contexts

To understand better the existence and perpetuation of health disparities, it is important to consider the historical contexts related to social determinants of health. For example, for African Americans, Jim Crow racial segregation laws and the threat of lynchings in the South resulted in the Great Migration of the 20th century, in which African Americans sought better opportunities in cities in the Northeast, Midwest, and West. Even though Jim Crow laws were abolished through the Civil Rights Act of 1964, African Americans still faced employment discrimination and wage restrictions for generations, which barred them from obtaining critical assets and wealth through home and land ownership. Common in cities such as Boston, the practice of redlining perpetuated lending discrimination and restricted African Americans to purchasing homes in certain areas and communities, which often lacked resources, including supermarkets. The practice of redlining persisted as late as the late 1970s in cities throughout the United States.

Similarly, policies targeting Native Americans have historically resulted in reliance on government food subsidies and lack of food sovereignty, and today contribute to the limited access to foods that make up a nutritious diet.[61] As in the case of the Pima Indians, policies that limited access to natural resources precluded the practice of traditional hunting, farming, and gathering. In the Navajo nation, the government-designated reservation structure necessitates leaving the reservation for grocery shopping for over half of the residents.[62]

Socioeconomic Status and Class

Socioeconomic status and social class are contributing factors for diet-related health outcomes for a variety of reasons. Over the past 40 years, industrialization of the food system has resulted in an increase in inexpensive, energy-dense, processed foods that tend to be high in fat, sodium, and added sugars. Industrialization also has led to reductions in the time-cost of food.[63] Paralleling these changes were increased costs of foods promoted for a healthy diet, such as fruit, vegetables, and fatty fish.[64,65] Consequently, studies show that individuals of lower socioeconomic status have poorer diet quality and food purchasing behavior in comparison with those of higher socioeconomic status.[52-56]

According to 2014 PEW Research Center data, the median income for Black and Hispanic households in the United States was about $43,300 in 2014, compared with $77,900 for Asian households, and $71,300 for white

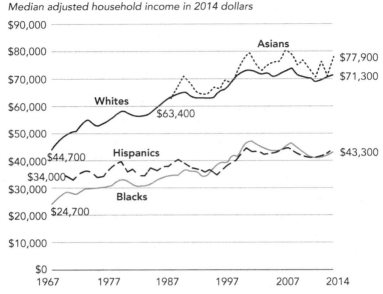

Racial gaps in household income persist

Median adjusted household income in 2014 dollars

FIGURE 4.5 Trends in household income by race, 1967–2014.
Pew Research Center.

households.[66] (See Figure 4.5 and Box 4.4). Although educational attainment is associated with higher income, the black–white income gap persists across all educational levels. Data from the Federal Reserve's Survey of Consumer Finances from 2013 suggested that the total worth of white households was

---

BOX 4.4

Case Study: Wealth Gap in Boston

Main findings of *The Color of Wealth in Boston* report

- White households had a median wealth of $247,500
- Dominicans and U.S. blacks have a median wealth of close to zero
- Of all nonwhite groups (for which estimates could be made), Caribbean Black households had the highest median wealth with $12,000 (5% of wealth of white households)

Original report: Muñoz, A.P., Kim, M., Chang, M., Jackson, R., Hamilton, D. and Darity, W.A., 2015. *The Color of Wealth in Boston.*

$144,200, nearly 13 times that of black households and 10 times that of Hispanic households.[66]

Although the terms social stratum, income, social class, and socioeconomic status often are used interchangeably, they are, in fact, different constructs, and there is a lack of consensus regarding their definitions. Mean income, for example, does not fully account for social class and generational wealth given the potential influence of family support in the acquisition of wealth (i.e., assistance with down payment for first home or family contributions to college and graduate education).

Being of lower socioeconomic status increases the likelihood of exposure to life circumstances that result in greater levels of psychosocial stress; for example, financial instability, job insecurity, family dysfunction, discriminatory acts, neighborhood violence, and limited access to health care.

Employment

Employment status, income, and socioeconomic status often are considered interchangeably and are clearly interrelated. There are, however, several issues specific to employment and working conditions that are important in the consideration of diet-related health inequities. In the United States women and racial minorities are more likely to face precarious employment as well as unemployment.[67,68] Employment-related inequities are considered to have roots in historical policies and practices that were unfair to Blacks and women (e.g., redlining, which weakened the tax base in neighborhoods and led to lower wages and decreased employment,[69] and the exclusion of women's interests in the labor movement).[67] Employment itself is therefore increasingly recognized as a social determinant of health.

Consideration of the effects of precarious employment is relatively new. The term encompasses a range of employment situations that fall short of secure full-time, year-round, well-compensated, and socially protected employment, including temporary employment, underemployment, acute threat of layoff, persistent perceived job insecurity, "working poor" (workers with incomes below the poverty line), and migrant labor.[70] Benach et al. propose defining it as "a multidimensional construct encompassing dimensions such as employment insecurity, individualized bargaining relations between workers and employers, low wages and economic deprivation, limited workplace rights and social protection, and powerlessness to exercise workplace rights."[70] Some epidemiological evidence exists for an association between precarious employment and health outcomes. A body of work with British civil servants links low-ranking, low-autonomy positions with prevalence of angina, electrocardiogram evidence of ischemia, and other health outcomes.[71] In more recent studies, job insecurity in terms of acute threat of layoff was associated with an increase in cardiovascular risk factors such as increased BMI and hypertension;[72,73] and persistent perceived job insecurity was associated with lower self-rated health.[73-76]

Conceptual models have been proposed that link precarious employment and unemployment with health inequities by limiting the resources available to purchase healthy foods and engage in other health behaviors, increasing psychosocial stress, and by limiting access to health care.[69,70,77,78] Temporary employees often have lower pay and less access to benefits, which may lead to negative health behaviors and outcomes.[77,79] Empirical support is needed, however, for these proposed mechanisms. Additional evidence will be critical to crafting appropriate solutions, which may include policies related to minimum wage or guaranteed annual income.[80]

Psychosocial: Discrimination and Chronic Stress

Psychosocial factors such as exposure to and perception of racism and discrimination, perceived stress and stress coping styles, internalized anger, and socioeconomic-based stress may contribute to poor diet quality and elevated risk for hypertension among minority groups.[81-87] Racism in its multiple forms (personally mediated, internalized, and institutionalized)[88] is often an insidious, inescapable, distressing reality of everyday life for many racial/ethnic minorities. In a U.K.-based study, the Fourth National Survey of Ethnic Minorities, more than 12% of the study participants reported having experienced harassment during the previous year.[89] Data from the same study showed a positive association between reported experience of racism and self-report of poor health.[90] A community-based participatory research study among American Indians with type 2 diabetes found reports of race-based microaggressions to be correlated with self-reported heart attack history and poorer health outcome overall.[91]

Several U.S.-based studies have examined the psychosocial factors contributing to hypertension among Blacks. In one review, the authors discussed suppressed hostility and an active stress coping style (coined "John Henryism"[92]) in response to environmental stressors as associated factors in the development of high blood pressure.[85] Similarly, the work of the social epidemiologist Nancy Krieger has shown differences in high blood pressure outcomes based on whether a person challenges perceived unfair treatment, with those who do not challenge discriminatory treatment more likely to have elevated blood pressure compared with those who do challenge it.[93,94]

There is evidence that chronic stress contributes to physiological dysregulation, diminished physical and mental health, and chronic disease.[95] The concept known as allostatic load has been used to describe the physiological burden of stress and represents a potential mechanism underlying the racial/ethnic differences in mortality and morbidity from chronic diseases.[96] It specifically relates to the brain's response when exposed to an experience that is perceived as stressful and the physiological responses that occur to adapt to these exposures (see Figure 4.6). Over time, the overexposure to stress and the neural, endocrine, and immune responses can have a detrimental impact on various organ systems in the body, resulting in diseases such as hypertension and cardiovascular disease.[96] Although there are inconsistencies in how the load is measured, studies generally suggest that Blacks present with higher allostatic loads than whites, irrespective of socioeconomic status. Results are less consistent for other racial/ethnic groups. For example, in a study based on data from the National Health and Nutrition Examination survey, U.S.-born Mexican Americans had higher allostatic load scores than whites, while foreign-born Mexicans had lower allostatic load scores than their white counterparts.[97]

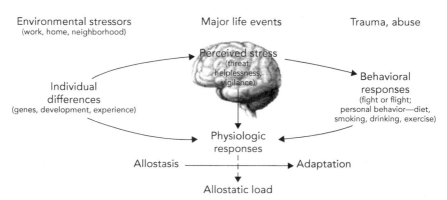

FIGURE 4.6 Allostatic load framework.

Source: McEwen, Bruce S., and Teresa Seeman. "Protective and damaging effects of mediators of stress: elaborating and testing the concepts of allostasis and allostatic load." *Annals of the New York Academy of Sciences 896.1* (1999): 30–47.

Environmental

Environmental factors such as inaccessibility of affordable, nutritious food, together with the overabundance of fast food retail chains in certain communities, are a contributing factor to diet-related health disparities. "Food desert" is a term used to describe an area of low access to healthy food. According to the United States Department of Agriculture, a food desert is a "low-income census tract where either a substantial number or share of residents has low access to a supermarket or large grocery store." [II,98] Another term used to describe communities with low access to healthy, affordable food is "supermarket desert"; conversely, "food swamps" is used to describe communities with an overabundance of fast food restaurant chains.

Previous studies have found that predominately Black and Hispanic neighborhoods have fewer supermarkets and less accessibility to grocery stores compared with white neighborhoods.[99-101] Low-income neighborhoods are likewise shown to have fewer supermarkets compared with middle-income neighborhoods.[100] One study, based on Census data from a variety of locations across the country (Jackson City, Mississippi; Forsyth County, North Carolina; Washington County, Maryland; and selected suburbs of Minneapolis, Minnesota) found that white neighborhoods had four times more supermarkets than Black neighborhoods.[99] For historical context, one theory as to why food deserts formed relates to the demographic shifts in major U.S. cities in the late 1970s and 1980s, in which more affluent, white households migrated from the inner cities to suburban areas. The decrease in both overall population and average income level in the inner cities resulted in the closure of large supermarket chains.[102] For example, it is reported that around 40% of the supermarkets in Los Angeles, Chicago, Brooklyn, and Manhattan shut down during this period as a result of the demographic shift.[102]

Availability and affordability of culturally appropriate foods is also a consideration for immigrant groups. Ethnic enclaves based on migration and settlement patterns of various ethnic groups contribute to growth in the demand for cultural foods. Based on sociological research, ethnic enclaves may

---

II. Low-income tracts are considered to be those where at least 20% of the people have income at or below the federal poverty levels for family size, or where median family income for the tract is at or below 80% of the surrounding area's median family income. Tracts qualify as "low access" tracts if at least 500 persons or 33% of their population live more than a mile from a supermarket or large grocery store (for rural census tracts, the distance is more than 10 miles).

stave off acculturation, reinforce norms and health behaviors, and contribute to resource sharing based on social networks, which ultimately facilitates adherence to diets of the culture of origin.[103] As evidenced in the model of dietary acculturation in Figure 4.3, changes in environmental factors such as the availability, accessibility, and affordability of restaurants and grocery stores, and food purchasing and preparation behaviors, as well as time constraints, factor into dietary intake patterns and whether individuals will preserve their cultural cuisine.

Advertising and Multicultural Marketing

The advertising of unhealthy foods and multicultural marketing tactics of multibillion-dollar food companies may play a role in influencing behavior and purchasing habits, which ultimately contribute to diet-related health disparities. Described as "consumers that are transforming the U.S. mainstream," minority groups such as Hispanics, Blacks, and Asians have strong purchasing power and an increasing proportion of marketing dollars is spent targeting these groups[104] For example, it is estimated that McDonald's spent $111.4 million on food marketing to Hispanics in 2013.[105]

Studies consistently show disproportionate advertisement of unhealthy foods to minority groups.[106-109] A 2005 study examining advertising in women's magazines showed that a greater percentage of the food advertisements in Hispanic- and Black-targeted magazines were for unhealthy food and beverages. Specifically, overtly unhealthy food and drink ads made up 52% of food and beverage advertisements in Hispanic magazines, compared with 32% in Black magazines and 29% in mainstream magazines.[108] Similar trends are seen in advertisements targeting children. In August 2015, the Rudd Center for Food Policy & Obesity released a report examining marketing expenditures of restaurant, food, and beverage companies in the United States with some of the highest advertising spending ($100 million or more) targeting youth.[109] Combined, the 26 companies included in the analysis spent $675 million in food advertisements on Spanish-language TV. The data also indicated that most companies in this analysis placed some advertising on Black-targeted TV networks, which totaled $161 million and represented 75% of all food-related advertising on these networks. Overall, the report concluded that the majority of food advertisements targeting Hispanic and Black youth consumers were for food of poor nutritional quality, and that these marketing practices likely contribute to observed diet-related health disparities.[109]

Access to Health Care

Interaction with the healthcare system affects an individual's knowledge about risk for disease as well as access to resources for behavior change to reduce risk, such as consultation with a registered dietitian. Historically there have been substantial inequities in access to health care by race/ethnicity, socioeconomic status, and sexual orientation and gender identity.[110-113]

From a socio-ecological perspective, consideration of the factors that influence access to health care have been focused at the level of the individual.[114] A key individual-level factor is health insurance coverage, which is critical to financial access. The Affordable Care Act (ACA) has resulted in increased coverage overall; for example, before implementation of the ACA, trends in coverage were worsening, but implementation resulted in nearly 20 million Americans gaining coverage by 2016.[115,116] By design, the ACA led to the largest improvements among racial/ethnic minorities.[117,118] Nonetheless, inequities have persisted, particularly among Blacks, Hispanics, and individuals in low-income households.[119]

There is increasing recognition, however, of the critical role of factors beyond the individual level in reducing inequities in healthcare access.[114] There are several provisions within the ACA itself to address these factors. For example, the policy option for states to expand Medicaid helps address coverage for low-income households. Additional strategies, however, are needed. A concept that is gaining increasing support within the public health community is "Health in All Policies," which is "a collaborative approach to improving the health of all people by incorporating health considerations into decision-making across sectors and policy areas."[120] Examples include involving the transportation sector in determining how public transportation affects physical access to healthcare facilities,[121] or involving the education sector in addressing issues related to health literacy. By focusing broadly, Health in All Policies promises to address persistent inequities more fully.

Global Health Disparities

When examining health disparities worldwide, differences in diet-related disease outcomes can be considered as within-country disparities or between-countries disparities. This section will predominately focus on between-country differences, yet within-country disparities and inequities are worth a brief mention. Although some examples beyond the United States were introduced, this chapter has predominately focused on U.S.-centered disparities. It should be noted, however, that differences in diet-related diseases on the basis of race/ethnicity, immigration status, and socioeconomic status are common in many countries. For example, these disparities could relate to a history of ethnocentrism and nationalism within a country or region; or in the case of Brazil, relate to race, which is intricately connected to skin complexion and roots in the sociopolitical system of slavery (See Box 4.5). The health and socioeconomic status of Australia's indigenous aboriginals is yet another example. According to the World Health Organization, the average Aboriginal household earns only about 55% of an average Australian family (i.e., US$ 316 a week compared with US$ 575), and the Aboriginal population is three times more likely to contract diabetes and nearly twice as likely to suffer heart disease between the ages of 35 and 44 compared with the total Australian population.[122]

Between-country differences include wide-ranging disparities in diet-related diseases, ranging from undernutrition and insufficient protein and energy intake to excessive energy intake and over nutrition related to

---

BOX 4.5

Case Study: Race/Skin Color-Based Disparities in Brazil

Unlike the United States and other countries across the world, absolute deaths from cerebrovascular disease are higher in Brazil than deaths from coronary disease. Brazil also has a more nuanced system for defining race. A study based on 2010 data from the Mortality Information System of the Brazilian Ministry of Health found differences in mortality from stroke based on race/skin color. The study showed that differences by race were significant for men and women. Mortality rates adjusted for age (per 100,000) for men were 44.4, 48.2, and 63.3 for whites, browns, and blacks, respectively. For women, the trends in cerebrovascular disease mortality were similar in that the age-adjusted mortality rates were 29.0, 33.7, and 51.0 for whites, browns, and blacks, respectively. Rates of related risk factors such as hypertension also differed by race/skin color. Overall, the study demonstrated that the burden of stroke mortality is highest among blacks compared to their brown and white counterparts.

Source: Lotufo, Paulo Andrade, and Isabela Judith Martins Bensenor. "Race and stroke mortality in Brazil." *Revista de saude publica* 47, no. 6 (2013): 1201–1204.

obesity. Based on United Nations International Children's Emergency Fund (UNICEF) data from 2010 to 2016, undernutrition (wasting, stunting, and micronutrient deficiencies), which is common throughout Asian and African countries, contributes to almost half of the deaths of children under 5 years of age. As shown in Figure 4.7, 33.5% of children under 5 years old are stunted in Western and Central Africa and 35.8% are stunted in South Asia. Comparatively, 11% of children under 5 years of age experience stunting in Latin America and the Caribbean and 9.8% and 8.9% in Central and Eastern Europe (see Figure 4.7)[123,124].

Gender-based disparities also have been noted globally. In nearly all countries and regions with available data, stunting rates are shown to be higher among boys than girls (Figure 4.8).[123] Although research is still needed to ascertain the underlying causes for this phenomenon, initial review of the literature suggests that this sex-based disparity is driven by the higher risk for preterm birth among boys (linked with lower birth weight) in comparison with girls.[123,124]

Juxtaposed against these high levels of undernutrition, low- and middle-income countries simultaneously have a high incidence of obesity and other non-communicable diseases, in what is called the "double burden of disease." In an address in the early 2000s, the Assistant Director-General of Non-Communicable Diseases and Mental Health of the WHO stated, "Non-communicable diseases are imposing a growing burden upon low- and middle-income countries, which have limited resources and are still struggling to meet the challenges of existing problems with infectious diseases."[125] This phenomenon is a manifestation of the changing globalized food system combined with increased urbanization, in which unhealthy foods are more readily available and sedentary lifestyles are becoming more prevalent. For example, in Accra, Ghana, while communicable diseases are the main cause of disability and death, especially among poor communities, there is an increased occurrence of non-communicable disease, particularly among wealthy city dwellers.[126] The "nutrition (epidemiological) transition" is a term used to describe complex changes in the patterns of health outcomes and disease and the demographic and socioeconomic factors contributing to these shifts in disease.[127] Specifically, the nutrition transition was characterized in the early 1970s, and included the "Age of Pestilence and Famine," "Age of Receding Pandemics," and the "Age of Degenerative and Man-made Diseases," which includes a shift in factors such as lifestyle, diet, education, and income. Ultimately, the double burden is experienced during a country's transition from the "Age of Receding Pandemics" to the "Age of Degenerative and Man-made Diseases."

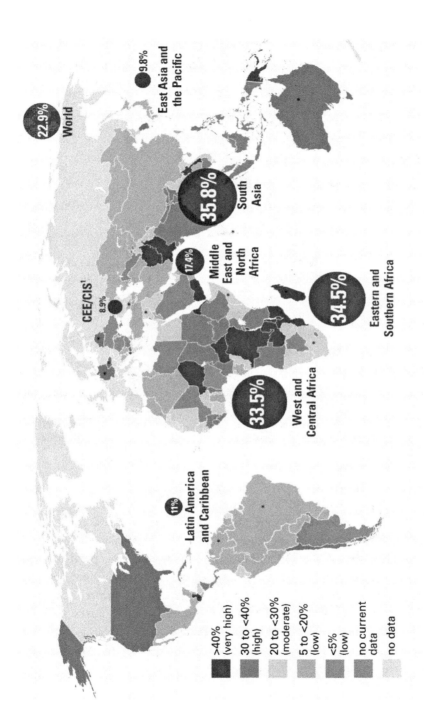

FIGURE 4.7 Percentage of children under 5 years of age who are stunted (global rates from 2010 to 2016). Source: UNICEF.

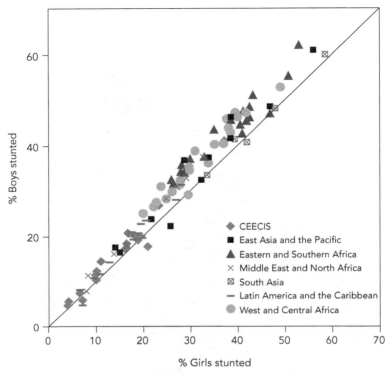

FIGURE 4.8 Percentage of boys under 5 years of age who are stunted vs. percentage of girls (by region, 2012).

Source: UNICEF global nutrition database, 2014, based on Multiple Indicator Cluster Surveys (MICS), Demographic and Health Surveys (DHS) and other nationally representative surveys.

The highest burden of non-communicable, "man-made" diseases is in the United States, where obesity, heart disease, diabetes, and related complications are some of the leading causes of mortality in the country. Of the members of the Organisation for Economic Co-operation and Development, the United States is followed by Mexico and New Zealand for the highest rates of obesity, where 38.2%, 32.4%, and 30.7% of those in the United States, Mexico, and New Zealand, respectively, are considered obese (see Figure 4.9). The non-communicable diseases of obesity and type 2 diabetes are also growing concerns in the Gulf Region of the Middle East, particularly in Kuwait, Saudi Arabia, Bahrain, Qatar, and the United Arab Emirates.

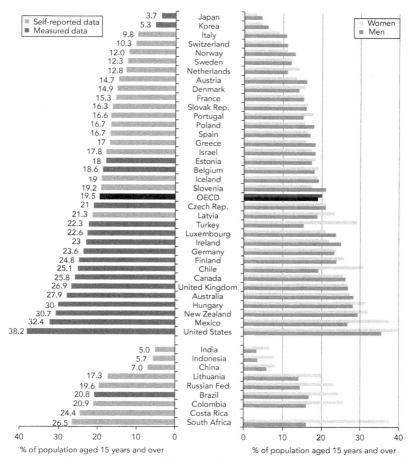

FIGURE 4.9 Obesity among population aged 15 years and over (2015 or nearest year).
Source: OECD (2017), OECD Health Statistics 2017. http://www.oecd.org/health/health-data.htm.

Conclusion

Diet- and nutrition-related health disparities and inequities are issues in the United States and globally. Several factors play a role in differences in disease risk between groups, including historically based inequities and differences in the social determinants of health, such as educational level, employment status, environmental factors, access and affordability of healthy food, neighborhood segregation, chronic stress, discrimination, and access to health care. Targeting dietary behaviors alone cannot adequately address these diet- and nutrition-related disparities. Instead, the other relevant contributing factors described in this chapter need to be recognized and addressed.

Quiz Questions

1. Health inequity and health disparity are interchangeable terms. True or false?
2. Social determinants of health that contributor to health disparities include all of the following except:
   a. Income
   b. Neighborhood segregation
   c. Ethnicity
   d. Educational attainment
   e. Discrimination
3. Current classifications of race were developed based on a scientific understanding of genetics. True or false?
4. In the United States, death rates have been highest among:
   a. American Indian Alaska Native
   b. Non-Hispanic Black
   c. Hispanic
   d. Pacific Islander
   e. Non-Hispanic White
5. Acculturation is a process of cultural and physical change resulting from intercultural contact and the extent to which ethnic minorities and immigrant groups participate in the dominant culture's values, beliefs, assumptions, and practices. True or false?
6. Measures used to estimate levels of acculturation include:
   a. Date of birth
   b. Mother's ethnicity
   c. Language
   d. Income
   e. All of the above
7. Cultural Niche Construction describes the interrelationship among:
   a. Genes, acculturation, and obesity
   b. Culture, obesity, and hunger
   c. Genes, hunger, and acculturation
   d. Genes, culture, and food choice
8. Today the income gap is largest between:
   a. Whites and Blacks
   b. Whites and Hispanics

    c.   Asians and Blacks

    d.   Asians and whites

    e.   None of these; there is no income gap.

9. The impacts of precarious employment include:

    a.   Divorce

    b.   Teen pregnancy

    c.   Substance abuse

    d.   Hypertension

    e.   Animal welfare abuses

10. Psychosocial factors are an important cause of hypertension. True or false?

Discussion Questions

1. What is the difference between health disparities and health inequities?
2. What is race? How is it conceptualized in the United States and in other parts of the world?
3. What are the limitations and social implications of using race as an identifier?
4. Describe some health disparities based on race/ethnicity.
5. Discuss what is known about health inequities based on sexual orientation.
6. What health disparities exist by gender? What are underlying causes? Could these be considered inequities? Why or why not?
7. What are social determinants of health? How do social determinants of health contribute to health disparities?
8. What is allostatic load? How does stress contribute to diet-related health disparities?
9. What are the different types of racism and how might this relate to the perpetuation of nutrition-related health disparities?
10. What is a food desert? How is the formation of modern-day food deserts in both urban and rural settings shaped by historical practices?
11. Describe some of the historical factors related to modern-day health disparities in the United States.
12. Define the concept of "Health in All Policies" and provide examples of how it may be used to address some of the diet-related health disparities described in this chapter.
13. What are global health disparities?
14. Describe the double burden of disease. What is the nutrition/epidemiological transition?

Additional Resources

PBS Series. Unnatural Causes: Is inequality making us sick? http://unnaturalcauses.
org/episode_descriptions.php?page=1

Food Desert Locator: https://www.fns.usda.gov/tags/food-desert-locator

Global Health Observatory (GHO) data, Overweight and Obesity http://www.who.
int/gho/ncd/risk_factors/overweight/en/

References

1. Yudell M, Roberts D, DeSalle R, Tishkoff S. Taking race out of human genetics. *Science.* 2016;351(6273):564–565.

2. Bennett C. Racial categories used in the decennial censuses, 1790 to the present. *Government Information Quarterly.* 2000;17(2):161–180.

3. Lin SS, Kelsey JL. Use of race and ethnicity in epidemiologic research: concepts, methodological issues, and suggestions for research. *Epidemiologic Reviews.* 2000;22(2):187–202.

4. Jones CP. Invited commentary: "race," racism, and the practice of epidemiology. *American Journal of Epidemiology.* 2001;154(4):299–304.

5. Registrar F. Revisions to the standards for the classification of federal data on race and ethnicity. *Federal Registrar.* 1997;62:58781–58790.

6. U.S. Department of Health and Human Services OoMH. Hispanic/Latino. https://www.minorityhealth.hhs.gov/omh/browse.aspx?lvl=3&lvlid=64. Accessed July 2017.

7. Zsembik BA, Fennell D. Ethnic variation in health and the determinants of health among Latinos. *Social Science & Medicine.* 2005;61(1):53–63.

8. Ruiz JM, Steffen P, Smith TB. Hispanic mortality paradox: a systematic review and meta-analysis of the longitudinal literature. *American Journal of Public Health.* 2013;103(3):e52–e60.

9. Ribble F, Keddie M. Understanding the Hispanic paradox. *Ethnicity & Disease.* 2001;11:496–518.

10. Kennedy S, McDonald JT, Biddle N. The healthy immigrant effect and immigrant selection: evidence from four countries. SEDAP; 2006.

11. Markides KS, Eschbach K. Aging, migration, and mortality: current status of research on the Hispanic paradox. *The Journals of Gerontology Series B: Psychological Sciences and Social Sciences.* 2005;60(Special Issue 2):S68–S75.

12. Markides KS, Rote S. Immigrant health paradox. *Emerging Trends in the Social and Behavioral Sciences: An Interdisciplinary, Searchable, and Linkable Resource.* 2015.

13. Abraido-Lanza AF, Dohrenwend BP, Ng-Mak DS, Turner JB. The Latino mortality paradox: a test of the" salmon bias" and healthy migrant hypotheses. *American Journal of Public Health.* 1999;89(10):1543–1548.

14. Jasso G, Rosenzweig MR. Estimating the emigration rates of legal immigrants using administrative and survey data: The 1971 cohort of immigrants to the United States. *Demography.* 1982;19(3):279–290.

15. U.S. Department of Health and Human Services OoMH. Black/African Americans. https://www.minorityhealth.hhs.gov/omh/browse.aspx?lvl=3&lvlid=61. Accessed July 27, 2017.

16. Schiller JS, Lucas JW, Ward BW, Peregoy JA. Summary health statistics for US Adults: National health interview survey, 2010. *Vital and Health Statistics Series 10, Data from The National Health Survey.* 2012(252):1–207.

17. Go AS, Mozaffarian D, Roger VL, et al. Heart disease and stroke statistics–2014 update. *Circulation.* 2014;129(3).

18. Go AS, Mozaffarian D, Roger VL, et al. Executive summary: heart disease and stroke statistics–2014 update: a report from the American Heart Association. *Circulation.* 2014;129(3):399.

19. U.S. Department of Health and Human Services OoMH. American Indian/Alaska Native. https://www.minorityhealth.hhs.gov/omh/browse.aspx?lvl=3&lvlid=62. Accessed July 27, 2017.

20. U.S. Department of Health and Human Services OoMH. Asian Americans. https://www.minorityhealth.hhs.gov/omh/browse.aspx?lvl=3&lvlid=63. Accessed July 27, 2017.

21. U.S. Department of Health and Human Services OoMH. Native Hawaiians/Pacific Islanders. https://www.minorityhealth.hhs.gov/omh/browse.aspx?lvl=3&lvlid=65. Accessed July 27, 2017.

22. J ZJaB. Frequently Requested Statistics on Immigrants and Immigration in the United States. March 8, 2017: http://www.migrationpolicy.org/article/frequently-requested-statistics-immigrants-and-immigration-united-states/ - CurrentHistoricalNumbers. Accessed July 21, 2017.

23. Abraído-Lanza AF, Armbrister AN, Flórez KR, Aguirre AN. Toward a theory-driven model of acculturation in public health research. *American Journal of Public Health.* 2006;96(8):1342–1346.

24. Berry JW. *Conceptual approaches to acculturation.* American Psychological Association; 2003.

25. Berry J. W. Acculturation as varieties of adaptation. *Acculturation: Theory, models, and some new findings.* 1980;9–25.

26. Berry JW. Immigration, acculturation, and adaptation. *Applied psychology.* 1997;46(1):5–34.

27. Ryder AG, Alden LE, Paulhus DL. Is acculturation unidimensional or bidimensional? A head-to-head comparison in the prediction of personality, self-identity, and adjustment. *Journal of Personality and Social Psychology.* 2000;79(1):49.

28. Cabassa LJ. Measuring acculturation: Where we are and where we need to go. *Hispanic Journal of Behavioral Sciences.* 2003;25(2):127–146.

29. Satia-Abouta J, Patterson RE, Neuhouser ML, Elder J. Dietary accultura-
    tion: applications to nutrition research and dietetics. *Journal of the American
    Dietetic Association.* 2002;102(8):1105–1118.
30. Bermúdez OL, Falcon LM, Tucker KL. Intake and food sources of macronutrients
    among older Hispanic adults: association with ethnicity acculturation, and length
    of residence in the United States. *Journal of the American Dietetic Association.*
    2000;100(6):665–673.
31. Gordon-Larsen P, Harris KM, Ward DS, Popkin BM. Acculturation and
    overweight-related behaviors among Hispanic immigrants to the US: the
    National Longitudinal Study of Adolescent Health. *Social Science & Medicine.*
    2003;57(11):2023–2034.
32. Salant T, Lauderdale DS. Measuring culture: a critical review of accultura-
    tion and health in Asian immigrant populations. *Social Science & Medicine.*
    2003;57(1):71–90.
33. Cho Y, Frisbie WP, Hummer RA, Rogers RG. Nativity, duration of residence, and
    the health of Hispanic adults in the United States. *International Migration Review.*
    2004;38(1):184–211.
34. Sundquist J, Winkleby MA. Cardiovascular risk factors in Mexican American
    adults: a transcultural analysis of NHANES III, 1988–1994. *American Journal of
    Public Health.* 1999;89(5):723–730.
35. Messerli F, Ventura H, Glade L, Sundgaard-Riise K, Dunn F, Frohlich E. Essential
    hypertension in the elderly: haemodynamics, intravascular volume, plasma renin
    activity, and circulating catecholamine levels. *The Lancet.* 1983;322(8357):983–986.
36. Neuhouser ML, Thompson B, Coronado GD, Solomon CC. Higher fat intake and
    lower fruit and vegetables intakes are associated with greater acculturation among
    Mexicans living in Washington State. *Journal of the American Dietetic Association.*
    2004;104(1):51–57.
37. Woodruff S, Zaslow K, Candelaria J, Elder J. Effects of gender and acculturation
    on nutrition-related factors among limited-English proficient Hispanic adults.
    Ethnicity & Disease. 1996;7(2):121–126.
38. Elder JP, Castro FG, de Moor C, et al. Differences in cancer-risk-related behaviors
    in Latino and Anglo adults. *Preventive Medicine.* 1991;20(6):751–763.
39. Ayala GX, Baquero B, Klinger S. A systematic review of the relationship between
    acculturation and diet among Latinos in the United States: implications for future
    research. *Journal of the American Dietetic Association.* 2008;108(8):1330–1344.
40. Opie FD. *Hog and hominy: Soul food from Africa to America.* Columbia University
    Press; 2010.
41. Sharma S, Cruickshank J. Cultural differences in assessing dietary intake and pro-
    viding relevant dietary information to British African–Caribbean populations.
    Journal of Human Nutrition and Dietetics. 2001;14(6):449–456.
42. Sharma S, Sharma S, Yacavone MM, et al. Nutritional composition of com-
    monly consumed composite dishes for Afro-Caribbeans (mainly Jamaicans)

in the United Kingdom. *International Journal of Food Sciences and Nutrition.* 2009;60(S7):140–150.

43. Control CfD. Body-weight perceptions and selected weight-management goals and practices of high school students—United States, 1990. *MMWR: Morbidity and Mortality Weekly Report.* 1991;40(43):741, 747.

44. Akan GE, Grilo CM. Sociocultural influences on eating attitudes and behaviors, body image, and psychological functioning: A comparison of African American, Asian American, and Caucasian college women. *International Journal of Eating Disorders.* 1995;18(2):181–187.

45. Kumanyika S, Wilson JF, Guilford-Davenport M. Weight-related attitudes and behaviors of black women. *Journal of the American Dietetic Association.* 1993;93(4):416–422.

46. Mosca L, Barrett-Connor E, Wenger NK. Sex/gender differences in cardiovascular disease prevention. *Circulation.* 2011;124(19):2145–2154.

47. Valanis BG, Bowen DJ, Bassford T, Whitlock E, Charney P, Carter RA. Sexual orientation and health: comparisons in the women's health initiative sample. *Archives of Family Medicine.* 2000;9(9):843.

48. Hatzenbuehler ML, McLaughlin KA, Slopen N. Sexual orientation disparities in cardiovascular biomarkers among young adults. *American Journal of Preventive Medicine.* 2013;44(6):612–621.

49. Saydah S, Lochner K. Socioeconomic status and risk of diabetes-related mortality in the US. *Public Health Reports.* 2010;125(3):377–388.

50. Rabi DM, Edwards AL, Southern DA, et al. Association of socio-economic status with diabetes prevalence and utilization of diabetes care services. *BMC Health Services Research.* 2006;6(1):124.

51. Connolly V, Unwin N, Sherriff P, Bilous R, Kelly W. Diabetes prevalence and socioeconomic status: a population based study showing increased prevalence of type 2 diabetes mellitus in deprived areas. *Journal of Epidemiology & Community Health.* 2000;54(3):173–177.

52. Guenther PM, Casavale KO, Reedy J, et al. Update of the healthy eating index: HEI-2010. *Journal of the Academy of Nutrition and Dietetics.* 2013;113(4):569–580.

53. Galobardes B, Morabia A, Bernstein MS. Diet and socioeconomic position: does the use of different indicators matter? *International Journal of Epidemiology.* 2001;30(2):334–340.

54. Darmon N, Drewnowski A. Does social class predict diet quality? *The American Journal of Clinical Nutrition.* 2008;87(5):1107–1117.

55. Wang DD, Leung CW, Li Y, et al. Trends in dietary quality among adults in the United States, 1999 through 2010. *JAMA Internal Medicine.* 2014;174(10):1587–1595.

56. Raffensperger S, Kuczmarski MF, Hotchkiss L, Cotugna N, Evans MK, Zonderman AB. Effect of race and predictors of socioeconomic status on diet quality in the HANDLS Study sample. *Journal of the National Medical Association.* 2010;102(10):923–930.

57. Feeding America. Poverty and Hunger in America. http://www.feeding-america.org/hunger-in-america/hunger-and-poverty-facts.html?gclid=CjwKCAjwzMbLBRBzEiwAfFz4gRVvRsVy5g-IEhAN5kEAf4gZJG4vkrovuddZnBp34JNuXYt587mgThoCg4MQAvD_BwE?referrer=https://www.google.com/. Accessed July 21, 2017.

58. Sobal J, Stunkard AJ. Socioeconomic status and obesity: a review of the literature. *Psychological Bulletin.* 1989;105(2):260.

59. McLaren L. Socioeconomic status and obesity. *Epidemiologic Reviews.* 2007;29(1):29–48.

60. Camargo Jr KRd. *Closing the gap in a generation: health equity through action on the social determinants of health.* Taylor & Francis; 2011.

61. O'Connell M, Buchwald DS, Duncan GE. Food access and cost in American Indian communities in Washington State. *Journal of the American Dietetic Association.* 2011;111(9):1375–1379.

62. Institute DP. Diné Food Sovereignty: A Report on the Navajo Nation Food System and the Case to Rebuild a Self Sufficient Food System for the Diné People. April 2014; http://www.dinecollege.edu/institutes/DPI/Docs/dpi-food-sovereignty-report.pdf.

63. Monsivais P, Drewnowski A. The rising cost of low-energy-density foods. *Journal of the American Dietetic Association.* 2007;107(12):2071–2076.

64. Swinburn BA, Sacks G, Hall KD, et al. The global obesity pandemic: shaped by global drivers and local environments. *The Lancet.* 2011;378(9793):804–814.

65. Jetter KM, Cassady DL. The availability and cost of healthier food alternatives. *American Journal of Preventive Medicine.* 2006;30(1):38–44.

66. Pew Research Center. June 27, 2016.

67. Menéndez M, Benach J, Muntaner C, Amable M, O'Campo P. Is precarious employment more damaging to women's health than men's? *Social Science & Medicine.* 2007;64(4):776–781.

68. Solis HL, Galvin JM. Labor force characteristics by race and ethnicity, 2011. *Bureau of Labor Statistics.* 2012.

69. Doede MS. Black jobs matter: Racial inequalities in conditions of employment and subsequent health outcomes. *Public Health Nursing.* 2016;33(2):151–158.

70. Benach J, Vives A, Amable M, Vanroelen C, Tarafa G, Muntaner C. Precarious employment: understanding an emerging social determinant of health. *Annual Review of Public Health.* 2014;35.

71. Marmot MG, Stansfeld S, Patel C, et al. Health inequalities among British civil servants: the Whitehall II study. *The Lancet.* 1991;337(8754):1387–1393.

72. Mattiasson I, Lindgärde F, Nilsson JA, Theorell T. Threat of unemployment and cardiovascular risk factors: longitudinal study of quality of sleep and serum cholesterol concentrations in men threatened with redundancy. *BMJ.* 1990;301(6750):461–466.

73. Ferrie JE, Shipley MJ, Marmot MG, Stansfeld SA, Smith GD. An uncertain future: the health effects of threats to employment security in white-collar men and women. *American Journal of Public Health.* 1998;88(7):1030–1036.

74. Fullerton AS, Anderson KF. The role of job insecurity in explanations of racial health inequalities. Paper presented at: Sociological Forum; 2013.

75. Campos-Serna J, Ronda-Pérez E, Artazcoz L, Moen BE, Benavides FG. Gender inequalities in occupational health related to the unequal distribution of working and employment conditions: a systematic review. *International Journal for Equity in Health.* 2013;12(1):57.

76. Landsbergis PA, Grzywacz JG, LaMontagne AD. Work organization, job insecurity, and occupational health disparities. *American Journal of Industrial medicine.* 2014;57(5):495–515.

77. Benach J, Muntaner C, Solar O, Santana V, Quinlan M. Employment, work, and health inequalities: a global perspective. *Geneva: WHO.* 2007.

78. Lipscomb HJ, Loomis D, McDonald MA, Argue RA, Wing S. A conceptual model of work and health disparities in the United States. *International Journal of Health Services.* 2006;36(1):25–50.

79. Keuskamp D, Ziersch AM, Baum FE, LaMontagne AD. Precarious employment, psychosocial working conditions, and health: Cross sectional associations in a population based sample of working Australians. *American Journal of Industrial Medicine.* 2013;56(8):838–844.

80. Benach J, Vives A, Tarafa G, Delclos C, Muntaner C. What should we know about precarious employment and health in 2025? Framing the agenda for the next decade of research. *International Journal of Epidemiology.* 2016;45(1):232–238.

81. Clark R, Anderson NB, Clark VR, Williams DR. Racism as a stressor for African Americans: A biopsychosocial model. *American Psychologist.* 1999;54(10):805.

82. Krieger N, Kosheleva A, Waterman PD, Chen JT, Koenen K. Racial discrimination, psychological distress, and self-rated health among US-born and foreign-born Black Americans. *American Journal of Public Health.* 2011;101(9):1704–1713.

83. Williams DR, Neighbors HW, Jackson JS. Racial/ethnic discrimination and health: findings from community studies. *American Journal of Public Health.* 2003;93(2):200–208.

84. Peters RM. Racism and hypertension among African Americans. *Western Journal of Nursing Research.* 2004;26(6):612–631.

85. Anderson NB, Myers HF, Pickering T, Jackson JS. Hypertension in blacks: psychosocial and biological perspectives. *Journal of Hypertension.* 1989;7(3):161–172.

86. Anderson ES, Winett RA, Wojcik JR. Self-regulation, self-efficacy, outcome expectations, and social support: social cognitive theory and nutrition behavior. *Annals of Behavioral Medicine.* 2007;34(3):304–312.

87. Williams DR, Neighbors H. Racism, discrimination and hypertension: evidence and needed research. *Ethnicity & Disease.* 2001;11(4):800–816.

88. Jones CP. Levels of racism: a theoretic framework and a gardener's tale. *American Journal of Public Health.* 2000;90(8):1212.

89. Modood T. *Ethnic minorities in Britain: diversity and disadvantage: the fourth national survey of ethnic minorities.* Policy Studies Institute; 1997.

90. Karlsen S, Nazroo JY. Relation between racial discrimination, social class, and health among ethnic minority groups. *American Journal of Public Health.* 2002;92(4):624–631.

91. Walls ML, Gonzalez J, Gladney T, Onello E. Unconscious biases: racial microaggressions in American Indian health care. *The Journal of the American Board of Family Medicine.* 2015;28(2):231–239.

92. James SA. John Henryism and the health of African-Americans. *Culture, medicine and psychiatry.* 1994;18(2):163–182.

93. Krieger N. Racial and gender discrimination: risk factors for high blood pressure? *Social Science & Medicine.* 1990;30(12):1273–1281.

94. Krieger N, Sidney S. Racial discrimination and blood pressure: the CARDIA Study of young black and white adults. *American Journal of Public Health.* 1996;86(10):1370–1378.

95. Beckie TM. A systematic review of allostatic load, health, and health disparities. *Biological Research for Nursing.* 2012;14(4):311–346.

96. McEwen BS, Seeman T. Protective and damaging effects of mediators of stress: elaborating and testing the concepts of allostasis and allostatic load. *Annals of the New York Academy of Sciences.* 1999;896(1):30–47.

97. Peek MK, Cutchin MP, Salinas JJ, et al. Allostatic load among non-Hispanic Whites, non-Hispanic Blacks, and people of Mexican origin: effects of ethnicity, nativity, and acculturation. *American Journal of Public Health.* 2010;100(5):940–946.

98. Ver Ploeg M. *Access to affordable and nutritious food: measuring and understanding food deserts and their consequences: report to Congress.* Diane Publishing; 2010.

99. Morland K, Wing S, Roux AD, Poole C. Neighborhood characteristics associated with the location of food stores and food service places. *American Journal of Preventive Medicine.* 2002;22(1):23–29.

100. Powell LM, Slater S, Mirtcheva D, Bao Y, Chaloupka FJ. Food store availability and neighborhood characteristics in the United States. *Preventive Medicine.* 2007;44(3):189–195.

101. Zenk SN, Schulz AJ, Israel BA, James SA, Bao S, Wilson ML. Neighborhood racial composition, neighborhood poverty, and the spatial accessibility of supermarkets in metropolitan Detroit. *American Journal of Public Health.* 2005;95(4):660–667.

102. Alwitt LF, Donley TD. Retail stores in poor urban neighborhoods. *Journal of Consumer Affairs.* 1997;31(1):139–164.

103. Osypuk TL, Roux AVD, Hadley C, Kandula NR. Are immigrant enclaves healthy places to live? The Multi-ethnic Study of Atherosclerosis. *Social Science & Medicine.* 2009;69(1):110–120.

104. Company TN. The Multicultural edge: Rising Super Consumers. 2015.

105. Wentz L. McDonald's Is Marketer of the Year at AHAA's Hispanic Conference. http://adage.com/article/hispanic-marketing/mcdonald-s-marketer-year-ahaa-conference/292979/. Accessed July 27, 2017.

106. Grier SA, Kumanyika SK. The context for choice: health implications of targeted food and beverage marketing to African Americans. *American Journal of Public Health.* 2008;98(9):1616–1629.

107. Deurenberg P, Deurenberg Yap M, Guricci S. Asians are different from Caucasians and from each other in their body mass index/body fat per cent relationship. *Obesity Reviews.* 2002;3(3):141–146.

108. Duerksen SC, Mikail A, Tom L, et al. Health disparities and advertising content of women's magazines: a cross-sectional study. *BMC Public Health.* 2005;5(1):85.

109. Harris J, Shehan C, Gross R. Food advertising targeted to Hispanic and Black youth: Contributing to health disparities. *Rudd Report.* 2015.

110. Nelson AR, Stith AY, Smedley BD. *Unequal treatment: confronting racial and ethnic disparities in health care (full printed version).* National Academies Press; 2002.

111. Adler NE, Newman K. Socioeconomic disparities in health: pathways and policies. *Health Affairs.* 2002;21(2):60–76.

112. Ranji U, Beamesderfer A, Kates J, Salganicoff A. *Health and access to care and coverage for lesbian, gay, bisexual, and transgender individuals in the US.* Henry J. Kaiser Family Foundation; 2014.

113. Hughto JMW, Reisner SL, Pachankis JE. Transgender stigma and health: a critical review of stigma determinants, mechanisms, and interventions. *Social Science & Medicine.* 2015;147:222–231.

114. Derose KP, Gresenz CR, Ringel JS. Understanding disparities in health care access—and reducing them—through a focus on public health. *Health Affairs.* 2011;30(10):1844–1851.

115. Avery K, Finegold K, Whitman A. *Affordable Care Act has led to historical, widespread increase in health insurance coverage.* United States Department of Health and Human Services; 2016.

116. Uberoi N, Finegold K, Gee E. *Health insurance coverage and the Affordable Care Act, 2010–2016.* United States Department of Health and Human Services; 2016.

117. Sommers BD, Gunja MZ, Finegold K, Musco T. Changes in self-reported insurance coverage, access to care, and health under the Affordable Care Act. *JAMA.* 2015;314(4):366–374.

118. Chen J, Vargas-Bustamante A, Mortensen K, Ortega AN. Racial and ethnic disparities in health care access and utilization under the Affordable Care Act. *Medical Care.* 2016;54(2):140.

119. Agency for Healthcare Research and Quality. 2015 national healthcare quality and disparities report and 5th anniversary update on the national quality strategy. 2016.

120. Rudolph L, Caplan J, Ben-Moshe K, Dillon L. *Health in All Policies: A guide for state and local governments.* American Public Health Association; 2013.

121. Heiman HJ, Artiga S. Beyond health care: the role of social determinants in promoting health and health equity. *Health.* 2015;20(10). https://www.kff.org/disparities-policy/issue-brief/beyond-health-care-the-role-of-social-determinants-in-promoting-health-and-health-equity/

122. Dart J. Australia's disturbing health disparities set Aboriginals apart. World Health Organization; 2008.

123. UNICEF. *Progress for Children beyond Averages: Learning from the MDGS.* eSocialSciences; 2015.

124. UNICEF. Undernutrition contributes to nearly half of all deaths in children under 5 and is widespread in Asia and Africa. https://data.unicef.org/topic/nutrition/malnutrition/.

125. Marshall SJ. Developing countries face double burden of disease. *Bulletin of the World Health Organization.* 2004;82(7):556.

126. Agyei-Mensah S, Aikins Ad-G. Epidemiological transition and the double burden of disease in Accra, Ghana. *Journal of Urban Health.* 2010;87(5):879–897.

127. Omram A. The epidemiologic transition theory. A preliminary update. *Journal of Tropical Pediatrics.* 1983;29(6):305–316.

5

Healthy Food Marketing

Allison Karpyn

Chapter Highlights

- Four P's of marketing
- Marketing in supermarkets
- "Junk" food marketing to kids including online advertising
- School food and marketing

Introduction

Food and beverage marketing is responsible for driving consumer demand for much of what we eat. Although considerable efforts have been made to limit "junk" food marketing to kids, it remains the case that the products most heavily marketed to youth are those high in sugar, fat, and/or sodium.[1] And, given the fast pace of Internet content and the swiftly changing media environment, past regulation efforts are becoming less able to regulate predatory advertising effectively. At the same time, efforts to utilize marketing strategies originated by industry for public health promotion are underway.

In this chapter, we will first review recent efforts to curb unhealthy marketing to kids while illuminating emerging challenges. In the second part of the chapter, we will discuss current efforts to apply marketing strategies for health promotion.

Food Marketing to Kids

From packaging, to in-store marketing approaches, to TV websites and downloadable Internet content, the landscape of food marketing is dynamic and quickly changing. The food industry spends more money than any other industry on advertising. In 2009, $280 million was spent on healthy-food marketing to kids while $1.7 billion was spent on marketing unhealthy food to kids.[2] Among the unhealthy items of greatest concern are sugary drinks, snack foods, and fast food. As America becomes more and more diverse, public health officials are increasingly paying attention to how and when marketing activities target specific cultural subgroups. Concerns regarding greater exposures to unhealthy marketing strategies targeting African American and Hispanic children are of particular concern given evidence of disproportionate risk for obesity and diet-related disease. Early research shows that the majority of foods and drinks advertised to kids on Spanish TV (84%) are unhealthy and that African American children see more than twice as many advertisements for sugar-sweetened beverages than do white children.[2,3]

Advertisements for fast foods are responsible for more than a third of food industry advertising expenditures.[1,4] It should be no surprise then that McDonald's and Coca-Cola top the list of advertising among all companies worldwide. Children are constantly exposed to marketing messages, and one approach to improving the food environment is to set limits on the amount of advertising to which children are exposed. Looking at Nielsen data, researchers believe that children aged 2 to 11 years see 25,600 TV ads per year[5] (more than 73 per day), and on average, see 14 food or beverage ads daily.[6] Adolescents see slightly more. A more recent study found that in 2009, 3 billion advertisements for food and beverages were found on children's websites.[7]

Beginning in 2006, the children's food and beverage advertising initiative was launched by the Council of Better Business Bureaus. Later, at the end of 2013, updated criteria were introduced as a way to further improve the nutritional quality of foods marketed to children.

In its 2012 report, the Federal Trade Commission found that advertising quick-service restaurant foods, carbonated beverages, and breakfast cereals represented the largest portion of youth-directed expenditures by industry.[1] Together they account for 72% of the $1.29 billion spent on youth food advertising in 2009. Carbonated beverage companies reported $395 million in direct advertising costs, of which 97% was directed toward the teenage market. Of note, 21% of the carbonated beverage marketing was spent in schools. Breakfast cereal companies more evenly distributed their expenditures between children and teens, spending $186 million in 2009. In 2009, the majority of food marketing dollars were spent on television advertising, totaling about 35% of expenditures.

Breakfast cereals continue to represent the most highly advertised packaged food on child-targeted television, and advertisements are predominately for products high in sugar. Ready-to-eat cereals have included notable icons on the front of their boxes, ranging from General Mills' Trix the Rabbit to Kellogg's Tony the Tiger, and some even have used licensed media characters such as SpongeBob SquarePants. Cereals that are targeted for kids are also more likely to have greater quantities of sugar than cereals that are marketed to adults. On average, children's cereals have about 57% more sugar.[8] Furthermore, advertising is effective, and research has found that more marketing does translate to more family purchases. Nielsen food purchasing data found that households were 13 times more likely to purchase TV-advertised cereal products directed toward youth.[8]

New Media Environment and Marketing

The media environment has changed dramatically in the past 10 years. In the past, children would sit down to watch a scheduled program with intermittent advertising. Today, however, most programming is on-demand, and children can watch the programs they want at any time. Programming is streamed or downloaded, and mobile devices enable children to view content from almost anywhere. As online content grows, questions remain about how best to manage marketing to children within this environment.[9]

YouTube, launched in 2005, is now one of the most popular platforms for watching video. The service, along with Netflix, Amazon, and Hulu allows children to watch video programming without any subscription to cable or satellite services. In the case of YouTube in particular, marketing becomes far more personalized and is increasingly part of the content of the show itself. Professional YouTube celebrities, "YouTubers," have become increasingly popular and, according to a recent study, are likely as influential or even more influential than traditional celebrities. Advertisers have capitalized on this trend and now use YouTubers as a mechanism for marketing products to younger audiences (Figure 5.1).

One such strategy is called *unboxing* and encompasses an advertising strategy wherein people open a box of product to get a feel for it, often in a highly dramatic and sensualized way. The approach attempts to tell the story of a brand and builds relationships with consumers while taking on a playful, fun, and often quirky spirit. Content now often is driven by YouTube creators who work directly with multi-channel networks (MCNs) brokering relationships between advertisers and influencers to reach audiences.[9] Today, more

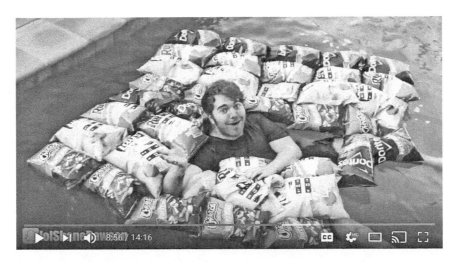

TRYING DUMB SUMMER LIFE HACKS

FIGURE 5.1 Screen shot of YouTuber Shane Dawson in his June post, "Trying Dumb Summer Life Hacks." The YouTube celebrity has 9 million followers and 1,790 videos.

than half of the content on YouTube is professionally produced by MCNs. In fact, 2016 reports suggest that spending on digital advertisements in the United States will soon, if not already, surpass TV advertising expenditures.

Because YouTube celebrities are influencing product brands, while at the same time doing skits, it can be difficult to determine when a program is paid for by industry and when it is not. The inability to distinguish programming from advertising is a key legal threshold and a historic dividing line between predatory marketing and non-predatory marketing. The subsequent lack of delineation has now brought formal complaints to the Federal Trade Commission (FTC).[10]

Two agencies help to regulate advertising to kids in the media: The Federal Trade Commission (FTC) and The Federal Communications Commission (FCC). The FTC has the power to prevent deceptive and unfair marketing practices regardless of the medium employed, while the FCC applies only to television delivered by broadcast cable or satellite. A study published in 2017, using 2013–2014 data, found that children spend an average of 21.5 hours per week using electronic media and half of that time is spent on regular cable or satellite television.[9]

Younger children are also regularly exposed to online marketing and YouTube. Among children aged 8 to 10 years, 69% use smart phones or tablets when available in the home, and children generally prefer these devices to TV. Some programs, such as YouTube, explicitly state the service is not for children under the age of 13. A 2014 survey revealed that 72% of 6- to 8-year-olds visit YouTube daily as do 66% of children ages 6 to 12. Programs such as Toy Freaks are directly targeted to young children and at the same time have become the most watched YouTube channel with more than 661 million views in August of 2016.[9] In response to trending use among children, Google launched a YouTube kids app in February 2015 in order to give children their own place to "discover videos channels and playlists they love."[11]

Although many of the toy-based channels initially may seem unrelated to food advertising, many influencer videos feature candy and snack foods. From videos that teach children how to make a new Nutella milkshake to Twizzlers made out of Playdough and Snickers bar lip gloss, channels subtly yet strategically promote junk food to kids.[10]

Efforts to Apply Marketing Strategies for Health Promotion

Marketing's 4 Ps

The key elements of marketing are commonly defined by 4 P's: Product, Price, Promotion, and Place (or distribution). An effective marketing strategy ideally combines all four of the P's of the marketing mix.

Product

The product, as one might expect, refers to the specific food, good, or service offered by a company to its customers. The same product can vary in many ways. Let's take the grocery store itself as a product. Not all grocery stores are alike. A store could shift the variety or quality of its products, adopt a modern or traditional in-store design or layout, and vary its features such that it offers a pharmacy and a delicatessen or does not. The way that the store appears from the outside and its cleanliness all have a role in your perception. How you feel about this product, in this case the grocery store, drives its demand.

This is an example of a store as a product; now let's take another example, something perhaps a bit more common, such as cereal.

Price

As one might expect, the product price, or the amount of money paid by customers to purchase the product is a critical factor in how food is marketed.

How the product is priced and whether discounts are offered plays an important role in how customers value the product.

Promotion

Promotion refers to the activities that communicate the product features and benefits and can be used to persuade customers to purchase the product. Although these strategies may include advertising of a price, they are distinct from a price.

Place (or Distribution)

Place refers to the placement of the product and the activities that make the product available to the consumer. Where and on which shelf a product is placed, the kinds of stores where it is sold, the locations or regions where it is available, and the transportation and logistics required to sufficiently supply the product, all fall within the marketing category of place.

In-store Marketing

Just as the content on the web represents a seemingly endless selection of options, today's grocery stores are a sea of products.

According to The Food Marketing Institute, an umbrella organization for food retailers, the average supermarket carries an average of 40,000 distinct products. Together these items account for average weekly grocery sales of over $355,000 per store in the United States alone. Americans still spend most of their food dollar on purchases intended for home consumption (5.5% of disposable income) though the trend is increasing when it comes to spending on food away from home (currently 4.5% of disposable income). Figures 5.2 to 5.4 provide an overview of expenditure trends.

Efforts to understand better the ways in which marketing strategies in grocery stores can influence healthier decisions have been a growing focal point of public health research globally. A variety of studies have examined marketing strategies specific to categories of the grocery store, such as candy at checkout, cereal, frozen food, grab-and-go beverage containers, milk and dairy products, salty snacks, and bread. Findings suggest that various strategies work better in some categories than in others. For example, strategies such as increasing the number of facings a product has on the shelf may be better suited for the milk category than for cereal.[12,13]

In addition researchers have compiled healthy in-store strategies into a list, called the supermarket scorecard. On it, retailers are able to score themselves

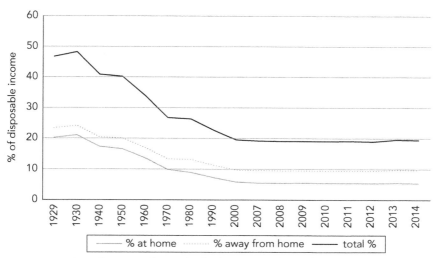

FIGURE 5.2 Trends in expenditures for food eaten at and away from home, by percentage of disposable income, 1929–2014.

on the extent to which the store layout and positioning of products is aligned with the strategies shown to have an impact on purchasing.[14]

One early informational strategy used by retailers to help consumers identify healthier items in the store is a nutritional scoring system. The concept is relatively simple; tags are provided on the shelf edge next to products and

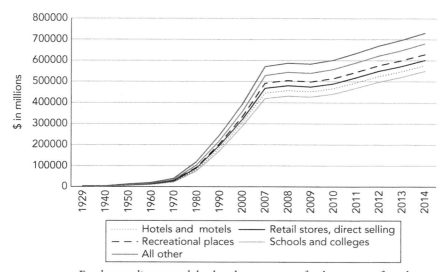

FIGURE 5.3 Food expenditure trends by decade, 1929–2014, food eaten away from home.

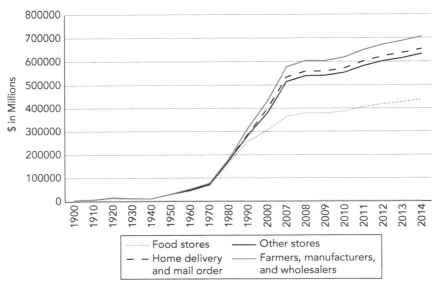

FIGURE 5.4   Trends by decade in food purchased for home consumption, 1900–2014.

each is scored according to its nutrient profile. Available systems include Guiding Stars, developed by Hannaford Supermarkets (see Figure 5.5). Other strategies include placing produce at the store entrance, widening aisles where healthy foods are displayed, maintaining lighting on healthier products, offering products in more than one place in the store (i.e., secondary placement), removing candy at checkout, and offering in-store taste-testing for healthier items, to name a few.[14]

Although Americans continue to rely on local grocery stores and supermarkets for the majority of their food purchases, purchases from other stores, home delivery and mail order, farmers markets and wholesalers, as well as increased amounts of food produced at home, account for an increasingly dynamic and complex web of mechanisms to obtain food.

New efforts to understand how online ordering for food to be consumed at home influences the healthfulness of the shopping basket are in nascent phases. SNAP (Supplemental Nutrition Assistance Program) customers wishing to make online purchases for home delivery face some challenges in doing so, though the U.S. Department of Agriculture (USDA) and others are now in the process of understanding how technology would need to change in order to accommodate purchases from services such as Peapod and Amazon. The ways in which marketing strategies can be applied to online and in-app purchases are relatively unstudied by public health experts, but represent a new area of potential research.

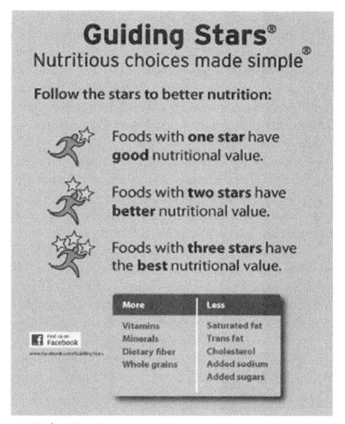

FIGURE 5.5 Guiding Stars image.

School Food Environments and Marketing

I recently was in a position to review an elementary school wellness policy wherein cupcakes were a centerpiece of debate. Two competing issues created tension: One was the position that all kids should be able to have a treat on their birthdays. Parents fondly recalled their childhoods, when they celebrated birthdays alongside their classmates with homemade treats they were proud to show off to the class. These memories, however, stood in stark contrast to the conflicting reality that with 25 kids in a classroom this meant 25 birthday celebrations, in addition to the candy given as occasional rewards, plus the various holiday celebrations and school fundraisers. With 180 days in the school year, this quickly added up to extra calories on a larger proportion of school days than was intended. It meant school children were eating many more treats than most people realized.

What regulated the conversation, however, was the reality that schools face in their efforts to effectively limit some unhealthy items and keep track of what and how much was allowed into the building. They also were concerned about managing child safety in a building where 10% of children have a food allergy. Although most of those concerned believed that some restriction on food in schools was reasonable, exactly where to draw the line was a constant source of debate, and enforcement seemed like a nightmare for teachers and principals alike.

Despite new policy put forth in the Healthy Hunger Free Kids Act, the issue continues to generate discussion at the local level. Indeed, although the local and organic food movements have become a central theme in many communities, most of today's parents grew up in classrooms where they as children brought cupcakes to share and to celebrate their birthdays. After all, if the cupcake was fine for them, why is it not fine for their children?

The food that is served and advertised at school represents an important part of a child's food and marketing environment. Schools can be places where children have unique experiences with new foods by learning about and tasting school garden-grown products through local farm-to-school programs,[15] or places where the default items and the marketing that goes alongside them are subtly encouraging the over-consumption of foods low in nutrients and high in calories, sugar, and salt (Box 5.1). Compounding the impact is a social

---

BOX 5.1

The Farm-to-School Movement

One approach to exposing children to healthy food at a young age is Farm to School. Farm to School has grown to become a relatively large national movement that addresses issues of local procurement of foods for consumption in the cafeteria or classroom, advances local educational activities related to agriculture, nutrition, and health, and incorporates school gardens, which help children see where their food comes from and participate in growing it. Reports of its impact are wide ranging and reveal that farm-to-school programs have increased student meal participation, increased economic activity at community and state levels, and have stimulated an additional $2.16 to $.60 more for every dollar spent. Farm-to-School program research also has shown improvements in knowledge, attitudes, and nutrition behaviors, wherein children increase fruit and vegetable consumption and experience improved household food security. Benefits also include decreased food waste and improved sustainability and community engagement.

environment where students are closely nested with peers, often feeling pressure to look and act cool.

Children on average consume half of their calories at school.[16] Schools often participate in a variety of child nutrition programs offered by the USDA, such as the national school lunch program (NSL), the school breakfast program (SBP), the fresh fruit and vegetable program (FFVP), the special milk program (SMP), summer food service program (SFSP), and supper programs (Box 5.2).

Several significant federal efforts were undertaken in the last 15 years to improve the quality of food available and the healthfulness of marketing to children in schools in the United States. In 2004, the Child Nutrition and Special Supplemental Nutrition Program for Women, Infants, and Children, otherwise known as the WIC Reauthorization Act, required that all local education agencies (such as school districts) that were participating in NSLP or other child nutrition programs develop a local school wellness policy. Nearly all school districts complied, and by 2006 most had some kind of wellness policy in place.

BOX 5.2

Partnership for a Healthier America

The Partnership for a Healthier America (PHA) is a nonprofit organization supported by an honorary chair, the former First Lady Michelle Obama. Its mission is to work with the private sector to solve the childhood obesity crisis and ensure that the nation's youth remain healthy. Supporting the *Let's Move*! initiative, which among other things works to provide healthy food in schools and to provide access to healthy affordable foods, the partnership distinguishes itself by bringing together public, private, and non-profit leaders to commit to develop strategies that will support progress toward a healthier generation. Among its initiatives is FNV, a marketing campaign that aims to promote fruits and vegetables in the same way that other big brands market their products. The partnership also has worked on a healthier campus initiative to support colleges and universities in promoting healthier foods and physical activity on college campuses. Another initiative of note is Active Design Verified, in which efforts are focused on making health a priority in the way affordable housing communities are built.

Policy approaches to address school wellness were further developed when Congress passed the Healthy Hunger Free Act of 2010, which added new stipulations for school wellness policies to further enhance requirements for the implementation of evaluation and reporting on the progress of the policy itself. Later in 2014, FNS advanced an even more comprehensive final rule, which was published in 2016. The final rule ultimately further strengthened the requirements to limit the availability of less healthy, higher calorie products. Among a number of requirements, by June 2017 schools were required to specify their own policy for nutrition promotion and education, physical activity, and other school-based activities to promote student wellness. Schools also were required to have clear policies in place for all *other* foods and beverages available on the school campus during the school day. These included policies regulating the kinds and quantities of foods allowed in schools for classroom parties, fundraisers, birthday celebrations, classroom snacks brought in by parents, and foods given as rewards or incentives by teachers. Food and beverage marketing policies are also included in the requirements, and local education agencies or LEAs are required to stipulate that food and beverage marketing only be allowed on those foods and beverages that meet "Smart Snacks in School Nutrition Standards."[17]

The Smart Snacks in School Nutrition Standards were first rolled out in 2014–2015 and applied to all food sold at school during the school day. This included foods that were available on the lunch line, items sold separately (also referred to as à la cart foods), items in the school store, foods in vending machines, and food sold to students at any other location in the building. The standards, however, did not apply to teachers or places where students did not go. Foods that are "Snack Smart" contain a calorie content of 200cal or less for a snack, 200 mg of sodium or less, 35% of calories from fat or less, 10% of calories from saturated fat or less, zero trans-fat, and 35% or less sugar content by weight. Entrées must have equal to or less than: 350cal, 480mg of sodium, 35% of calories from fat, less than 10% of calories from saturated fat, zero trans-fat, and 35% or less sugar by content weight.

An average store-bought cupcake (with frosting) has about 300cal, 14g of fat, and 5g of saturated fat; and, as you might expect, it does not meet healthy school snacks standards.

Smarter School Lunchrooms

What is a smarter school lunchroom? The smarter school lunchroom movement began in response to the policy initiatives underway to improve the quality of school meal programs. The Cornell Food and Brand Lab, the USDA, and other organizations came to realize that in order to successfully transition schools away from high-fat, high-salt food to healthier items, additional research on how and why children choose the foods they do was needed. The school lunchrooms movement sought to provide schools with the knowledge and resources needed to change the way products appear to children, ultimately shifting their appeal.[18]

An important foundation of the Smarter School Lunchroom effort is to apply principles of behavioral economics to healthy eating. Behavioral economics works to explain our economic decisions with psychological insights. For example, humans generally react poorly and rebel when they feel as though they are being coerced into doing something, and they are more likely to enjoy themselves when they feel they have an influence over decisions. In the case of school food, this means giving children healthy choices and allowing them choice in that decision. Such principles also have led to shifts in displays to make them more convenient and attractive and to normalize healthier eating behaviors. The goal is to influence food choices in a way that, with the support of subtle cues, creates nudges toward selection of the healthier items while not restricting food choices. Smarter School Lunchrooms also operate on an underlying principle that changes should be low cost.

The program developed a 60-point score card, which is used to seed new ideas and encourage schools to adopt new strategies, reflect small changes in the way things are packaged, where they are placed, how images appear, the types of names given to products, and the way that cafeteria staff prompt students to make selections. Changes such as these have resulted in increased selection and consumption of fruits and vegetables even when a variety of less healthy and starchy foods are available.

In one study, for example, the smarter lunchroom makeover increased fruit consumption by 18% and vegetable consumption by 25%.[18,19,20,21] Further, the movement has successfully encouraged food service operations in schools to undertake a self-assessment in the form of a scorecard to determine strategies that could increase the appeal of healthier foods for children. Since 2009 the smarter lunchroom assessment has been administered in over 15,000 schools in the United States.[22]

Conclusions

What we eat is influenced by a myriad of factors, many of which are beyond our immediate control; our desires are motivated by much more than individual will and logic. Although most of us are drawn to food that is tasty, inexpensive, and convenient, we also are influenced by our culture, the way we identify ourselves, social norms, diets, and our emotions, in addition to our nutrition knowledge. These factors further interact with one another to create a complex set of circumstances that surround each purchase and eating decision. Marketing communications, including how and where products are advertised and placed, the nutrition and health claims of the products, and the ways in which consumers expect to experience products are all important influencers.

Only in the past 10 years has a serious and concentrated look at the school food environment been undertaken with an eye toward improving the dietary quality of meals while regulating marketing. Such efforts will need to continue in order to maintain and continue progress in the fight against obesity. Programs such as Farm to School and the Partnership for a Healthier America have made meaningful contributions to the integration of changes into the school culture and curriculum.

The food retail environment also is changing, with more and more on-line purchases driving sales. As our ability to receive delivered food becomes more and more convenient, public health experts will need to shift the way in which they approach the food retail marketing environment. Indeed, a healthy food basket is increasingly becoming a virtual reality. As the rapidly changing media environment responds to new and unforeseen ideas and demands, so too will marketing efforts on the part of industry. Public health will likely face mounting challenges to keep up with tactics and apply what works to influence healthful decisions. Efforts will also likely require ongoing legal challenges in order to keep up with new media marketing strategies aimed toward kids.

Quiz Questions

1. What percentage of foods and drinks advertised to kids on Spanish TV are unhealthy?
   a. 32%
   b. 54%
   c. 84%
   d. 92%
2. In 2009, how much was spent on healthy marketing to kids?
   a. $28 million
   b. $108 million

   c. $280 million
   d. $1.8 billion
3. The Partnership for a Healthier America is a governmental organization that works to regulate food industry marketing practices. True or false?
4. Which of the following is not one of the 4 P's of marketing?
   a. Planning
   b. Product
   c. Price
   d. Profit
5. The average supermarket carries 40,000 products. True or false?

Discussion Questions

- How can the 4 P's of marketing be applied to online content such as YouTube?
- In what ways was your school cafeteria influenced by the 4 P's of marketing?
- What tactics do you see used by industry marketers today that could be applied to promote healthier food?

References

1. Schwartz MB, Kunkel D, DeLucia S. Food marketing to youth: Pervasive, powerful, and pernicious. *Communication Research Trends.* 2013;32:4–13.
2. Robert Wood Johnson Foundation. Recommendations for Responsible Food Marketing to Children; 2014.
3. Grier S. African American & Hispanic youth vulnerability to target marketing. Public Health Institute: Center for Digital Democracy, Berkley Media Studies Group; 2013.
4. Graff S, Kunkel D, Mermin SE. Government can regulate food advertising to children because cognitive research shows that it is inherently misleading. *Health Affairs (Project Hope).* 2012;31:392–398.
5. Holt D, Ippolito P, Desrochers D, Kelley C. Children's exposure to TV advertising in 1977 and 2004: Information for the obesity debate. Federal Trade Commission; 2007.
6. Rudd Center for Food Policy & Obesity. Trends in television food advertising to young people: 2011; update 2012.
7. Ustjanauskas A, Harris J, Schwartz M. Food and beverage advertising on children's web sites. *Pediatric Obesity.* 2014;9:362–372.

8. Page R, Montgomery K, Ponder A, Richard A. Targeting children in the cereal aisle: Promotional techniques and content features on ready-to-eat cereal product packaging. *American Journal of Health Education.* 2008;39:272–282.

9. Campbell AJ. *Rethinking Children's Advertising Policies for the Digital Age. Vol 29.* Georgetown University Law Center; 2017:55.

10. Kang C. YouTube kids app faces new complaints over ads for junk food. *New York Times.* November 24, 2015.

11. Google I. Description of YouTube Kids App2017.

12. Foster GD, Karpyn A, Wojtanowski AC, et al. Placement and promotion strategies to increase sales of healthier products in supermarkets in low-income, ethnically diverse neighborhoods: a randomized controlled trial. *American Journal of Clinical Nutrition.* 2014;99:1359–1368.

13. Glanz K, Bader MD, Iyer S. Retail grocery store marketing strategies and obesity: an integrative review. *American Journal of Preventive Medicine.* 2012;42:503–512.

14. Wansink B, Brumberg A, Gabrielyan G. Slim by design shopping: Assessing the reliability of a grocery retailer scorecard for healthy shopping. *Journal of Nutrition Education and Behavior.* 2015;47:S45–S46.

15. National Farm to School Network. *The Benefits of Farm to School*; 2017.

16. Institute of Medicine FaNB. The Food Environment in Schools. *Hunger and Obesity: Understanding a Food Insecurity Paradigm Workshop Summary*: National Academies Press; 2011.

17. United States Department of Agriculture FaNS. A guide to Smart Snacks in school: Help make the healthy choice the easy choice for kids at school. Vol FNS-6232016:14.

18. Hanks AS, Just DR, Wansink B. Smarter lunchrooms can address new school lunchroom guidelines and childhood obesity. *The Journal of Pediatrics.* 2013;162:867–869.

19. Wansink B, Just DR, Payne CR. The behavioral economics of healthier school lunch payment systems. *The FASEB Journal.* 2011;25:232.

20. Andrew S, Hanks DRJ, Smith LE, Wansink B. Healthy convenience: nudging students toward healthier choices in the lunchroom. *Journal of Public Health*; 2012;34(3):370–376. doi:10.1093/pubmed/fds003. Epub 2012 Jan 31.

21. Wansink B, Devereaux J. Slim by design for schools. *Child Obesity.* 2014;10:445–447.

22. Wright M. Smarter lunchroom movement fights childhood obesity. *Cornell Chronicle*; 2014.

6

Policy Efforts Supporting Healthy Diets for Adults and Children

Courtney A. Parks, Eric E. Calloway, Teresa M. Smith, and Amy L. Yaroch

Chapter Highlights

- Describe how legislation or ordinances can be expected to influence behaviors and health outcomes.
- Describe two ways in which the U.S. "farm bill" impacts dietary behaviors.
- Discuss the pros and cons of one potential change to the farm bill in terms of potential impact on dietary behaviors.
- Describe two ways in which the dietary guidelines impact dietary behaviors.
- Discuss how you would modify the dietary guidelines product or process in order to improve health, including the pros and cons, and why you think this approach would be beneficial.
- Describe two ways in which food assistance programs impact dietary behaviors.
- Discuss the pros and cons of block grants for food assistance programs.
- Describe any changes you would make to the current food assistance landscape to improve health, including the pros and cons, and why you think this approach would be beneficial.
- Discuss a few of the ways that public health professionals can influence the policy process.

Introduction

Dietary patterns are not solely reliant on individual behavior, they also are influenced at multiple levels.[1] Eating behavior is highly complex and results from the interplay of multiple influences across various contexts. The Social Ecological Model is an adaptation of Bronfenbrenner's Ecological Systems Theory, which states that in order to understand human behavior one also must understand the social and environmental context in which it takes place.[2] In Ecological Systems Theory, behavior exists in environmental systems or layers that can influence each other bidirectionally. In this model, as applied to dietary behaviors, these layers often include *individual factors* (personal knowledge, skills, beliefs, etc.), *social environment* (family, friends, peers, etc.), *physical environment* (physical setting in which behaviors take place), and *macro-level environment* (public policy, laws, and cultural context).[3]

Little is known about the mechanisms and causal pathways by which specific environmental influences might interact with individual factors to influence eating behaviors.[4] This macro level is the focus of this chapter, specifically the impact that policy has on food access and ultimately dietary patterns. Figure 6.1 shows an ecological model depicting the multiple influences on what people eat.[3] The macro level and physical environments are the two outer-most levels (i.e., "macro-level environments (sectors)" and "physical environments (sectors)"). These are the levels toward which policy change is targeted. According to this model, if policy change is successful in positively modifying these outer levels (e.g., improving access to healthy affordable foods or places to be physically active), then this will influence the inner two levels that relate to lifestyles of individuals and their social networks.[3,5]

Health policy advocacy organizations attempt to affect change on the macro and physical environment levels by influencing policy. This approach was widely utilized by tobacco cessation advocacy organizations in the 1990s and 2000s. Tobacco control advocacy efforts began in the 1970s, following increased public health focus on the detrimental effects of smoking.[6] By the 1980s, advocacy efforts became more pronounced and focused. Many types of organizations advocated for policies, such as banning advertising to children; banning smoking in many public or communal areas such as restaurants, planes, and work places; launching government-funded anti-smoking advertising campaigns; and levying high taxes on cigarettes. In the context of the Social Ecological Model, in response to tobacco policy changes affecting the macro and physical environments, the social and individual levels began to shift in a more positive direction, namely smoking prevalence began to drop.

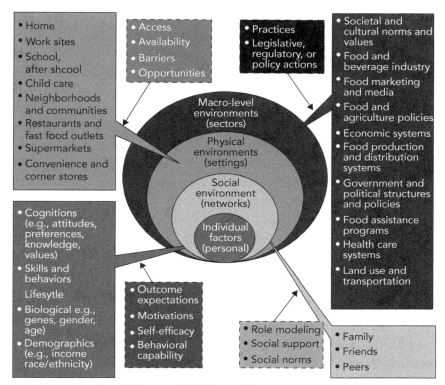

FIGURE 6.1 Ecological framework for dietary behaviors.

Now public health professionals are taking lessons learned from tobacco control and applying them to diet and physical activity, to address obesity.[7]

Why Policy is Important in Shaping Food Environments

Policy approaches target the primary components that help to shape the food environment, and they can be influential across populations and settings.[8] Particular to dietary patterns, challenges exist with regard to access to affordable, quality, and culturally appropriate fruits and vegetables,[9–11] which can be addressed, at least in part, through policy and advocacy efforts. Frieden's Health Impact Pyramid highlights the broad impact that policies can have on population health, in comparison to individual behavior change efforts.[12] However, policies that promote a more healthful diet and improved lifestyles in general are in conflict with the individualistic orientation that dominates American legal, cultural, and social discourse.[13] Fostering policies that improve conditions for everyone to reduce health disparities, and create a more equitable environment, can be cost effective and is the right thing to do, especially using a health equity and/or social justice lens.[14] Addressing obesity as a societal problem, rather than an individual problem, could save hundreds of billions of dollars in healthcare costs.[15]

Popular opinion is that dietary patterns are an individual choice, which assumes that everyone lives in an environment where healthy choices are readily available, and fresh produce can be purchased in their neighborhoods. Unfortunately, this is not the case, but policy efforts aim to achieve this type of utopia of equitable access to more healthful (e.g., fruits and vegetables) foods. Policy can influence dietary patterns and other health behaviors through creating conditions and environments that *make the healthy choice the easy choice or the default choice.*[16] These policies can alter the *choice architecture*, which leads individuals to decisions through default options.[17] One way to move policy and choice architecture is through policy levers, which can be considered the "control knobs" of the health system, and through which governments can utilize specific tools for reform and system-wide change.[18,19] Policy levers include mechanisms by which this influence occurs and can be grouped into the following broad categories of legal powers of governments to promote and protect the public's health: (a) Taxing and spending on specific programs; (b) Direct regulation of persons, professionals, and businesses; (c) The power to alter built, socioeconomic, and informational environments; and (d) Deregulation when laws act as barriers to health.[20,21]

One other policy strategy is to consider the role that preemption plays in policy implementation. Preemption is a legal principle that provides that a higher level of government may limit, or even override, the power of a lower level of government to regulate a certain issue. Although the term is often used to describe federal laws that eliminate the states' ability to act, preemption also can occur when state laws prevent localities from legislating on specific issues.[22]

Healthy Hunger Free Kids Act of 2010

Prior to implementation of the Healthy Hunger Free Kids Act of 2010 (HHFKA), school meals did not provide sufficient fruits and vegetables to meet Dietary Guidelines recommendations.[23] In 2008, a study using a nationally representative sample found only half of schools participating in the National School Lunch Program (NSLP) offered fresh fruits and vegetables on a daily basis.[24] In addition, many children rely on school meals for the majority of their caloric intake and provision of quality nutrition is important.[25] The HHFKA of 2010, a reauthorization of the Child Nutrition Act, provides funding for federal school meal and child nutrition programs, increases access to healthy food, and promotes overall student wellness. The HHFKA included $4.5 billion in new funding for its programs and provisions over a 10-year period. For schools to receive federal funding for school lunch and breakfast, they must meet the new nutrition standards.

Overall, the changes to nutrition standards provide guidelines, such as the number of meal components served (e.g., fruits, vegetables, grains, meat/meat alternative, and milk), calorie ranges for different age groups, and foods sold outside of the school meal program to meet the Dietary Guidelines for Americans (DGA).[26] Since the implementation of the new NSLP guidelines, policymakers, school food service personnel, parents, students, and others across the country have expressed mixed reactions.[26] One of the main critiques of the new nutrition standards was that there would be increased waste due to students being required to choose a fruit or vegetable and specifications for portion sizes. Empirical evidence has demonstrated, however, that there has not been a substantial change from pre- to post-implementation of the new standards in terms of waste. In fact, these studies have shown an increase in consumption of fruits and vegetables following new nutrition standards implementation.[27–29] In addition, when the new nutrition standards were implemented, selections of foods that are higher in nutrients increased.[30] Furthermore, several states have passed laws setting school nutrition standards that are stronger than the federal standards. Researchers examining these state laws found that stricter nutrition standards were associated with lower obesity rates.[31]

HHFKA is important because it addresses both childhood hunger and health and obesity (Table 6.1).

Farm Bill

Overview

The U.S. "farm bill" has gone by many official names since the first bill of its type was proposed in 1933 (Agriculture Adjustment Act of 1933). The farm bill covers a wide range of areas (i.e., omnibus) from farming subsidies, to conservation, to food assistance programs. There are 12 areas, or "titles," covered in the current iteration of the farm bill (Agricultural Act of 2014),[32] which are designed to fund programs that oversee functions related to food and nutrition, environment and energy, and the rural/farming economy.

Table 6.1 Healthy Hunger Free Kids Act

Childhood Hunger: HHFKA addresses by expanding before/after school meals for at-risk children, expanding universal meal service through community eligibility, and connecting more eligible low-income children with school meals through expanding direct certification	Health and Obesity: HHFKA addresses by establishing national nutrition standards for all foods sold in school during the school day,[1] strengthening local school wellness policies and school food safety programs, and developing model product specifications for USDA commodity foods used in school meals

[1]includes á la carte and vending machines

Approximately every five years, Congress votes on a new farm bill.[33] The process of drafting a new farm bill starts years before the deadline to renew when the House and Senate Agricultural Committees meet to discuss potential revisions to, and future directions for, the farm bill. Concurrently, members of Congress hold meetings with farm bill stakeholders (e.g., farm lobbyists and trade organization representatives) and constituents. Also, the U.S. Department of Agriculture (USDA) reviews the scientific evidence and generates policy proposals and recommendations for Congress as they consider the new farm bill legislation. The Agricultural Committees then hold hearings, debates take place on the floor among members of Congress, and the House and Senate separately draft their versions of the new farm bill. A joint version of the bill is negotiated in conference committee and sent to the residing president to sign or veto.

After the farm bill is passed, and made into an Act, the funding phase begins. The farm bill legislation authorizes certain programs, sets eligibility requirements and benefit levels, and sets other parameters around various pieces of the bill. For some pieces of the farm bill, funding is mandatory, but for others it is not. The larger pieces of the farm bill, such as many federal nutrition assistance programs, including the largest one, the Supplemental Nutrition Assistance Program (SNAP) (formerly known as food stamps), commodity programs, and some conservation programs, generally receive mandatory funding. Other programs must compete for funding during the Congress's annual budget appropriations process.

Since its inception, the priorities of the farm bill have changed, as evidenced by funding allocation. The first farm bill originated after the Great Depression to stabilize farm incomes and promote conservation of farm lands. Today, although considerations related to farming are major pieces of the Agricultural Act of 2014, the vast majority of funding goes toward nutrition assistance programs, as has been the case for most years since the early 1990s and especially since 2009.[33,34] The Agricultural Act of 2014 was funded for approximately $489 billion total for fiscal years 2014–2018.[33] Table 6.2 shows the allocation of funds with Titles I, II, IV, and XI accounting for 99% of funding.

Directly and indirectly, the farm bill plays a large role in determining what is grown and eaten in the United States. Provisions in the farm bill impact many levels of the food system. For example, the Specialty Crop Research Initiative (SCRI)[35] authorized under Title VII in the Agricultural Act of 2014 supports research on ways to improve yields, farming technologies, and pest prevention for specialty crops (e.g., non-commodity-crop fruits and vegetables, tree nuts, and nursery crops); and the Value-Added Agricultural Product Market Development Grants program[36] authorized under Title VI in the Agricultural Act of 2014 provides funding to pursue processing and marketing of farm products for small- and mid-sized farms, beginning farmers, or

Table 6.2 Projected Proportion of Funding for Each Title in the Agricultural Act of 2014

Agricultural Act of 2014 Titles	Projected Total Funding FY 2014-2018	Proportion of Funding
Title IV: Nutrition Assistance	$390,650,000,000	79.9%
Title XI: Crop Insurance	$41,420,000,000	8.5%
Title II: Conservation	$28,165,000,000	5.8%
Title I: Commodity Programs	$23,555,000,000	4.8%
Title III: Trade	$1,782,000,000	0.4%
Title XII: Miscellaneous	$1,544,000,000	0.3%
Title X: Horticulture and Organic Agriculture	$874,000,000	0.2%
Title VII: Research	$800,000,000	0.2%
Title IX: Energy	$625,000,000	0.1%
Title VI: Rural Development	$218,000,000	0.0%
Title VIII: Forestry	$8,000,000	0.0%
Title V: Credit	−$1,011,000,000	−0.2%

Source: Congressional Research Service (CRS), using the Congressional Budget Office (CBO) cost estimate of the Agricultural Act of 2014 (January 28, 2014), and the CBO Budget and Economic Outlook, "10-Year Budget Projections," January 2017.

farmers considered to be from a socially disadvantaged group. However, the two components in the Agricultural Act of 2014 that have the biggest direct impact on the diet quality of Americans include the commodity programs (Title I) and nutrition assistance (Title IV).

Commodity Programs (Title I)

Title I covers financial protections against crop price fluctuations (i.e., subsidies) for farmers who grow any of the selected "commodity crops" (i.e., specific crops classified as commodities, which include several types of grains, legumes, oil seeds, and cotton). Between 1996 and 2013, farmers were provided fixed direct payments to grow commodity crops, but in the Agricultural Act of 2014, this changed to subsidies that are triggered only when commodity crop prices drop below a statutory or historical (e.g., last five years of crop prices and yields) threshold.[37] There are about two dozen commodity crops covered, but 90% of payments (from 2005 to 2014) went toward corn, cotton, wheat, rice, and soybeans (however, cotton is now covered under Title XI).[37] Although there is a federal crop insurance program available for more than 100 non-commodity crops, including fruits and vegetables, farmers must purchase a policy and it covers the farmer only in cases of unavoidable loss of yield (e.g., adverse weather conditions), and not typically in cases of market price fluctuations, and only after a deductible is paid.[38]

Because of these subsidies, growing commodity crops has low financial risk and can be very profitable. One unintended consequence of these programs is that the number of small- and mid- sized farms is decreasing in favor of large commercial farms. Also, the vast majority of farmland is used to grow commodity crops, leading to large supplies and low prices. These factors make corn, wheat, rice, and soybeans, and ingredients derived from these crops, very attractive (and ultimately "cheaper") to food manufacturers, which, in turn, affects our food supply and diet quality.

Nutrition Assistance (Title IV)

Title IV covers domestic food assistance programs (as opposed to international food aid, which is covered in Title III).[39] Approximately 80% of funding in the Agricultural Act of 2014 goes to Title IV, and the vast majority of Title IV funding goes to SNAP.[40] Individuals are eligible for SNAP if their income and assets are below a specified level based on family size, or they can be "categorically eligible" if all members of the household receive certain other governmental assistance. Stipulations on eligibility requirements, benefit amounts, and how benefits can be used are outlined in the farm bill. Other food assistance programs in the farm bill include the Emergency Food Assistance Program (TEFAP), which provides food to food banks and food pantries; Commodity Supplemental Food Program (CSFP), which provides monthly food packages to low-income elderly people; the Fresh Fruit and Vegetable Program (FFVP), which provides grants to schools to purchase fresh fruits and vegetables; and two smaller programs called the Senior Farmers Market Nutrition Program (SFMNP) and the Community Food Projects (CFP).

SNAP alone covers approximately 43 million people and issues $5.3 billion in benefits per month,[41] which are spent on food and beverages. SNAP is by far the largest food assistance program and unlike the Special Supplemental Nutrition Program for Women, Infants, and Children (WIC), for example, it has few restrictions on the types of foods and beverages it covers. This impacts supply and demand in our food economy, given that consumer demand is partially driven by the types of foods and beverages covered by food assistance programs, which, in turn, impacts the food supply of all Americans. There is potential to restrict SNAP purchases to certain foods (e.g., restrict sugar-sweetened beverages) as a means to impact public health; however, this is still highly controversial.

Another impact of food assistance programs on the food system is through "commodities."[39] These are bulk foods that the USDA purchases and distributes through several food assistance programs, such as TEFAP and CSFP. The USDA decides which foods and how much to purchase, partially based on the needs of the agricultural producer community. In doing so, the USDA can artificially create demand and "prop up" the price of foods when there is surplus.

Next Steps for the Farm Bill

The provisions under the current farm bill (Agricultural Act of 2014) end September 30, 2018. Prior to this date, the agriculture committees of each chamber of Congress will meet and draft their versions of the bill, and the process of devising a new farm bill will begin again. Some pieces up for debate include aspects of SNAP, such as the funding structure (e.g., block grants) and work requirements, the future of several pilot programs funded under the 2014 farm bill, and the partisan issue of potentially splitting the farm bill into two pieces (e.g., one for the nutrition assistance programs and the other for the rest of the components), as well as many other issues that likely will be debated.[42] See the *How to Get Involved* section later in this chapter for more information.

Dietary Guidelines

Brief History

In 1977, the U.S. Senate Select Committee on Nutrition and Human Needs issued the first "dietary guidelines," called the Dietary Goals for the American People.[43] These guidelines covered energy balance, as well as nutrient-based and food-based guidelines. There was controversy, however, over the scientific rigor underlying the recommendations, and so in 1980, new guidelines were issued. These new guidelines were a joint effort by the USDA and the Department of Health, Education, and Welfare (now known as the Department of Health and Human Services [DHHS]) along with outside expertise from the scientific community. The 1980 dietary guidelines (*Nutrition and Your Health: Dietary Guidelines for Americans*)[44] presented seven main recommendations focusing on variety, weight maintenance, moderation of less healthful dietary components (e.g., sugar, saturated fat, and sodium), and promotion of high-fiber foods. Even though these straightforward recommendations were extrapolations of the available science, and remain core principles of healthful diets today, they again met with some resistance from industry and scientific groups. After this iteration of guidelines, for subsequent guidelines the two departments formed advisory committees made up of outside scientific experts who weighed the science and fielded formal and informal comments/advice. Since 1980, the USDA and DHHS convene every five years to review, update, and add to the dietary guidelines, with outside consultation from scientific experts.

Process for Creating the Dietary Guidelines

Although both groups collaborate, the USDA and DHHS take turns leading the effort to develop the new dietary guidelines every five years.[45] The most recent dietary guidelines came out in 2015, led by the USDA. The process begins by forming a scientific advisory committee. The scientific advisory committee for the 2015 dietary guidelines was made up of 15 scientists and medical doctors, primarily from academia, public health, nutrition, and medicine. They are selected based on their contributions to their fields and geographic, demographic, and disciplinary diversity, and they are thoroughly vetted for financial conflicts of interest. The scientific advisory committee first devises formal research questions (e.g., what is the relationship between dietary patterns and colorectal cancer?) based on reviewing the last guidelines and discussions of the current state of nutrition science. Then, research staff at the USDA and DHHS identify existing meta-analyses/systematic reviews, conduct de novo systematic literature reviews, and conduct food pattern modeling/analyses of national data to answer these questions. Additionally, the public can make comments at public hearings and online. The scientific advisory committee then takes the evidence and public comments under consideration, and guides the production of a scientific report outlining its recommendations (*Scientific Report of the 2015 Dietary Guidelines Advisory Committee*).[46]

The second stage is to translate the scientific report into the Dietary Guidelines "policy document" (*Dietary Guidelines for Americans 2015–2020*).[45] Experts from various agencies within the USDA and DHHS, other federal policy and communication experts, and outside content area experts review the scientific report for rigor and considerations in translating the science to policy. In addition, the public is again allowed to make comments. Finally, the policy document is peer-reviewed anonymously by non-federal experts who examine it for clarity, accuracy, and the fidelity with which the evidence from the scientific report was translated into policy. Once the policy document is finalized, it is the Dietary Guidelines for Americans for the next five years. The policy document also is translated into a lay version of the dietary guidelines and disseminated to practitioners and other relevant stakeholders.

Impact on Diet

The dietary guidelines serve as the evidence-based foundation from which government nutrition policy, programing, and educational materials are created.[45] All federal nutrition educational materials and publications are bound by law to be consistent with the dietary guidelines. Also, the guidelines directly inform the foods served via food assistance programs such as the National School Lunch Program and the Special Supplemental Nutrition Program for Women, Infants, and Children (WIC). By influencing school lunches, the guidelines also affect food manufacturers who must reformulate products to remain in compliance so they can continue to supply school cafeterias. For SNAP, the largest food assistance program, the guidelines indirectly influence allotment amounts, which are based on the USDA's Thrifty Food Plan (i.e., the lowest cost food plan that can still meet the dietary guidelines). Outside of the government, nutrition and health professionals use the guidelines to inform their practice; and the public, although not the intended audience, is influenced by the guidelines directly through governmental communication efforts and indirectly by dietary advice they receive from health professionals.

Food Assistance Programs

The Supplemental Nutrition Assistance Program (SNAP)

As mentioned previously, SNAP is by far the nation's largest food assistance program, providing for 43 million people annually and issuing about $125 per month per person on Electronic Benefit Transfer (EBT) cards (similar to debit cards) to purchase food and drinks.[41] Allotment amounts are basically calculated by determining the minimum amount needed to meet the Dietary Guidelines for a family of a given size (i.e., the Thrifty Food Plan), minus non-deductible household income. Though SNAP has relatively few restrictions on the types of foods and drinks that can be purchased, participants cannot use their benefits for prepared/cooked foods, alcohol/tobacco, and household items or other non-food products.[47] The overall goal of SNAP is to reduce food insecurity among very low-income groups.

To qualify for SNAP, families and single individuals must meet several financial and work requirements.[48] They must have a gross household income less than 130%, and a net household income less than 100%, of the federal poverty line. Households also must have less than $2,250 in assets (e.g., bank account and vehicle), or $3,250 if a person 60 years of age or older, or who is disabled, lives in the household. Additionally, participants must be working (without reducing their number of hours worked), be applying for work, or be participating in an employment training program.

Due to the flexibility given to SNAP participants in how to use their benefits, there is some debate over potential changes to SNAP allotments. Opponents of this "flexibility" granted to SNAP participants insist that it contributes to poor diet quality, particularly sugar-sweetened beverage (SSB) consumption.[49] Some argue that because so many people use SNAP, there is an opportunity to improve the diets of low-income Americans by restricting foods covered by SNAP to only healthful foods—similar to the WIC model. In fact, many local governments have applied for waivers from the USDA to restrict purchases of certain products, but all requests have been denied up to this point.[50,51] Proponents argue that because lower-income Americans are at greater risk for diet-related chronic disease compared to more affluent Americans, SNAP can be used as a tool to improve public health of vulnerable populations. Opponents of SNAP restrictions argue that such changes are too authoritarian and all people should have free will over their food choices, regardless of their income level.[52] Also, implementing such restriction would likely increase administrative costs of the program; in addition, there is limited evidence such proposed restrictions would even impact diets of SNAP participants, given that they could always use their own resources for any foods that might be restricted by SNAP.[53] The evidence indicates that SNAP participants actually consume similar or only slightly less healthful diets compared to their income-matched peers,[54–56] and in fact, few Americans consume healthful diets.[55,57,58]

An alternative to SNAP restriction is an incentive-based approach. Largely based on a model called "Double-Up Food Bucks,"[59] these allotment structures add a certain amount of benefits back to the electronic benefit transfer (EBT) cards of SNAP participants when they purchase healthful foods, such as fresh fruits and vegetables. SNAP is currently funding pilot projects through the Food Insecurity Nutrition Incentive (FINI) Grant Program,[60] outlined in the 2014 farm bill, to test various approaches to incentive-based allotments to promote healthful diets. This is appealing in many ways in that it is a reward system, rather than a punishment, to low-income SNAP participants.

Another change that has been proposed to SNAP is funding through "block grants" to states, rather than the current funding structure (i.e., entitlement funding) that allows SNAP to be guaranteed to anyone who applies and meets eligibility requirements; funding, therefore, adjusts with participation. From a funding perspective, the current model has the disadvantage of being somewhat unpredictable and making cost cutting difficult. Block granting SNAP, on the other hand, involves awarding states an a priori amount based on anticipated need—an approach primarily intended to help rein in costs. Opponents to this method argue that because about 93% of all SNAP funds go toward food for poor families and individuals,[41] there is little room to cut costs. Additionally, it has been shown that programs (e.g., TANF) using the block granting structure have a difficult time responding to increases in need such as was seen during the 2008 economic crisis (Figure 6.2).[61]

Figure 6.2 shows how SNAP, being entitlement funded, increased participation rates coinciding with the increase in unemployment rates (used as a proxy metric for the level of need in the population). Conversely, TANF (another federally funded assistance program for the poor), which is funded

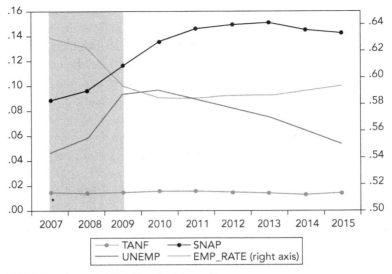

SNAP: Supplemental Nutrition Assistance Program
TANF: Temporary Assistance for Needy Families

FIGURE 6.2 Trends in SNAP and TANF participation rates compared to employment and unemployment (2007–2015).

Source: Washington Post article from 2016, based on data from the USDA, TANF, and Bureau of Labor Statistics.

through predetermined block grants to states, showed little to no response in participation rates when unemployment rose.

The Special Supplemental Nutrition Program for Women, Infants, and Children (WIC)

WIC, now the nation's third largest (by funding level) food assistance program, started as a pilot program in 1972 and became permanent in 1975 with the passage of Public Law 94-105. It was reauthorized in 1998 by the William F. Goodling Child Nutrition Reauthorization Act and in 2004 by the Child Nutrition and WIC Reauthorization Act. Today, the program provides nutrient-rich foods, infant formula, and nutrition and breastfeeding counseling to nearly 8 million low-income (set by states, but between 100% and 185% of the federal poverty line) pregnant or postpartum (up to 1 year if breastfeeding, < 6 months if not) women and children aged 0–5 who are at risk for poor nutrition.[62] On average, WIC provides families with $42 per month in benefits that can be redeemed for approved types of healthful foods and beverages.[41] Approximately 53% of all infants born in the United States are served by WIC.[63] The specific foods and beverages are decided at the state level in accordance with the Dietary Guidelines and the American Academy of Pediatrics. These food packages currently include certain types of 100% fruit juice, infant food/formula, milk, breakfast cereal, cheese, eggs, fruits and vegetables, whole grain products, canned fish, legumes, and peanut butter. Overall, the WIC model of food distribution provides a healthful supplement to the diets of a low-income nutritionally vulnerable population.

National School Lunch Program (NSLP) and School Breakfast Program (SBP)

The NSLP and SBP are the second and fourth largest (by funding level) food assistance programs in the United States, respectively. They were established and evolved through a series of legislation that included the National School Lunch Act of 1946, the Child Nutrition Act of 1966, the Child Nutrition and WIC Reauthorization Act of 2004, and the HHFKA. The NSLP and SBP are the largest of a set of programs known as the Child Nutrition programs,[64] which also include the Child and Adult Care Food Program, which provides food for child care centers and homes, as well as senior centers; the Summer Food Service Program, which provides meals at local sites in low-income areas when school is not in session; Fresh Fruit and Vegetable Program, which provides fruits and vegetables as snacks to students in participating schools; and the After-School Snacks and Suppers program, which provides healthful snacks to students in after-school care.

The NSLP provides healthful lunches, in line with the Dietary Guidelines, to over 30 million students each school day.[65] Of these lunches, approximately 66% are free to qualifying students and 7% are offered at a reduced price.[41] To qualify for free lunch, household income must fall below 130% of the federal poverty line, and below 185% for a reduced price lunch.[64] Also, schools with 40% or more of students who meet these income thresholds have universal free lunch eligibility for all students who attend the school. As mentioned above, the HHFKA further increased the nutrition standards for breakfasts and lunches provided by schools in an effort to improve the diets of school children. School guidelines state lunches must provide daily 0.5–1.0 cups of fruits (at least half must be whole fruits), 0.75–1.0 cups of a variety of vegetables, 1–2 oz. of grains (at least half whole grains), and also a certain amount of milk and meat/meat alternatives and limit calories, saturated fat, trans-unsaturated fat, and sodium.[66] Research suggests these high standards can have a positive impact on the nutritional quality of foods selected by children without negatively impacting school lunch participation rates. They also may have a smaller, though still positive, impact on the nutritional quality of foods the children actually consume at lunch.[27,30,67,68]

The SBP provides nearly 15 million healthful breakfasts to students each school day.[69] Of these breakfasts, 79% are free of charge and 6% are offered at a reduced price to qualifying students. Eligibility standards are the same as for the NSLP. Breakfast can be served in the cafeteria or in the classroom and must provide a daily cup of fruits (at least half must be whole fruits), 1 oz. of grains (at least half whole grains), and 1 cup of low-fat or fat-free milk. It also must meet standards for calories, saturated fat, trans-unsaturated fat, and sodium.[66]

How You Can Get Involved

This chapter describes a few areas of legislation and policy of potential interest to public health professionals. It is also important to highlight how public health professionals can get involved in education and advocacy related to relevant legislative areas through professional associations and coalitions.

1. Stay updated on the issues, follow listservs and other communications from professional organizations and other recognized entities.
2. Identify legislation that is currently being discussed in committees (e.g., Senate Agriculture Committee).
3. Identify potential public health impacts of proposed legislative changes.
   a. Impacts on access to food assistance programs (e.g., SNAP, WIC), either through changes in eligibility, accessibility in terms of maintaining benefits, or restrictions/incentives offered on eligible foods.
   b. Changes to commodity crops, crop insurance, and so forth dictate which types of foods farmers are growing (e.g., vegetables as specialty crops) versus promotion of local and regional food systems.
   c. Changes to guidelines for school food or other publicly funded programs.
   d. Support for programs that increase opportunities for underserved and underrepresented communities (e.g., rural, racial/ethnic minority groups).
   e. Support for programs that increase food access in underserved communities.

4. Connect with your professional organizations and determine their endorsement for various issues and how your views align.
5. Form larger coalitions—write letters, develop one-pagers, go to Capitol Hill and speak with representatives.
6. Utilize technical assistance available through campaigns and other organizations.
7. Find out if members of Congress are hosting a town hall or other constituent meetings in your community or state.
8. Provide testimony before local councils and state legislatures.
9. Once bills are approved by the Senate and House of Representatives, and approved by the President, final rules are open to the public, so provide comments on proposed rules.

Lobbying versus Non-Lobbying

Depending on the source of funding and where you work, you may need to consider the fine line between lobbying and advocacy.

Two Types of Lobbying

Direct lobbying involves communicating directly to a legislator about a particular view on specific legislation. By contrast, grassroots lobbying involves communicating a view on specific legislation to the public and also includes a call to action that supports that view.

You can modify an activity that would be considered lobbying to transform it into an activity that is considered to be educational under Internal Revenue Service (IRS) rules (Box 6.1). For example, organizations can release public communication stating their support of a particular bill, and as long as they do not include a call to action in this communication, the organization is safely in the non-lobbying realm.

BOX 6.1

Specifically, the IRS defines a communication as lobbying if it is made either: (1) directly to a legislator or legislative staffer and reflects a view on specific legislation; or (2) to the public, reflects a view on specific legislation, and includes a call to action.

In addition, the "subsequent use" rule, that is, all costs for purely educational materials are presumed to be grassroots lobbying if the materials are used for grassroots lobbying within six months of being produced. To avoid this issue and maximize non-lobbying dollars, organizations can develop and produce their educational materials well in advance of the six-month cut-off, in order to legally demonstrate that the materials' primary purpose was not lobbying. Alternatively, organizations may avoid having these costs treated as lobbying by distributing the materials broadly to the public for educational purposes, prior to using them for lobbying, and ensuring that the subsequent lobbying use is minimal compared to the more robust educational use.

Innovative Policy Approaches
Sugar-Sweetened Beverage (SSB) Tax

A great deal of research has demonstrated a link between consumption of sugar-sweetened beverages (SSBs; e.g., sodas, sports drinks, sweetened tea, fruit drinks and punches, and other sweetened beverages) and obesity.[70-74] A 2007 meta-analysis of the relationship between SSB intake and nutrition and health concluded that SSB intake was associated with greater energy intake and body weight, as well as lower intake of other important nutrients and poorer health outcomes.[75] A later study demonstrated that a reduction in SSB intake led to weight loss among study participants.[76] SSB consumption is believed to displace healthier, more nutrient-dense beverages such as milk, 100% fruit juice, and water among children, adolescents, and adults.[74] Higher SSB consumption and associated health concerns are especially prominent among low-income communities and racial and ethnic minority communities,[74,77] who have the highest intake of SSBs.[74]

Emerging studies are showing that increasing the price of SSBs may lead to a reduction in consumption, and subsequently, overall caloric intake when there is not a substituted beverage.[78,79] With tobacco, an increase in taxes on tobacco products is believed to have been the single most effective policy approach to reducing tobacco use, and the revenues gained from these taxes have been used for other comprehensive tobacco control programs, which has led to further reductions in tobacco use.[74] Similarly, several communities across the United States have been working to enact an SSB tax in an effort to reduce consumption and promote health. These efforts are further supported by evidence showing a relationship between price and general food-purchasing behaviors.[74]

Proponents of a SSB tax say that it will reduce consumption of unhealthy beverages and promote public health while also generating revenue.[74] They often mention that the estimated annual cost of obesity in the United States is about $150 billion and that about one-half of this is paid by Medicare and Medicaid, which suggests that taxpayers are paying the price.[74] It is estimated that there would be a 8.5% reduction in Medicare costs and 11.8% reduction in Medicaid costs if obesity-related costs were eliminated. Medicaid proponents are also mindful that an SSB tax would need to work alongside other public health obesity prevention efforts in order to effectively promote healthier lifestyles and save on obesity-related costs.[74]

Opponents of an SSB tax argue, however, that the tax is regressive, meaning it will disproportionately affect lower-income individuals.[77] Others have argued that the evidence linking SSBs to obesity or other poor health outcomes is not strong enough to warrant policy intervention.[77,80] For example, Dr. Maureen Storey, senior vice president of science policy for the American Beverage Association, commented on a 2011 study linking SSB consumption to hypertension, stating, "the study does not show that drinking sugar-sweetened beverages in any way causes hypertension."[81] A 2008 meta-analysis concluded that among children, there was insufficient evidence of an association between consumption of SSBs and body weight.[82] Additionally, an intervention study that aimed to reduce SSB consumption among adolescents also found no significant change in body mass index between the adolescents who reduced their SSB intake and those who did not.[83] Findings from these studies should be interpreted with caution, though, as both were funded by the beverage industry, and there is other evidence that demonstrates a link between SSBs and obesity.[77] Lastly, opponents claim that it is unknown whether taxes would lead to reduced consumption, and that other high-calorie beverages may be substituted.[84] Evaluation of implementation of an SSB tax should consider measuring intake of other high-calorie beverages (e.g., milk) alongside SSBs in order to determine whether this is truly a concern.

Genetically Modified Organism (GMO) Labeling

Genetically modified organisms (GMOs) are organisms in which the genes have been altered in a way that does not occur naturally.[85] GMOs have been used in crops in the United States throughout their history for their herbicide tolerance (HT) and insect resistance.[86] Although U.S. Senator Chuck Grassley, an Iowa Republican, has said, "the science has proven that GMO foods are safe and equivalent to non-GMO foods from a safety perspective," [87] others have raised numerous concerns regarding the health and environmental implications of GMOs.[85,88] Consequently, it has been proposed that foods containing GMOs be labeled as such in order to help consumers make choices.[89] Many countries across the globe currently do require GMO labeling (e.g., Australia, France, and Germany).

The entire U.S. food system is affected by GMOs, but it is especially problematic for local food systems. GMOs are largely commodity crops, utilize large amounts of land, are shipped across the county, and are not directly eaten by consumers. GMO crops have potential to reduce the amount of land available for growing nutritious foods, such as "specialty" fruits and vegetables. Opponents of the wide use of GMOs postulate that when land is used for fruits and vegetables rather than commodity crops, they can be eaten directly by consumers, especially those in the immediate area, reducing nutrient-loss during transport[90] and promoting the local economy.

Proponents of growing GMO crops commonly cite their potential to help reduce food insecurity by increasing crop yields.[91] Opponents, however, assert that increases are seen in crops such as corn and soybeans, which are used in high-calorie, non-nutritous foods, in ethanol, and as feed for livestock. Additionally, most research in support of GMOs has been funded by organizations whose interests are economic and policy-related.[91] It is important to note that food-insecure families may lack quality in their diets,[92] so in order to increase food security, Americans need access to healthful foods (e.g., fruits and vegetables), as opposed to high-calorie, non-nutritous foods. Additionally, several GMO crops are only approved for animal feed and deemed unhealthy for human consumption. When these crops are used, there is a high risk for cross-contamination into "human food," reducing the amount of land availabile to be used to grow human food.[85] Finally, no conclusive evidence has been found that GMO crops help to increase food supplies for developing countries.[93]

Also noteworthy is the suggestion that GMOs may be contributing to childhood obesity. Some GMO farmers are experiencing increased crop yields, and/or lower pesticide costs for corn and soybean seeds.[86] However, these crops are widely used to produce high-calorie, non-nutritous processed foods (such as sugar and refined grains).[94,95] The availability of cheap foods is one of several factors contributing to the nation's obesity epidemic.[96]

Overseeing the safety of GMOs in the United States falls under the authority of the U.S. Food and Drug Administration (FDA), the U.S. Environmental Protection Agency, and the USDA. The Center for Food Safety cites, however, that across these agencies, GMO regulations are contradictory and lack coordination, are almost all voluntary, and have loopholes.[89] In June 2016, two U.S. senators introduced a compromise bill for a mandatory, national labeling standard for GMO foods. This bill was passed by the

Senate and the House of Representatives and signed by President Obama on July 29, 2016. At the time of this writing, the USDA was then given two years to require food producers to use text, symbols, or QR codes to declare which products contain GMOs.[97,98]

Reactions to the GMO labeling legislation have been mixed. Those wanting to see stricter labeling, such as the Vermont Genetically Engineered Food Labeling Act, were left unsatisfied with this legislation.[87] In contrast to the national standards, Vermont required that foods be labeled as either "partially produced with genetic engineering" or "may be partially produced with genetic engineering" or "produced with genetic engineering."[99] Some proponents of labeling have claimed that this new federal law would solve the problem of a patchwork of state labeling laws.[87]

Nutrition Labeling

Research continues to link diet to health outcomes, and poor diet to obesity and chronic diseases such as cardiovascular disease.[100] Packaged foods in the United States currently feature nutrition labels, but several shortcomings of the labels have been identified, and the FDA therefore has recently revised the labels in order to help adults choose healthier foods. In 2016, the FDA announced a new Nutrition Facts label for packaged foods, aimed to facilitate consumers in making better-informed food choices.[100]

Proponents have advocated that nutrition labeling has the potential to shift norms and contribute to food and social environments that support healthful choices.[101] Although this appears to be a step in the right direction, there needs to be more frequent evolution of the labeling in order to reflect advances in the field of nutrition and consumer behaviors.[101]

Proposed Industry Standards

In some cases, the field of public health recognizes that a policy may not be practical, and, therefore, voluntary regulations may be a viable alternative. As described earlier, obesity, especially among children, is problematic in the United States. Research has suggested that children are highly susceptible to food marketing, so much so that a 2006 Institute of Medicine report recommended that Congress enact legislation mandating changes in advertising practices to shift emphasis away from high-calorie and low-nutrient foods and beverages.[102] Congress has yet to enact this legislation, but evidence has led to some members of the food and beverage industry engaging in self-regulation efforts. Groups leading the charge include the Children's Food and Beverage Advertising Initiative (CFBAI), the Alliance for a Healthier Generation, the Healthy Weight Commitment Foundation, the Partnership for a Healthier America, and the Balance Calorie Initiative from the American Beverage Association.

Proponents, however, have identified a lack of transparency and objectivity in industry verifications, weaknesses in industry pledges, and interests rooted in tapping into consumer preferences for purchasing "healthy" foods rather than truly wanting to provide better foods.[103,104] Additionally, findings from evaluations have been inconsistent, with some suggesting positive outcomes and others not. A CFBAI evaluation stressed high compliance among advertising practices,[105] while an independent evaluation described compliance with self-regulation, but with seemingly little improvement in the nutritional quality of foods advertised to children via multiple media channels and settings.[106]

Summary

Policy is ever evolving as new legislation is implemented and the needs and opinions of society shift. As public health professionals, it is important to remain aware of the current policy issues that impact diet and ultimately health-related outcomes. Policy approaches help to shape the food environment and food systems and can have wide-ranging impacts across populations and settings. Policy levers are the control knobs through which governments can reform and influence system-wide changes, making the healthy choice the easy or default choice. With policy change, however, can come unintended consequences, which often adversely affect vulnerable populations. A considerate and evidence-based approach is necessary to guide the efforts of policymakers, advocates, and health professionals to ensure policy efforts remain positive and relevant.

Quiz Questions

1. In Ecological Systems Theory, behavior exists in environmental systems or layers that can influence each other bi-directionally. True or false?
2. We have a relatively good understanding of the causal pathways by which diet is influenced. True or false?
3. Obesity is a problem most effectively addressed through:
   a.   Education

    b. Policy

    c. Eliminating its stigma

    d. Improved health care

4. Making the *healthy choice the easy choice* is an example of:

    a. Marketing healthy food

    b. Choice architecture

    c. Change architecture

    d. Individual choice driving decisions

    e. The importance of healthy choices

5. Preemption was tried as a policy strategy, but lacks significant ability to shift the food environment. True or false?

6. SNAP stands for:

    a. Supplemental Nutrition Aid Program

    b. Standard Nutrition Assistance Program

    c. Supplemental Nutrition Assistance Program

    d. Standard Nutrition Assistance Plan

    e. Supplemental Nutrition Assistance Plan

7. The Farm Bill currently covers eight areas or "titles." True or false?

8. The vast majority of funding for the Farm Bill goes toward farm subsidies for corn. True or false?

9. The cost of the Farm Bill is approximately:

    a. $80 billion

    b. $500 billion

    c. $800 billion

    d. $1 trillion

    e. $1.2 trillion

10. Fruit and vegetable crops for consumption by people are called "specialty crops." True or false?

References

1. Story M, Kaphingst KM, Robinson-O'Brien R, Glanz K. Creating healthy food and eating environments: policy and environmental approaches. *Annu Rev Public Health*. 2008;29:253–272. doi:10.1146/annurev.publhealth.29.020907.090926.

2. Bronfenbrenner U. Ecology of the family as a context for human development: research perspectives. *Dev Psychol*. 1986;22:723–742.

3. Story M, Kaphingst KM, Robinson-O'Brien R, Glanz K. Creating healthy food and eating environments: policy and environmental approaches. *Annu Rev Public Health*. 2008;29(1):253–272. doi:10.1146/annurev.publhealth.29.020907.090926.

4. Ball K, Timperio AF, Crawford DA. Understanding environmental influences on nutrition and physical activity behaviors: where should we look and what should we count? *Int J Behav Nutr Phys Act.* 2006;3(1):33.

5. Sallis JF, Owen N, Fisher EB. Ecological models of health behavior. In: Glanz K, Rimer BK, Viswanath K, eds. *Health Behavior and Health Education: Theory, Research, and Practice (4th ed.).* Jossey-Bass; 2008:465–485.

6. *50 Years of Tobacco Control.* Robert Wood Johnson Foundation http://www.rwjf.org/maketobaccohistory. Accessed April 15, 2015.

7. Yach D, McKee M, Lopez AD, Novotny T. Improving diet and physical activity: 12 lessons from controlling tobacco smoking. *BMJ.* 2005;330(7496):898.

8. Wiley LF. The struggle for the soul of public health. *J Health Polit Policy Law.* 2016;41(6):1083–1096.

9. Moore LV, Thompson FE. Adults meeting fruit and vegetable intake recommendations—United States, 2013. *MMWR Morb Mortal Wkly Rep.* 2015;64(26):709–713.

10. Satia JA. Diet-related disparities: understanding the problem and accelerating solutions. *J Am Diet Assoc.* 2009;109(4):610.

11. Kirkpatrick SI, Dodd KW, Reedy J, Krebs-Smith SM. Income and race/ethnicity are associated with adherence to food-based dietary guidance among US adults and children. *J Acad Nutr Diet.* 2012;112(5):624–635.

12. Frieden TR. A framework for public health action: the health impact pyramid. *Am J Public Health.* 2010;100(4):590–595. doi:10.2105/AJPH.2009.185652.

13. Wallack L, Lawrence R. Talking about public health: developing America's "second language." *Am J Public Health.* 2005;95(4):567–570.

14. Dorfman L, Wallack L. Moving nutrition upstream: the case for reframing obesity. *J Nutr Educ Behav.* 2007;39(2):S45–S50.

15. Finkelstein EA, Trogdon JG, Cohen JW, Dietz W. Annual medical spending attributable to obesity: payer-and service-specific estimates. *Health Aff (Millwood).* 2009;28(5):w822–w831.

16. Ashe M, Graff S, Spector C. Changing places: policies to make a healthy choice the easy choice. *Public Health.* 2011;125(12):889–895.

17. Thaler RH, Sunstein CR, Balz JP. *Choice Architecture.* Social Science Research Network; 2014. https://papers.ssrn.com/abstract=2536504. Accessed March 24, 2017.

18. Grace FC, Meurk CS, Head BW, et al. An analysis of policy levers used to implement mental health reform in Australia 1992–2012. *BMC Health Serv Res.* 2015;15(1):479.

19. Bemelmans-Videc M-L, Rist RC, Vedung EO. *Carrots, Sticks, and Sermons: Policy Instruments and Their Evaluation.* Vol 1. Transaction Publishers; 2011.

20. McGinnis JM, Williams-Russo P, Knickman JR. The case for more active policy attention to health promotion. *Health Aff (Millwood).* 2002;21(2):78–93.

21. Gostin LO. *Public Health Law: Power, Duty, Restraint.* University of California Press; 2000.

22. Preemption: What It Is, How It Works, and Why It Matters for Public Health. | ChangeLab Solutions. http://www.changelabsolutions.org/publications/preemption-memo. Accessed March 9, 2017.

23. Stallings VA, Suitor CW, Taylor CL. *School Meals: Building Blocks for Healthy Children.* National Academies Press; 2010.

24. Finkelstein DM, Hill EL, Whitaker RC. School food environments and policies in US public schools. *Pediatrics.* 2008;122(1):e251–e259.

25. Briefel RR, Wilson A, Gleason PM. Consumption of low-nutrient, energy-dense foods and beverages at school, home, and other locations among school lunch participants and nonparticipants. *J Am Diet Assoc.* 2009;109(2):S79–S90.

26. Byker CJ, Pinard CA, Yaroch AL, Serrano EL. New NSLP guidelines: challenges and opportunities for nutrition education practitioners and researchers. *J Nutr Educ Behav.* 2013;45(6):683–689.

27. Cohen JF, Richardson S, Parker E, Catalano PJ, Rimm EB. Impact of the new US Department of Agriculture school meal standards on food selection, consumption, and waste. *Am J Prev Med.* 2014;46(4):388–394.

28. Byker CJ, Farris AR, Marcenelle M, Davis GC, Serrano EL. Food waste in a school nutrition program after implementation of new lunch program guidelines. *J Nutr Educ Behav.* 2014;46(5):406–411.

29. Cullen KW, Chen T-A, Dave JM, Jensen H. Differential improvements in student fruit and vegetable selection and consumption in response to the new National School Lunch Program regulations: a pilot study. *J Acad Nutr Diet.* 2015;115(5):743–750.

30. Johnson DB, Podrabsky M, Rocha A, Otten JJ. Effect of the healthy hunger-free kids act on the nutritional quality of meals selected by students and school lunch participation rates. *JAMA Pediatr.* 2016;170(1):e153918–e153918.

31. Taber DR, Chriqui JF, Powell L, Chaloupka FJ. Association between state laws governing school meal nutrition content and student weight status: implications for new USDA school meal standards. *JAMA Pediatr.* 2013;167(6):513–519.

32. *Agricultural Act of 2014*; 2014.

33. Johnson R, Monke J. What is the Farm Bill? *Curr Polit Econ U S Can Mex.* 2013;15(3):413.

34. Chite RM. The 2014 Farm Bill (PL 113-79): Summary and side-by-side. *CRS Rep.* 2014;43076.

35. Specialty Crop Research Initiative (SCRI) | National Institute of Food and Agriculture. https://nifa.usda.gov/funding-opportunity/specialty-crop-research-initiative-scri. Accessed April 3, 2017.

36. Value Added Producer Grants | USDA Rural Development. https://www.rd.usda.gov/programs-services/value-added-producer-grants. Accessed April 3, 2017.

37. Shields DA. *Farm Commodity Provisions in the 2014 Farm Bill (P.L. 113-79)*. Congressional Research Service; 2014.

38. History of the Crop Insurance Program. http://www.rma.usda.gov/aboutrma/what/history.html. Accessed April 3, 2017.

39. Aussenberg RA, Colello KJ. *Domestic Food Assistance: Summary of Programs*. Congressional Research Service; 2017.

40. Aussenberg RA. *SNAP and Related Nutrition Provisions of the 2014 Farm Bill (P.L. 113-79)*. Congressional Research Service; 2014.

41. *Program Information Report: U.S. Summary, FY 2016–FY 2017*. United States Department of Agriculture; 2016.

42. Good K. 2018 Farm Bill. *Farm Policy News*. December 2016. http://farmpolicynews.illinois.edu/2016/12/2018-farm-bill/. Accessed April 3, 2017.

43. History of Dietary Guidance Development—DGAC Meeting 1—health.gov. https://health.gov/dietaryguidelines/2015-binder/meeting1/historycurrentuse.aspx. Accessed April 3, 2017.

44. U.S. Department of Agriculture and U.S. Department of Health and Human Services. *Dietary Guidelines for Americans*. U.S. Government Printing Office; 2010.

45. U.S. Department of Health and Human Services, U.S. Department of Agriculture. *2015–2020 Dietary Guidelines for Americans*; 2015. http://health.gov/dietaryguidelines/2015/guidelines/. Accessed November 16, 2016.

46. Office of Disease Prevention and Health Promotion, Office of the Assistant Secretary for Health, Office of the Secretary, U.S. Department of Health and Human Services. *Scientific Report of the 2015 Dietary Guidelines Advisory Committee*. Department of Health and Human Services and United States Department of Agriculture; 2015. http://health.gov/dietaryguidelines/2015-scientific-report/.

47. *Determining Product Eligibility for Purchase with SNAP Benefits*. United States Department of Agriculture; 2010. https://www.fns.usda.gov/sites/default/files/eligibility.pdf.

48. Eligibility | Food and Nutrition Service. https://www.fns.usda.gov/snap/eligibility. Accessed April 3, 2017.

49. Daines RF, Farley TA. No food stamps for sodas. *New York Times*. October 7, 2010. http://www.nytimes.com/2010/10/07/opinion/07farley.html. Accessed April 3, 2017.

50. SNAP and Restrictions | Snap To Health. https://www.snaptohealth.org/snap-innovations/snap-and-restrictions/. Accessed April 3, 2017.

51. Waivers of Rules | Food and Nutrition Service. https://www.fns.usda.gov/snap/waivers-rules. Accessed April 3, 2017.

52. Berg J. Food stamps soda ban: the wrong way to fight obesity. *Huffington Post*. December 2010. http://www.huffingtonpost.com/joel-berg/food-stamps-soda-ban-the-_b_791863.html. Accessed April 3, 2017.

53. Implications of Restricting the Use of Food Stamp Benefits. Scribd. https://www.scribd.com/doc/299817488/Implications-of-Restricting-the-Use-of-Food-Stamp-Benefits. Accessed April 3, 2017.

54. Gregory C, Ver Ploeg M, Andrews M, Coleman-Jensen A. Supplemental Nutrition Assistance Program (SNAP) participation leads to modest changes in diet quality. *US Dep Agric Econ Res Serv*. 2013;ERR-147:1–36.

55. Gu X, Tucker KL. Dietary quality of the US child and adolescent population: trends from 1999 to 2012 and associations with the use of federal nutrition assistance programs. *Am J Clin Nutr*. November 2016:ajcn135095. doi:10.3945/ajcn.116.135095.

56. Leung CW, Ding EL, Catalano PJ, Villamor E, Rimm EB, Willett WC. Dietary intake and dietary quality of low-income adults in the Supplemental Nutrition Assistance Program. *Am J Clin Nutr*. 2012;96(5):977–988.

57. Hiza HA, Casavale KO, Guenther PM, Davis CA. Diet quality of Americans differs by age, sex, race/ethnicity, income, and education level. *J Acad Nutr Diet*. 2013;113(2):297–306.

58. Wang DD, Leung CW, Li Y, et al. Trends in dietary quality among adults in the United States, 1999 through 2010. *JAMA Intern Med*. 2014;174(10):1587–1595.

59. Double Up Food Bucks. http://www.doubleupfoodbucks.org/. Accessed April 3, 2017.

60. FINI Grant Program | Food and Nutrition Service. https://www.fns.usda.gov/snap/FINI-Grant-Program. Accessed April 3, 2017.

61. Block-Granting SNAP Would Abandon Decades-Long Federal Commitment to Reducing Hunger. Center on Budget and Policy Priorities; 2017. http://www.cbpp.org/research/food-assistance/block-granting-snap-would-abandon-decades-long-federal-commitment-to. Accessed April 3, 2017.

62. WIC Eligibility Requirements | Food and Nutrition Service. https://www.fns.usda.gov/wic/wic-eligibility-requirements. Accessed April 3, 2017.

63. About WIC—WIC at a Glance | Food and Nutrition Service. https://www.fns.usda.gov/wic/about-wic-wic-glance. Accessed April 3, 2017.

64. USDA Economic Research Service—Child Nutrition Programs. https://www.ers.usda.gov/topics/food-nutrition-assistance/child-nutrition-programs. Accessed April 3, 2017.

65. National School Lunch Program (NSLP) | Food and Nutrition Service. https://www.fns.usda.gov/nslp/national-school-lunch-program-nslp. Accessed April 3, 2017.

66. Final Rule: National School Lunch Program and School Breakfast Program: Nutrition Standards for All Foods Sold in School as Required by the HHFKA of 2010 | Food and Nutrition Service. https://www.fns.usda.gov/school-meals/fr-072916d. Accessed April 3, 2017.

67. Bergman EA, Englund T, Taylor KW, Watkins T, Schepman S, Rushing K. School lunch before and after implementation of the Healthy Hunger-Free Kids Act. *J Child Nutr Manag*. 2014;38(2).

68. Schwartz MB, Henderson KE, Read M, Danna N, Ickovics JR. New school meal regulations increase fruit consumption and do not increase total plate waste. *Child Obes*. 2015;11(3):242–247.

69. School Breakfast Program (SBP) | Food and Nutrition Service. https://www.fns. usda.gov/sbp/school-breakfast-program-sbp. Accessed April 3, 2017.

70. Bachman CM, Baranowski T, Nicklas TA. Is there an association between sweetened beverages and adiposity? *Nutr Rev.* 2006;64(4):153–174.

71. Malik VS, Schulze MB, Hu FB. Intake of sugar-sweetened beverages and weight gain: a systematic review. *Am J Clin Nutr.* 2006;84(2):274–288.

72. Johnson L, Mander AP, Jones LR, Emmett PM, Jebb SA. Is sugar-sweetened beverage consumption associated with increased fatness in children? *Nutr Burbank Los Angel Cty Calif.* 2007;23(7-8):557–563. doi:10.1016/j.nut.2007.05.005.

73. Palmer JR, Boggs DA, Krishnan S, Hu FB, Singer M, Rosenberg L. Sugar-sweetened beverages and incidence of type 2 diabetes mellitus in African American women. *Arch Intern Med.* 2008;168(14):1487–1492. doi:10.1001/archinte.168.14.1487.

74. Chaloupka F, Powell L, Chriqui J. *Sugar-Sweetened Beverage Taxes and Public Health.* Robert Wood Johnson Foundation; 2009. http://www.rwjf.org/en/library/research/2009/07/sugar-sweetened-beverage-taxes-and-public-health. html. Accessed March 7, 2017.

75. Vartanian LR, Schwartz MB, Brownell KD. Effects of soft drink consumption on nutrition and health: a systematic review and meta-analysis. *Am J Public Health.* 2007;97(4):667–675. doi:10.2105/AJPH.2005.083782.

76. Chen L, Appel LJ, Loria C, et al. Reduction in consumption of sugar-sweetened beverages is associated with weight loss: the PREMIER trial. *Am J Clin Nutr.* 2009;89(5):1299–1306. doi:10.3945/ajcn.2008.27240.

77. *Model Sugar-Sweetened Beverage Tax Legislation.* ChangeLab Solutions; 2011. http://www.changelabsolutions.org/publications/ssb-model-tax-legislation. Accessed March 7, 2017.

78. Andreyeva T, Chaloupka FJ, Brownell KD. Estimating the potential of taxes on sugar-sweetened beverages to reduce consumption and generate revenue. *Prev Med.* 2011;52(6):413–416. doi:10.1016/j.ypmed.2011.03.013.

79. Finkelstein EA, Zhen C, Nonnemaker J, Todd JE. Impact of targeted beverage taxes on higher- and lower-income households. *Arch Intern Med.* 2010;170(22):2028–2034. doi:10.1001/archinternmed.2010.449.

80. Kaplan MG. Taxing sugar-sweetened beverages. *N Engl J Med.* 2010;362(4):368–369. doi:10.1056/NEJMc0911234.

81. Storey M. This Week, It's All About Hypertension… | American Beverage Association; 2011. http://www.ameribev.org/education-resources/blog/post/this-week-its-all-about-hypertension/. Accessed March 7, 2017.

82. Forshee RA, Anderson PA, Storey ML. Sugar-sweetened beverages and body mass index in children and adolescents: a meta-analysis. *Am J Clin Nutr.* 2008;87(6):1662–1671.

83. Ebbeling CB, Feldman HA, Osganian SK, Chomitz VR, Ellenbogen SJ, Ludwig DS. Effects of decreasing sugar-sweetened beverage consumption on body weight

in adolescents: a randomized, controlled pilot study. *Pediatrics.* 2006;117(3):673–680. doi:10.1542/peds.2005-0983.

84. Williams R, Christ K. Taxing Sin. Mercatus Center. https://www.mercatus.org/publication/taxing-sin. Published July 2009. Accessed March 7, 2017.

85. World Health Organization. 20 questions on genetically modified foods. WHO; 2013. http://www.who.int/foodsafety/publications/biotech/20questions/en/. Accessed November 1, 2013.

86. U.S. Department of Agriculture. Biotechnology. USDA; 2013. http://www.ers.usda.gov/topics/farm-practices-management/biotechnology/background.aspx#.UnQkk1OwWKg. Accessed November 1, 2013.

87. GMO labeling. NPR.org. http://www.npr.org/tags/164598857/gmo-labeling. Accessed March 24, 2017.

88. Dona A, Arvanitoyannis IS. Health risks of genetically modified foods. *Crit Rev Food Sci Nutr.* 2009;49(2):164–175.

89. Center for Food Safety | Campaigns | Center for Food Safety. http://www.center-forfoodsafety.org/issues/976/ge-food-labeling/state-labeling-initiatives. Accessed March 24, 2017.

90. Non-GMO Project. GMO Facts. The Non-GMO Project; 2013. http://www.nongmoproject.org/learn-more/. Accessed November 4, 2013.

91. Qaim M. The economics of genetically modified crops. *Annu Rev Resour Econ.* 2009;1(1):665–694. doi:10.1146/annurev.resource.050708.144203.

92. Definitions of Food Security. USDA Economic Research Service; 2013. http://www.ers.usda.gov/topics/food-nutrition-assistance/food-security-in-the-us/definitions-of-food-security.aspx#. Accessed November 4, 2013.

93. Kiers ET, Leakey RR, Izac A-M, et al. Agriculture at a crossroads. *Sci-N Y THEN Wash-.* 2008;320(5874):320.

94. Pollan M. The (Agri)Cultural Contradictions of Obesity. *New York Times.* October 12, 2003. http://www.nytimes.com/2003/10/12/magazine/12WWLN.html. Accessed November 4, 2013.

95. Matthews CM. Exploring the obesity epidemic. *Proc Bayl Univ Med Cent.* 2012;25(3):276–277.

96. Sallis JF, Glanz K. Physical activity and food environments: solutions to the obesity epidemic. *Milbank Q.* 2009;87(1):123–154. doi:10.1111/j.1468-0009.2009.00550.x.

97. Rupert E. Senate passes bill to create federal labeling standard for GMO foods. TheHill. July 7, 2016. http://thehill.com/blogs/floor-action/senate/286949-senate-passes-bill-to-create-federal-labeling-standard-for-gmo. Accessed March 24, 2017.

98. Wicker R. Text—S.764 - 114th Congress (2015–2016): A bill to reauthorize and amend the National Sea Grant College Program Act, and for other purposes. https://www.congress.gov/bill/114th-congress/senate-bill/764/text. Published July 29, 2016. Accessed March 24, 2017.

99. Vermont GMO Labeling Act.pdf.

100. Nutrition C for FS and A. Labeling & Nutrition—Changes to the Nutrition Facts Label. https://www.fda.gov/Food/GuidanceRegulation/GuidanceDocumentsRegulatoryInformation/LabelingNutrition/ucm385663.htm. Accessed March 24, 2017.

101. Malik VS, Willett WC, Hu FB. The revised nutrition facts label: a step forward and more room for improvement. *JAMA*. 2016;316(6):583–584. doi:10.1001/jama.2016.8005.

102. Committee on Food Marketing and the Diets of Children and Youth. *Food Marketing to Children and Youth: Threat or Opportunity?* (McGinnis JM, Kraak VI, eds.). The National Academies Press; 2006. http://www.nap.edu/openbook.php?record_id=11514.

103. Mozaffarian D. The Healthy Weight Commitment Foundation Trillion Calorie Pledge. *Am J Prev Med*. 2014;47(4):e9–e10. doi:10.1016/j.amepre.2014.07.029.

104. Panjwani C, Caraher M. The public health responsibility deal: brokering a deal for public health, but on whose terms? *Health Policy Amst Neth*. 2014;114(2-3):163–173. doi:10.1016/j.healthpol.2013.11.002.

105. Kolish ED, Enright M, Oberdorff B. The Children's Food & Beverage Advertising Initiative. In: *A Report on Compliance and Progress During 2011*. Council of Better Business Bureaus; 2012.

106. Kunkel DL, Castonguay JS, Filer CR. Evaluating industry self-regulation of food marketing to children. *Am J Prev Med*. 2015;49(2):181–187. doi:10.1016/j.amepre.2015.01.027.

7

Food Insecurity and Public Health

Molly Knowles, Joanna Simmons, and Mariana Chilton

Chapter Highlights

- Food insecurity—lack of access to enough food for an active and healthy life—is a major public health issue, affecting the health and well-being of one in seven people in the United States.
- Food insecurity is related to economic, social, and political conditions, and is beyond the control of a single household. Structural inequalities and discrimination against people of color, LGBTQ people, immigrants, people with disabilities, and women drives disparities in food insecurity.
- Major policy interventions include raising wages, improving the Supplemental Nutrition Assistance Program, various programs of the Child Nutrition Reauthorization, and the Elder Nutrition Program, but these programs are not sufficient to fully address food insecurity.
- A human rights approach, which recognizes the right to food, and increasing civic participation among people from all sectors, offers new possibilities in addressing food insecurity in the United States.

Introduction

Joanna Cruz: When I first joined Witnesses to Hunger—a program where caregivers who have experienced hunger firsthand take photographs to teach the public, the press, and policymakers about food insecurity and ways to solve it—I was living with my children, aged 6 and 2, and their father. This is a photograph of my kitchen (Figure 7.1). I owned the house, which my mother had given me and was where I had grown up. But I didn't have enough money to make repairs to the plumbing, which had started to weaken over the years and was leaking sewage into the basement. When I got a quote, they told me that fixing the plumbing would cost at least $5,000. I didn't have that kind of money, so I had no choice but to turn off the water. Since I couldn't find a job, I was receiving $416 per month in cash assistance, which was hardly enough to cover heating and cooking gas, so they were often turned off. I also got food stamps, which could never stretch far enough, especially since I couldn't cook at home without water or gas. I was going through deep depression, frustration, and anxiety. When I joined Witnesses, I learned that what I'd been experiencing—not having enough money for food, which caused me to lose weight and miss meals for myself and occasionally my children—had

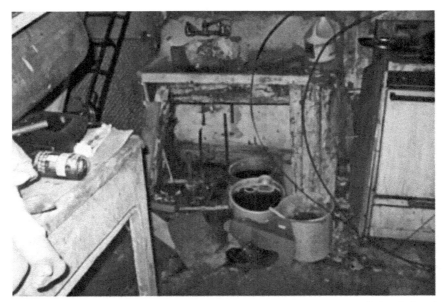

FIGURE 7.1 My Neighbor's Kitchen "You never know what goes on behind closed doors. Some people need to know exactly how we're living being single moms, being that we're on our own and we don't have that many opportunities. When something breaks, we may not be able to fix it because we have limited income. It's really hard to try to get everything fixed. How would my neighbor actually try to work with something like that? Being in a situation like that, your kids can stay hungry."– Barbie I., Witnesses to Hunger Philadelphia

another name: very low food security. Meanwhile, my children were often in the hospital with ear infections, colds, and rashes.

My neighbor, Barbie, who took this photo of my kitchen, explained it this way: "Sometimes things can get so bad, you are afraid to ask for help." I used to spend my days at Barbie's house, since she had water, gas, and electricity. I stored my food and cooked there, bathed the kids there, and just generally took my mind off of the problems at home. If it weren't for Barbie, I don't know what I would have done. Everybody needs somebody, and she was my somebody. But I didn't know how I was going to make it from one day to the next. I could barely focus on anything outside of moment to moment. When I woke up, I was thinking: *How am I going to wash my face and make sure the kids brush their teeth? Then, how am I going to get them ready for school? Do they look messy? Is the teacher going to think they're not being taken care of, or are the other kids going to make fun of them? Then, did they get enough to eat at school, and what am I going to feed them when they get home? Then, where are they going to sleep? If they sleep on the floor in the living room, there are bugs; but, if they sleep in their bedroom, there are leaks, which aren't safe either.* Then they'd go to sleep and we'd start the cycle all over again the next day. The stress was unbelievable. But I couldn't give up—I had to think about my kids.

After several months and some encouragement from a program I was in called Witnesses to Hunger, I was able to move out and sell the house, but under market value. Right now, I live with my mother, who helps me with living costs and child care. I work the overnight shift at a convenience store, which gives me time to spend with my children and lets me work on my cro- cheting and catering business, where I sell hats, baby booties, and cupcakes.

In this photograph of Joanna's kitchen, you can see the trade-offs that lead to poor mental and physical health of parents and children, public systems that fail to adequately support families, and fear in asking for help. Since that time in her life, she has made progress toward a better life. She now has access to a steady and stable job, opportunities for entrepreneurship, and overall, she's gaining a bit more control over her own future. In *Hunger and Public Action,* Jean Drèze and Amartya Sen suggest that hunger is about "who has control over what": The fact that a society can have plenty of food yet still have people dying of hunger suggests that hunger is not about lack of food but lack of *power.* It follows that if people had more control over their own lives, they would be able to secure the necessary food for themselves.[1] In the sections below, we describe the public health context of Joanna's experience of food insecurity: the health impacts, economic conditions, policy interven- tions, and need for civic participation.

Although focus on adequate nutrition is as old as the development of modern medicine and public health itself, there is a recent and robust 30-year history of food insecurity research that has identified the causes and consequences of food insecurity in the U.S. population. The United States also has over 50 years of history of concern for improving nutrition through the structural interventions of the Supplemental Nutrition Assistance Program (SNAP, formerly known as food stamps) and the Special Supplemental Nutrition Program for Women, Infants and Children (WIC), which, together with other policy interventions has eradicated widespread severe malnutrition and hunger in the United States. Currently, the United States does not have pervasive malnutrition in Appalachia, on American Indian reservations, or in urban enclaves, as we did up through the 1960s. However, we have a widespread obesity epidemic, a significant form of malnutrition, as well as widespread food insecurity affecting 13.4% of the population and costing our health, education, and prison systems almost $179 billion annually.[2,3] The disparities in food insecurity and hunger are quite stark: African American and Latino families have rates of food insecurity that are twice the rates of white families; Native American groups, immigrants, returning citizens, and people with disabilities also have very high rates of food insecurity.

In this chapter, we describe these disparities, as well as the determinants and consequences of food insecurity. With an eye to the public health ecological approach—which takes into account the individual, social, economic, institutional, and structural forces that affect health—we describe the systemic public health issues associated with food insecurity, including the economic trade-offs, as well as the other experiential issues described by those who know hunger firsthand. We then characterize policy and systems solutions involving the need for higher wages; changes to SNAP, WIC and other nutrition programs; and trauma-informed approaches. We end with a call for greater participation and inclusion of people who have experienced food insecurity in the development of policies and programs.

Major Topics
Food Insecurity Definition, Prevalence, and Disparities

The formal definition of food security as defined by the U.S. Department of Agriculture is, "access by all people at all times to enough food for an active, healthy life." By contrast, *food insecurity* is having inadequate economic resources to enable consistent access to safe, adequate, and nutritious food to support an active and healthy life for all household members. It has two levels: *low food security* (reduced quality, variety, and desirability of diet) and *very low food security* (multiple indications of disrupted eating patterns and reduced food intake).[4]

The U.S. Department of Agriculture's Economic Research Service (ERS) 18-item survey, the *Household Food Security Survey Module (HFSSM),* is considered the gold standard survey measure of severity and depth of food insecurity in the United States (see Table 7.1). This survey is embedded into the Current Population Survey, which also has

Table 7.1 Categorizations of Food Security Status as Measured by the U.S. Department of Agriculture

Category	Sub-category	Description
Food Security	**High Food Security**	No reported indications of food access problems or limitations among adults or children in household.
	Marginal Food Security Worried food would run out Food bought did not last	One or two reported indications; typically, anxiety over food sufficiency or shortage of food. Little or no indication of changes in diets or food intake.
Food Insecurity	**Low Food Security** Worried food would run out Food bought did not last Could not afford balanced meal Cut size of meal or skipped meal	Reports of reduced quality, variety, or desirability of diet among adults and/or children in the household. Little or no indication of reduced food intake.
	Very Low Food Security Cut or skipped meal Ate less than felt should Hungry but did not eat Lost weight Did not eat whole day Did not eat whole day, 3+ months	Reports of multiple indications of disrupted eating patterns and reduced food intake among adults and/or children in the household.

Derived from: http://www.ers.usda.gov/topics/food-nutrition-assistance/food-security-in-the-us/definitions-of-food-security.aspx questions about public assistance participation, employment, and other demographic characteristics. Researchers working with specific populations also use the HFSSM to investigate the relationship between food insecurity and outcomes such as low birth weight, child development,[5] anemia,[6] suicidal ideation,[7] social isolation, depression, diabetes,[8] and obesity.[9] According to the USDA, in 2015, more than 42 million people (13.4%) in the United States lived in food insecure households, including approximately 13.1 million children (17.9%). These rates were significantly higher during the recession and have only begun to decline significantly since 2014. Before the recession, the food insecurity rates hovered around 12% of the U.S. population without much change since the USDA ERS began measurement in 1995.[4]

National and state rates of food insecurity obscure stark racial, ethnic, gender, and age disparities. For instance, 30.3% of single female-headed households were food insecure as opposed to 22.7% of single male-headed households and 12.7% of all U.S. households in 2015.[4] Households with children under the age of six are also more likely to be food insecure than others, with nearly 16.9% of such households affected. Additionally, more than 21.5% of African American households and 19.1% of Hispanic households were food insecure. These rates are double those of white, non-Hispanic households, where the rate is 10%.[4] Rates among American Indians and immigrant populations are harder to document and vary regionally, though the rates can be quite high compared to the general U.S. population as we describe below. Why pay attention to such disparities? Because the health consequences of food insecurity are unrelenting, harsh, and long-lasting, and populations more vulnerable to food insecurity experience greater burden from its negative health effects.

Food insecurity is not solely an individual or household-level phenomenon. It is related to political, economic, and social contexts most often beyond control of the household. An *ecological approach*—a framework rooted in the notion that multiple factors such as economic, social, cultural, political, and institutional structures shape health outcomes—emphasizes the importance of the structural conditions that affect food insecurity. These can be educational attainment, employment opportunities, mortgage lending practices, corporate pay scales, labor laws, zoning laws, and other socioeconomic factors. The ecological approach creates a structure for us to see how policies, programs, and economic structures shape the contours of our social and political systems, our agriculture and food systems, and ultimately, our individual experiences.

The ecological approach also helps us to understand how marginalized groups such as American Indians and first generation immigrants, LGBTQ youth and adults, formerly incarcerated individuals and their families, and people with disabilities experience a high burden of food insecurity relative to the general population.

American Indians and Immigrants

Over one in five (23%) of American Indians and Alaska Natives experience food insecurity, more than twice the rate of non-Hispanic White households (11%).[10] In one study of the Navajo Nation, more than three-quarters of households (76.6%) were food insecure, the highest rate of food insecurity among any U.S. population.[11] Food insecurity is exacerbated by limited access to affordable, nutritious foods for American Indians living in their traditional homelands or reservations, who may need to travel long distances to reach a grocery store. In one study, 51% of members of the Navajo Nation reported traveling off-reservation to reach a grocery store; the shortest distance traveled was 155 miles.[11] In another study of American Indians in rural Oklahoma, 56% reported inadequate food quantity and 62% reported inadequate food quality. Health outcomes related to cardiovascular disease, including obesity, diabetes, and hypertension were higher among those with inadequate food quality after adjusting for age, gender, income, and education.[12] Diversity, geographic spread, and cultural differences make it more difficult to study and understand the magnitude of food insecurity among the variety of American Indian groups.

For similar reasons, it is also difficult to accurately measure food insecurity among immigrant households. Immigrants may live in mixed-citizenship households (e.g., citizen children and non-citizen parents); immigrant seasonal workers may move frequently; and undocumented immigrants, fearing deportation, may be less likely to participate in surveys and the Census. For these reasons, studies among immigrants are generally small scale and include participants from many different countries of origin, making it difficult to compare rates of food insecurity across groups and populations. One large study of 19,275 mothers of children under age four found that children of immigrants experience higher rates of food insecurity than children of U.S.-born mothers.[13] Another study found higher rates of food insecurity among children of non-citizens compared with children of citizens after introduction of legislation that barred non-citizen participation in SNAP.[14] Among immigrant farmworkers in Georgia, undocumented workers were nearly three times as likely to be food insecure compared with documented workers.[15]

LGBTQ Youth and Adults

Lesbian, gay, bisexual, transgender, and queer (LGBTQ) adults and youth face higher rates of poverty and other forms of economic insecurity. Despite poor documentation of food insecurity among the LGBTQ population, a few studies have shown higher rates of food insecurity and participation in SNAP among LGBTQ adults.[16] The most representative studies come from the Williams Institute, which combined data from three national population-based surveys to assess SNAP participation and food insecurity, as measured by an affirmative response to a question about not having enough money for food in the past year, among LGBTQ adults and same-sex couples.[17] Those identifying as lesbian, gay, or bisexual were 1.4 times as likely to participate in SNAP compared with people identifying as heterosexual. Although information on SNAP participation among transgender adults is not collected, transgender adults may face specific challenges in accessing nutrition assistance and other federal programs because of discrepancies between the identity-concordant name and gender listed on applications and the name and gender listed on birth certificates, state identification, and social security cards.[18] People identifying as LGBTQ reported not having enough money for food at higher rates than non-LGBT people (29% compared with 18%).[17] Within the LGBTQ population, women, people identifying as bisexual, and people of color experience higher rates of food insecurity.[17]

Despite a lack of studies assessing food insecurity of LGBTQ youth, it is likely that LGBTQ youth also face particular barriers to food security given their increased risk of homelessness compared with their non-LGBTQ peers.[16] As more LGBTQ youth come out to their parents, schools, and other service providers while they are still minors, they face rejection and harassment leading to an increase in runaway and homeless LGBTQ adolescents.[19,20] Barriers LGBTQ youth face in accessing housing and other resources is likely to increase their risk of food insecurity.[16]

Formerly Incarcerated and their Families

The United States has the largest incarcerated population of any country in the world, with over 2.1 million adults in jail or prison in 2015.[21] A disproportionate burden of incarceration among communities of color is well-documented;[22] more than 60% of people in prison are people of color.[23] Black men are 6 times and Latino men are 2.3 times as likely to be incarcerated compared with white men. Although women are less likely to be incarcerated overall, Black women are incarcerated at 6 times and Latina women at 2.5 times the rate of white women.[23] Approximately 650,000 people are released from prison each year, most without employment, stable housing, or family support. Those convicted of felony charges are ineligible to be primary leaseholders on subsidized housing, and in some states are prohibited from living in subsidized housing units. Those convicted of drug-related felonies, but not other types of felonies, including violent ones, are prohibited from receiving SNAP benefits. Although there are no nationally representative studies of returning citizens, one study of 101 individuals recently released from prison reported that 90% were food insecure, and 37% reported not eating for an entire day because they had no money for food.[24] Families of incarcerated individuals also face increased risk of food insecurity. In studies using data from the Fragile Families and Child Well-Being Study, households with children were more likely to report food insecurity after the incarceration of a parent.[25,26]

People with Disabilities

Low employment rates and high healthcare costs constrain the economic resources of people with disabilities, which can lead to food insecurity.[27] High rates of food insecurity among households with disabled members are poorly addressed by the federal government and community organizations alike. In a nationally representative study of over 420,000 adults, those with disabilities were 2.6 times as likely to be food insecure compared with adults without disabilities; working-age adults and adults with mental health disabilities experience even higher odds.[28] Among households reporting very low food security, 38% include an adult with a disability, and families with children who have special health care needs are more likely to experience both household and child food insecurity compared with families whose children do not have special health care needs.[29,30] Food insecurity can make coping with a disability difficult and potentially dangerous. One-third of chronically ill adults cannot afford both food and medicine.[31] In addition, people with disabilities may have health conditions that can be exacerbated by the negative health effects of food insecurity.

A Common Theme: Discrimination

The disparities in food insecurity described above reflect a common theme: each group highlighted has experienced oppression or discrimination. Structural racism in the United States, originating with European colonizers' enslavement of Africans and genocide of American Indians, has continued in various forms through to the present, resulting in health inequities between people of color and white Americans.[32,33] White Americans and the political institutions under their control have long oppressed African Americans, from slavery, legal segregation under Jim Crow, and federally supported housing discrimination through current police brutality and mass incarceration. Similarly, the U.S. government has conducted and supported genocide of American Indians and theft of their sovereign land, breaking treaties and enacting policies denying American Indians rights to traditional and sacred lands, farming and fishing, natural resources, and clean water.[34] Both documented and undocumented immigrants often lack worker protections; many are escaping violence or economic deprivation in their home countries; and increasing anti-immigrant sentiment results in harassment, detainment, and deportation of undocumented immigrants, breaking up families and creating fear and instability among immigrant communities.[35] LGBTQ people, particularly trans women of color, experience increased exposure to violence and discrimination in housing, education, and employment, despite growing legal protections in some states and cities.[36,37] High rates of incarceration and the nation's disparate sentencing laws have been recognized as yet another form of oppression of people of color.[22] In addition, prisoners are exposed to violence and loss of rights that have lifelong consequences,[38] increasing their vulnerability to food insecurity upon returning.[24] High rates of food insecurity among female-headed households with children suggest not only inequities in pay and access to adequate employment, but also a lack of care for families and a devaluation of women's unpaid work. Finally, people with disabilities face barriers to employment and accessing resources, often face high medical costs, and often are under-recognized in justice-seeking movements and organizations.

Once we recognize the patterns of disparity in U.S. food insecurity, we see that structural inequality and its mechanisms of discrimination are key drivers. Solutions to food insecurity, therefore, must go beyond ensuring access to more healthy food, and also focus on reducing and eliminating discrimination and oppression. These solutions also must be based on a solid understanding of food insecurity's impact on public health. Below we present the health effects of food insecurity across the life course, including effects on children, adolescents, adults, and seniors.

Public Health Impact of Food Insecurity

Children, Adolescents, and Families

The health effects of food insecurity are most pronounced among children, particularly in early childhood when significant growth and development are taking place. The majority of research assessing health effects of food insecurity has focused on households with children. In households with children, food insecurity can be measured at the household level or the child level, a more severe form in which food insecurity is reported to affect children directly. In 2015, 16.6% of households with children under 18 reported food insecurity, with 7.8% reporting food insecurity at the child level.[4] Food insecurity at either level has serious negative consequences for the health and development of infants, children, and adolescents. Inadequate or interrupted food intake, even for a short time, can cause long-lasting health effects. Among infants and toddlers under three years old, food insecurity is associated with increased hospitalization and poor health status,[39,40] iron deficient anemia,[41] and reduced cognitive, emotional, and social development.[42,43] Young children living in food insecure households have an increased developmental risk,[5,44,45] which has strong implications for a child's school readiness, subsequent well-being, and success later in life.[46]

Food insecurity is associated with poor academic performance and poor cognitive and social development among children and adolesecents.[47] Compared to low-income school-aged children living in food secure households, children in food insecure households were more likely to have repeated a grade, to have lower math and reading scores, and to report difficulty in social relationships.[48-50] Children who lived in homes experiencing food insufficiency were more likely to receive special education services or mental health counseling,[51] and children in food insecure households were more likely to exhibit both internalizing and externalizing behavioral problems.[50,52-54] Among adolescents and children, poor mental health and food insecurity are also strongly linked.[51,53,55-57] For example, family food insufficiency is positively associated with depression and suicidal ideation among adolescents.[7] Food insecurity is not explicitly associated with childhood obesity,[58,59] although it is associated with obesity in some adult populations, described in more detail in the following section.

Most research on child food insecurity is based on parental report, and much of the literature using caregivers' reports indicates that parents shield their children, especially young children, from experiencing food insecurity.[60-62] Research by Fram and colleagues, however, has shown that school-aged children are often aware of food insecurity, despite their parents' attempts to protect them from this knowledge.[63] In qualitative interviews, children and adolescents ages 9 to 16 reported distinct experiences of food insecurity, including managing immediate food resources for themselves and their parents, worrying about their parents' level of stress, and feeling angry and helpless when their families did not have enough food.

The health of children cannot be separated from the health and well-being of their caregivers. An alternative way to look at food security is through the lens of the *life course perspective*. The life course framework incorporates analysis of the relationships among social, behavioral, and biological factors as they develop throughout an individual's life and social context. By focusing on the ways early life events influence health behavior and health risks later in life, one can see how these risks can also be transmitted to the next generation,[64] the life course perspective provides additional avenues for intervention. For example, the intrauterine environment strongly affects fetal health and well-being, which later affects infants, and eventually plays out in children's health and well-being in their early years. When young children are food insecure, their social, cognitive, and emotional development falters, diminishing their ability to start school well-prepared. The negative consequences can proceed through the school years to adolescence, and can then translate into greater risk-taking behaviors, such as having many sexual partners; drug and alcohol abuse; greater exposure to violence; and high-risk pregnancy, affecting the next generation in turn.[65]

Food insecurity also is associated with poor mental health among children and adults (Box 7.1). Among mothers, food insecurity is associated with depressive symptoms, major depression, and anxiety, which negatively affect child health outcomes.[43,66–70] Among mothers, food insecurity

---

BOX 7.1

Ask Joanna: How did Food Insecurity Affect Your Health?

When I look at pictures of myself from the time when I lived in that house, I look completely unhealthy. I look like the stress was getting to me. Look at me now, compared to how I look then—my hair was falling out, I was skinny, I was pale. I wasn't healthy at all. But there was nothing doctors could really do about it if they weren't changing my situation. They can pump you up full of a bunch of pills to keep you from being so depressed and to calm you down, but they're not changing what the problem is. My problem is that I don't have food, so you can give me all the Xanax in the world, but it's still not changing what I'm going through. I don't want to go to the doctor for being depressed because I don't have any food. Unless you're giving me groceries, you're not doing anything for me. So, you can give those pills to somebody else.

and depressive symptoms may have a reciprocal relationship, in which each exacerbates the other. Mothers who report depressive symptoms experience more employment difficulties[67] that may be related to financial hardship and food insecurity.[71] In several studies, women who report experiencing post-traumatic stress disorder or associated symptoms are more likely to report household food insecurity.[54,72,73] Recent research has shown that exposure to violence and childhood trauma are important precursors to the mental health context of food insecurity, particularly among women. In studies of current and recent exposure to violence, intimate partner violence is associated with increased odds of food insecurity among women,[74,75] and depressive symptoms may mediate this association.[75] Exposure to abuse, neglect, or household instability in childhood is also linked with food insecurity in adulthood. In several studies, women exposed to childhood abuse and/or violence throughout their lives were more likely to report food insecurity compared with those who had not been exposed.[74,76,77] For example, compared with women who reported no childhood adversity, women with children who experienced neglect, abuse, or household instability in childhood were 12 times as likely to report household food insecurity in adulthood and 17 times as likely to report food insecurity among their own children.[78]

Adults and Seniors

Although there have been fewer studies of health effects on working-age adults (with and without children), research has shown that food insecurity among adults in this age group is associated with nutrient inadequacies,[79] poor diet quality,[80] and poor self-rated health.[81] Food insecurity also puts adults at risk for diet-sensitive chronic health conditions including diabetes.[8,82,83] Food insecure adults report "trade-offs" between paying for health care and medications or for food, which negatively affects overall health.[82] Food insecurity also is associated with lower adherence to treatment of chronic diseases, including HIV/AIDS,[84] diabetes,[85] and cancer.[86] In some studies, food insecurity reported among adults is associated with health risk factors such as obesity. Researchers have found that food insecurity is associated with obesity among women,[9,87,88] but evidence of the association among men is inconsistent and varies by race, ethnicity, age, and socioeconomic status.[89] Dinour and colleagues have suggested that obesity among food insecure individuals may be related to reliance on low-cost, energy-dense foods and to coping strategies for episodic food insufficiency linked to the monthly SNAP distribution cycle.[90]

In 2015, 8.3% of households with elderly people were food insecure, and this rate was higher (9.2%) for households consisting of elderly people living alone.[4] Among adults age 40 and older, living in multigenerational households is associated with higher rates of food insecurity.[91] For low-income seniors in particular, who often have difficulty obtaining adequate nutrient intake, food insecurity exacerbates nutritional deficiencies, including lower intake of macro and micronutrients.[92] Compared with seniors in food secure households, food insecure seniors are more likely to report limitations in their daily activities,[93] depression,[94] and fair or poor health overall.[95]

Economic Circumstances of Food Insecurity

Food insecurity occurs in a context in which people must make often impossible choices between paying for food and paying for other basic needs. Many of these trade-offs, such as paying for heat or for medicine by reducing money spent on food, or getting behind on rent in order to have enough money to pay for meals, have strong negative health consequences for children and adults.[96,97] Food insecure adults will often trade off paying for medical care or prescriptions in order to pay for food, or vice-versa, which may harm caregiver and child health.[82,98] Coping with food insecurity means that families may also struggle to pay for rent and utilities. These stressors, known as *housing insecurity* and *energy insecurity*, may exacerbate food insecurity and are associated with negative child health outcomes and poor child development.[96,99]

Food insecurity research often explores the associations among food insecurity, hardship, and poor child health, yet few studies investigate how children's poor health can place financial strain on the family, or the coping strategies that families adopt in response to it. The consequences of repeated or chronic child illnesses directly affect the caregivers' ability to maintain steady employment.[100,101] In Joanna's experience, her children's frequent illnesses, as well the lack of both paid and unpaid sick leave in many low-wage jobs, made it very difficult for her to find and keep a steady job.

The dynamic of hardships, illness, and difficulty finding and maintaining work can create even more vulnerability for families. Although consistent income is essential to buffering families from food insecurity, there is little investigation of the types of work that caregivers do to create income or find work. Qualitative research has demonstrated that to prevent or cope with food insecurity, families may find a second job, work overtime, or frequently change jobs. Quantitative research bears this out as well. Using the nationally representative Current Population Survey, research shows that most families with children that are food insecure are working in low-wage jobs, or jobs that have unpredictable or inconsistent hours, which makes it difficult to find and maintain child care or earn a stable income.[71]

Some studies have described ways that families generate income off the books through under-the-table work. This can include housekeeping and catering for small businesses or companies. Although such work does generate income, families take on risk, such as being injured on the job, forgoing worker protections, or triggering Internal Revenue Service (IRS) or public assistance investigations and sanctions. Other ways of generating additional income include what participants may call a "hustle" or side business. These businesses may include doing hair and nails for a nominal fee; selling dinners or desserts out of their homes or workplaces; or providing child care, housekeeping, or caretaking for neighbors, friends, and family. Other ad hoc income-generating techniques include selling blood, participating in research studies, collecting cans, and scrapping for metal.[102–104] Caregivers may not report these minor income increases out of fear of losing their benefits, whose dollar amount is often far greater than the small amount of money they make through other means to supplement income and public benefits.[105]

National Policies Addressing Food Security

Healthy People 2020 identifies national goals of reducing overall food insecurity to 6% and eliminating very low food insecurity among children,[106] yet there is no nationally recognized plan for ending food insecurity in the United States, despite several calls to do so.[107,108] Because the experience of poverty and food insecurity is multidimensional, numerous sectors of our society and our national and local structures have an impact on food security. These include, but are not limited to, our labor laws—including wages, family leave, child care support, and sick leave—nutrition-related policies, social support systems, and healthcare policy. Several federal policies and programs are designed explicitly to address food insecurity, including the farm bill and the Child Nutrition Reauthorization. Other policies that address food security do so indirectly by reducing related hardships, including housing insecurity and energy insecurity. Additionally, because of the strong relationship between food insecurity and health, healthcare policy also has a strong impact on food insecurity. Most recently, funding mechanisms structured into the 2010 Affordable Care Act also support food security by encouraging physicians and healthcare systems to address food insecurity as a means of preventing repeated hospitalizations. Nearly all programs that provide income or in-kind support to low-income families have an impact on food security rates. The following policies and programs are key to addressing and preventing food insecurity among children, adults, and seniors.

Labor Laws and Market Forces

Central to food security is the ability to pay for food or procure one's own food. The way the United States structures its workforce and labor laws have a major role in helping people put food on the table. During the Great Recession from 2007 to 2009, unemployment rates doubled from 7.1 million in 2007 to 14.3 million in 2009.[109] In response, food insecurity rates shot up to an all-time high of 14%.[110]

Globalization and America's massive loss of manufacturing and other types of jobs have kept wages low, especially for those without a college degree.[111,112] People without a college degree are often unable to secure jobs with higher wages and are also often forced to accept part-time, unstable, or seasonal employment. Such jobs offer few opportunities for career advancement and are less likely to provide fundamental work supports, such as paid sick leave or family leave.[100,113] Such employment also is associated with major income instability or sharp income fluctuations, which exacerbates food insecurity.[71,114] These fluctuations also affect eligibility for income supports and food assistance such as SNAP among people with low wages. Among SNAP participants of working age without disabilities, 82% worked in the year prior to receiving SNAP, and 58% worked full time for at least six months.[115] SNAP's ability to accommodate wage fluctuations effectively is still unclear: Evidence shows that even when SNAP participants see an increase in wages, and thus lose their benefits, their children are more likely to experience food insecurity because families may have less time to adapt.[71,116–118]

Given this sensitivity to labor laws and work supports, any type of legislation related to wages, family leave, sick leave, or child care will affect food insecurity.

Nutrition-Related Legislation

The farm bill, originally created in 1933 to provide subsidies to farmers during the Great Depression, authorizes most federal food and agriculture policies including nutrition assistance policy. Nutrition programs account for 80% of the farm bill's budget. Reauthorized approximately every five years, the bill provides funding for the Supplemental Nutrition Assistance Program (SNAP), formerly known as food stamps. SNAP is the nation's largest food assistance program and is one of the primary defenses against food insecurity.

In 2016, 44.2 million people participated in SNAP, nearly half of whom were children.[119] As an entitlement program, SNAP is responsive to economic downturns, supporting low-wage, unemployed, and underemployed workers as well as veterans, elderly people, and people with disabilities. In studies using the Supplemental Poverty Measure, SNAP has been shown to lift 4.6 million people out of poverty, including 2 million children.[120] SNAP participation has been shown to reduce food insecurity among children,[121] improve birth weight among infants born to mothers receiving SNAP,[122] and promote child health and reduce child hospitalizations.[123] An Institute of Medicine study, however, found that the SNAP allotment, based on the Thrifty Food Plan, does not reflect the true cost of a healthful diet,[124] particularly when accounting for regional differences in food prices (Box 7.2).[125]

The Child Nutrition and WIC Reauthorization Act authorizes programs that promote access to healthful and nutritious foods among children, primarily through the Special Supplemental Nutrition Program for Women, Infants, and Children (WIC) as well as the National School Lunch and School Breakfast programs. Originating with Lyndon B. Johnson's War on Poverty initiatives, the Child Nutrition Act is reviewed by Congress every five years. Although most of the programs it authorizes have been permanently implemented, Congress must review and approve their funding and structure. These programs also include the Child and Adult Care Food Program (CACFP), which reimburses child care providers for meals and

---

BOX 7.2

Ask Joanna: What Was It Like to Use SNAP to Feed Your Family?

When it was just me by myself, of course we ran out of food about a week before the food stamps came in. Whatever was in there, I would make it work. Oodles of noodles, cans of spaghetti, boneless chicken breasts shoved at the bottom of the freezer, macaroni and cheese and corn in a bowl. Trying to figure out something that my kids could eat real fast and not be hungry. A week is a long time to go when you don't have anything to eat. The same thing, oodles of noodles or cans of spaghetti, for days on end. That's why when you do get your food stamps you stock up on stuff like that, buying more than you think you need, because when the food runs out there's a backup. It's not the healthy stuff, but it'll fill them up.

snacks provided to children, the WIC Farmers Market Nutrition Program, which allows WIC recipients to purchase fresh fruits and vegetables at participating farmers' markets, and the Summer Food Service Program, which provides summertime meals to children who are eligible for free and reduced-price school breakfast and lunch. Under the National School Lunch Program, all children are able to receive lunch during the school day, and low-income children can qualify for free or reduced-price meals. Children who qualify for free or reduced-price school lunch are also eligible to receive breakfast at school through the School Breakfast Program. WIC provides nutritious foods, nutrition education, and healthcare referrals to low-income pregnant and postpartum women, infants, and children under 5 years of age who are determined to be at risk for poor nutrition. Widely regarded as one of the most effective social programs, WIC has been shown to reduce both food insecurity and poor child health and development outcomes. A longitudinal study demonstrated that longer participation in WIC was associated with reduced likelihood of household food insecurity.[126] Compared with eligible infants who did not receive WIC, infants receiving WIC benefits were less likely to be underweight and have a poor health status reported.[127] WIC also has been shown to improve school readiness.[128]

Seniors benefit from legislation that serves the general population, including SNAP and the Child and Adult Care Food Program (CACFP). CACFP provides meal and snack reimbursements to adult day care and senior centers that serve older adults who experience mental or physical impairments limiting daily activities.[129] Of households with at least one person over age 65, 8.3% participate in SNAP, including 9.2% of seniors living alone.[4] A far smaller proportion of eligible seniors participate in SNAP compared with the general eligible population, just 45% compared with 92% respectively. Mobility challenges, lack of information, difficulty completing the application, and stigma often act as barriers to participation for older adults.[130] In recognition of some of these limitations, additional legislation under the Older Americans Act also authorizes other nutrition programs for the elderly, including the Elderly Nutrition Program, which makes community-based meal services available to older adults through grants provided to states to fund group-setting and home-delivered meals. The meals, provided in churches, senior centers, adult day-care centers, as well as in participants' homes, must meet at least one-third of the recommended dietary allowances, but in practice often meet 40% to 50%.[131] Participants in Elderly Nutrition Program services must be at least 60 years old, and although there is no income eligibility requirement, services generally focus on older people with greatest economic and social need, including low-income seniors and seniors living in rural areas. The program often links to other community-based and in-home services that promote health among older adults.

Housing Policies and Energy Assistance Programs

Because many food-insecure households also experience energy and housing insecurity,[97] policies and programs that help with housing and utility costs can free up household resources to be spent on food. For low-income households with high energy costs, the Low-Income Heating and Energy Assistance Program (LIHEAP), administered by the Administration for Children and Families, provides grants to states to provide assistance with utility bills, weatherization services, and energy-related home repair to households under 150% of the federal poverty level.[132] Children whose families received LIHEAP were less likely to be at developmental risk, underweight, or hospitalized compared with children whose families did not receive energy assistance.[133] The three largest federal housing assistance programs, operated by the Department of Housing and Urban Development (HUD), are public housing, the housing choice voucher program, and the Low Income Housing Tax Credit (LIHTC). Public housing, in which residents live in buildings both owned/leased and subsidized by HUD, is the best known form of low-income housing. However, the voucher program and LIHTC have eclipsed it in size over the last few decades. The Housing Choice Voucher Program, formerly known as Section 8, assists recipients in paying rent in the private housing market. The Low Income Housing Tax Credit, the largest housing subsidy for low-income residents, is a provision of the Internal Revenue Code that offers tax-based financial incentives for investors to set aside a certain proportion of rental units for low-income tenants.[134] Because the number of families eligible for housing assistance far outstrips supply, a lottery system is in place to distribute both housing choice vouchers and public housing units; wait lists are often years long and have closed in many cities.[135] Compared with children living in subsidized housing, children whose families were wait-listed for a housing subsidy are more likely to be food insecure, underweight, and in poor health.[136] For households experiencing multiple hardships, co-enrollment in multiple benefits is associated with health benefits. For instance, young children whose families received WIC, SNAP, and a housing subsidy were less likely to be hospitalized or experience developmental risk.[137]

Healthcare Policy

The health consequences of food insecurity—including increased hospital-izations for children and seniors, exacerbation of chronic disease, and poor mental health—all are associated with increased healthcare costs that have been calculated to be at least $160 billion. An internal report created by the Research Training Institute for the National Commission on Hunger, a bi-partisan commission appointed by Congress to advise Congress and the United States Department of Agriculture on how to address hunger, found that food insecurity contributes to billions of extra dollars in Medicaid and Medicare spending, and that even a 10% reduction in food insecurity would decrease annual Medicaid expenditures by $1.3 billion and annual Medicare costs by more than $178 million.[138] The relationship between food insecu-rity and poor health can also be reciprocal: Not only does food insecurity in-crease healthcare costs, but healthcare costs often push families into poverty. In addition, families who experience food insecurity often describe how they may "trade off" seeking health care because they need money for food, or vice versa, an experience healthcare providers call "treat or eat."[31,85] Reduction in healthcare access for low-income families can have devastating consequences for food insecurity. Under the Affordable Care Act, nonprofit hospitals are required to engage in efforts improving community health to maintain their nonprofit status. New clarification states that addressing the social determi-nants of health [i.e., the conditions in which people are born, grow, live, work, and age that affect health and well-being], including food insecurity, counts toward this requirement, offering an opportunity for healthcare systems to address food insecurity among their patients and communities.

Civic Participation: How Professionals and Community Members Can Get Involved

The vast array of policies associated with treating food insecurity demon-strate how access to food crosses many sectors and policy arenas. On an even broader scale, the food industry itself has multiple stakeholders. There is no single government agency or sector that is responsible for ensuring our food system works efficiently from seed to table, effectively and sustainably. The food system includes five major areas: production, consumption, processing, distribution, and waste recycling. To address the gap in oversight of all these domains, local governments at the city, county, or regional level have begun to work with grassroots organizations. Some of these anti-hunger organi-zations, created to promote greater civic engagement on issues from local sustainability to access to food, helped to launch food policy councils to address policy-related food issues that cross all sectors. Food policy councils often create roadmaps for policy changes that can help to address a variety of goals, such as reducing food insecurity, creating more local sourcing of foods, shoring up emergency food supplies, addressing structural racism in access to food, creating more community gardens, and improving waste stream issues such as composting or identifying areas to prevent food waste.

The first food policy council of record launched in 1982 in Knoxville, Tennessee as a result of community action around hunger. In the 1980s, many new food policy councils emerged, addressing low wages in the farming and food industry, lack of access to food, and lack of opportunities for community members to engage with local government. Across the country, there are now almost 300 known food policy councils that have a variety of structures and many diverse and sometimes divergent goals.[139] The effectiveness of food policy councils varies, given that they often have few or no staff members and focus on "small wins" such as partnerships and contracts allowing school systems to source from locally grown foods and local businesses, completing food system assessments, and creating reports. They have no coordinated or consensus driven measure of outcomes.[140,141]

Sometimes, civic engagement occurs without government sanctioned involvement and support. Examples include "community food security" initiatives, where a variety of organizations may come together to create opportunities for community groups to address food security through raising awareness, helping to establish community gardens and community kitchens, or increasing access to local food markets or emergency food networks. These initiatives have helped to support greater access to SNAP benefits, or to supplement SNAP benefits to promote and increase access to fruits and vegetables.[142-144] These endeavors are usually driven by community organizations and have varying success in engaging families who are low income and who have experienced hunger firsthand.

One example of such civic engagement is Witnesses to Hunger, an ongoing advocacy program in which parents and caregivers who have firsthand experience with hunger and poverty share their expertise through photographs and written and oral testimony.[145,146] Beginning in 2008 in Philadelphia as a participatory action research program using the *Photovoice* methodology, Witnesses to Hunger has since grown to include several sites across the East Coast. Through photography, video, and written and oral commentary, members of Witnesses to Hunger share their experiences and hold elected officials accountable to their constituents on issues that impact family health and well-being, including access to healthful food, quality education, economic self-sufficiency, and living wages. Participants have displayed their photographs and spoken at over 30 exhibitions across the East Coast, including at the U.S. Senate, at the U.S. House of Representatives, and at multiple state capitol buildings and city halls. Members of Witnesses to Hunger frequently participate in media stories on hunger, poverty, housing, and other issues, including nutrition assistance policy or improvements to school nutrition programs. Witnesses to Hunger members also have spoken at forums, webinars, and panel discussions; have submitted written testimony that has been included in congressional hearings on poverty in the United States; and have been cited in the Congressional Record several times in Senate and House floor speeches. The members of Witnesses to Hunger regularly visit their elected representatives at the federal, state, and local levels. They speak out about the policy changes they want to see, and they are taking an active role in breaking the cycle of hunger and poverty (Box 7.3).

Other witnesses to experiences of hunger are healthcare professionals, who see the medical and health effects of food insecurity and hunger. Physicians and public health researchers documenting the experience of food insecurity,

---

BOX 7.3

Ask Joanna: What is it Like to Be a Member of Witnesses to Hunger?

It's a good way to get your voice out. Not even just your voice, but to be open and honest about what's real about the welfare system and all the other systems. It's a way to tell what really goes on, how things really work. If you can't speak out this week, how about next week? If you're afraid that someone might know who you are, you can be anonymous. When things were really bad with me, I didn't know what I was doing from one minute to the next. I couldn't even figure out what was wrong at that time, let alone how to fix it. If I couldn't fix me, how could I fix the whole system? After I was out of that situation, I felt like I could start speaking up. The worst of it was over and I could breathe now and think straight. We could take a bath and flush toilets and turn the stove on and cook a dinner in peace. I could leave my kids in the other room and know that they were safe; there wasn't something there to harm them. Now I could speak up and be a voice for some other mother who can't.

such as Children's HealthWatch, have been advocating for years to encourage the medical community to engage in efforts to screen for and refer for food insecurity (see Example in Practice).[147]

Example in Practice
Taking Action in a Healthcare Setting

An important strategy for addressing food insecurity in community settings involves identifying individuals and families at risk of food insecurity at the places they visit regularly and quickly connecting them to food assistance and other resources. In 2014, the American Academy of Pediatrics recommended that all pediatricians screen families for food insecurity during office visits and refer families at risk to necessary resources.[148] Several pediatric clinics across the country have begun screening people for food insecurity, with some offering referral to community resources.[149,150] In one example, at the Children's Hospital of Philadelphia, three primary care clinics implemented this screening for families of children under 5 years of age, using a two-item screener called the "Hunger Vital Sign" developed by Hager et al and based off of the Household Food Security Survey Module.[151] Families screening positive were then referred to an outreach organization for connection to public benefits and community resources.

Screener Questions:

1. Within the past 12 months, we worried whether our food would run out before we got money to buy more. (*Often, sometimes,* or *never true*)
2. Within the past 12 months, the food we bought just didn't last and we didn't have money to get more. (*Often, sometimes,* or *never true*)

Additionally, during the AIDS crisis in the 1980s and 1990s, community organizations and health professionals recognized the need for food delivery for medically compromised individuals. Examples include Manna in Philadelphia, God's Love We Deliver in New York City, and Community Servings in Boston. People with disabilities or multiple debilitating health conditions have an increased risk for hunger and poor nutrition status. As described earlier, homebound seniors often rely on home-delivered meal programs such as Meals on Wheels, which have been shown to improve seniors' nutritional intake and reduce healthcare costs.[152–158] Recognizing the medical necessity of food, some Medicare Advantage plans cover the cost of home-delivered meals, although this mechanism is not widely available. In addition, some physicians are taking matters into their own hands, making space for food pantries in their hospitals and clinics, or offering home-delivered meals for low-income people with diabetes, kidney disease, heart failure, AIDS, or other health conditions.[159]

Undergraduate students also can get involved in addressing hunger (Box 7.4). Research over the past several years has revealed that college students have significant rates of food insecurity in all types of colleges and universities—from Hawaii to New York, from rural to urban, from public to private, and from two-year to four-year colleges.[160–164] Food-insecure college students are more likely to struggle to afford textbooks and to miss or drop classes.[164] The USDA limits SNAP eligibility to college students who are working more than 20 hours per week, who are single caregivers of a young child, and who meet other highly restricted criteria. To address the gap in resources, college students have started to take matters into their own hands, creating food cupboards and pantries on campus, organizing ways to exchange meal card swipes to help low-income students, and planning conferences and summits to educate themselves and their college administrations. Not only do college and university students seek to help their fellow students, they also engage in community-based efforts to reduce food insecurity by working with their dining halls to donate leftover foods to soup kitchens and pantries, and they engage with other endeavors by volunteering in anti-hunger organizations or at community cafés.

Many different groups can become engaged in efforts to address food insecurity and hunger, including individuals, grassroots organizations,

---

BOX 7.4

Ask Joanna: What Should Students and Others Know About Addressing Food Insecurity?

Dealing with hunger is a really big and tough issue. It's not going to be easy. It's not going to change overnight. It's not going to change in a day, in a week, in a year. If you don't completely and wholeheartedly want to do it for the long-term, then find a food bank, or a soup kitchen—something for right now. But if you're going to join our advocacy, stick with it and be about it.

government at all levels, elders, healthcare providers, the healthcare financing industry, hospital administrators, grassroots activists, and students.

The Way Forward, a Rights-Based Approach

Although public assistance programs may buffer families from the health effects of severe deprivation, these programs alone cannot help families break the cycle of hunger and poverty. Given a public health, ecological approach that recognizes the institutional-level, systems-level, and policy-level factors associated with food insecurity, it is clear the United States must take broader, more systematic approaches to understanding and addressing food insecurity.

A human rights approach to food, according to the United Nations Economic and Social Council, aims to ensure that every person, alone or in community with others, has physical and economic access at all times to adequate food or means for its procurement. The right to food does not necessarily require governments to provide food directly. Rather, it obligates governments to respect the right (not prevent people from obtaining food), protect the right (ensure others do not prevent people from obtaining food), and fulfill the right (provide what is necessary for people to nourish themselves).[165] Viewing food security as a human rights issue means that ensuring good nutrition should not be left to benevolence or charity, but instead should be viewed as a duty and obligation of a country to its people.

The United States has not yet ratified the international covenant that covers the right to food, nor has it agreed with the rest of the international community that food is a basic human right.[166] However, food insecurity can and should be addressed with a rights framework. A rights approach demands that we place special emphasis on experiences of discrimination, and ensure that rights holders—meaning all of us—have an opportunity to demand our rights through participation in decision-making related to our security and well-being. Civic engagement can help to mobilize ordinary citizens, experts, and policymakers alike to create meaningful policy solutions that can reduce and ultimately put an end to food insecurity.[166] Such civic engagement can range from taking action to support people in our own surroundings in accessing food, to engaging with local food policy boards, engaging in advocacy around labor, nutrition, housing, and other supports, and demanding better, more accountable programming at all levels of government.

Remember Joanna Cruz's experiences. When she was living without running water, made little money, and suffered from depression, many of the circumstances of her life were beyond her control, leaving her little opportunity to participate in the national dialogue on hunger and poverty. Over the years, she has gained more stable employment and learned of opportunities to speak out. Through Witnesses to Hunger, she has engaged in local debates about hunger and poverty, had her photographs and testimonies featured in Congress, spoken directly to television, radio, and print news about her experiences, and has testified about the importance of SNAP benefits and work supports for her family in front of the National Commission on Hunger.[107] Her experience demonstrates that we all can get engaged on issues of poverty and hunger, and we all have the wisdom and expertise to insist on a healthier, more just life.

Conclusions

In this chapter we have covered the definition and distribution of food insecurity, focusing on the widespread racial, ethnic, gender, and other disparities in rates of hardship. We also have focused on how food insecurity affects the health and well-being of children, adults, and seniors, with problems such as poor overall physical health, diabetes, suicidal ideation, depression, and poor behavioral health. These problems are associated with poor school performance, increased yet avoidable healthcare costs and hospitalizations, lost days at work, and reduced income. Overall, food insecurity is a health, social, and political condition that is unnecessary and avoidable. It is an affront to the highest international standards for basic human rights and fundamental freedoms. Students and young people have the opportunity to engage, not only on their campuses, but also in their surrounding communities, as well as through direct engagement with those who have experienced hunger firsthand. Civic engagement goes far beyond voting to include volunteering and regularly advocating at the local, regional, and national level for better policies and programs that protect and promote resilience, good nutrition, and health. We have provided only a few examples here, but this kind of engagement can be carried forward in almost every profession. Even outside of health-related fields, all of us can find opportunities to create just social, economic, and political systems that provide all with the opportunity to control their own lives, to contribute to society, and to flourish.

Discussion Questions

(1) Describe how food insecurity is a significant public health problem. Is it a symptom of other public health or social issues? Or should it be something that is considered on its own?

(2) What are some ways in which public health professionals can be involved in addressing food insecurity? What is their obligation to engage?

Quiz Questions

1. Explain how the experience of Joanna Cruz and her family mirrors the importance of taking a systemic and an interpersonal approach to food insecurity.
2. What is the definition of food insecurity?
3. Describe the kinds of trade-offs people who are food insecure make, and why these trade-offs may have negative consequences for health.
4. What are some of the mechanisms through which food insecurity is associated with poor health?
5. What is the life course approach to food insecurity and why is it important?
6. Name three to five groups that are especially vulnerable to food insecurity and describe why.
7. What is the farm bill, and why is it important in setting food-related policy?
8. How did WIC start and what are its major goals?
9. Describe three ways in which health professionals can get involved in addressing food insecurity and hunger.
10. How would increasing the minimum wage and establishing consistent work hours have an impact on food insecurity and health? What groups would this help the most, and who might be left out?

References

1. Dréze J, Sen AK. *Hunger and Public Action.* Clarendon Press; 1989.
2. Cook J., Poblacion A. *Estimating the Health-Related Costs of Food Insecurity and Hunger, Appendix 2.* In 2016 Hunger Report: the Nourishing Effect: ending Hunger, Improving Health, and Reducing Inequality, Bread for the World Institute; 2016.

3. Coleman-Jensen A, Rabbit MP, Gregory C, Singh A. *Statistical Supplement to Household Food Security in the United States in 2015.* U.S. Department of Agriculture, Economic Research Service; 2016.

4. Coleman-Jensen A, Rabbitt MP, Gregory CA, Singh A. *Household Food Security in the United States in 2015.* U.S. Department of Agriculture, Economic Research Service; 2016.

5. Rose-Jacobs R, Black MM, Casey PH, et al. Household food insecurity: associations with at-risk infant and toddler development. *Pediatrics.* 2008;121(1):65–72.

6. Skalicky A, Meyers AF, Adams WG, Yang Z, Cook JT, Frank DA. Child food insecurity and iron-deficiency anemia in low-income infants and toddlers in the United States. *Matern Child Health J.* 2006;10(2):177–185.

7. Alaimo K, Olson CM, Frongillo EA, Jr. Family food insufficiency is associated with dysthymia and suicidal symptoms in adolescents: results from NHANES III. *Journal of Nutrition.* 2002;132:719–725.

8. Seligman HK, Bindman AB, Vittinghoff E, Kanaya AM, Kushel MB. Food insecurity is associated with diabetes mellitus: results from the National Health Examination and Nutrition Examination Survey (NHANES) 1999–2002. *Journal of General Internal Medicine.* 2007;22(7):1018–1023.

9. Adams EJ, Grummer-Strawn L, Chavez G. Food insecurity is associated with increased risk of obesity in California women. *Journal of Nutrition.* 2003;133(4):1070–1074.

10. Gundersen C. Measuring the extent, depth, and severity of food insecurity: an application to American Indians in the USA. *Journal of Population Economics.* 2008;21(1):191–215.

11. Pardilla M, Prasad D, Suratkar S, Gittelsohn J. High levels of household food insecurity on the Navajo Nation. *Public Health Nutrition.* 2014;17(01):58–65.

12. Blue Bird Jernigan V, Salvatore AL, Styne DM, Winkleby M. Addressing food insecurity in a Native American reservation using community-based participatory research. *Health Education Research.* 2012;27(4):645–655.

13. Chilton M, Black MM, Berkowitz C, et al. Food insecurity and risk of poor health among US-born children of immigrants. *Am J Public Health.* 2009;99(3):556–562.

14. Van Hook J, Balistreri KS. Ineligible parents, eligible children: Food Stamps receipt, allotments, and food insecurity among children of immigrants. *Social Science Research.* 2006;35(1):228–251.

15. Hill BG, Moloney AG, Mize T, Himelick T, Guest JL. Prevalence and predictors of food insecurity in migrant farmworkers in Georgia. *Am J Public Health.* 2011;101(5):831–833.

16. Research Triangle Institute. *Food Insecurity among LGBT Communities and Individuals.* Unpublished; 2015.

17. Gates GJ. *Food Insecurity and SNAP (Food Stamps) Participation in LGBT Communities.* Williams Institute, UCLA School of Law; 2014.

18. Family Equality Council and Center for American Progress. *All Children Matter: How Legal and Social Inequalities Hurt LGBT Families.* 2011.

19. Quintana NS, Rosenthal J, Krehely J. *On the Streets: The Federal Response to Gay and Transgender Homeless Youth.* Center for American Progress; 2010.

20. Corliss HL, Goodenow CS, Nichols L, Austin SB. High burden of homelessness among sexual-minority adolescents: findings from a representative Massachusetts high school sample. *Am J Public Health.* 2011;101(9):1683–1689.

21. Kaeble D, Glaze L. *Correctional Populations in the United States, 2015.* Bureau of Justice Statistics, U.S. Department of Justice; 2016.

22. Alexander M. *The New Jim Crow: Mass Incarceration in the Age of Colorblindness.* The New Press; 2012.

23. The Sentencing Project. *Fact Sheet: Trends in U.S. Corrections.* 2015.

24. Wang EA, Zhu GA, Evans L, Carroll-Scott A, Desai R, Fiellin LE. A pilot study examining food insecurity and HIV risk behaviors among individuals recently released from prison. *AIDS Education and Prevention.* 2013;25(2):112–123.

25. Turney K. Paternal incarceration and children's food insecurity: a consideration of variation and mechanisms. *Social Service Review.* 2015;89(2):335–367.

26. Cox R, Wallace S. Identifying the link between food security and incarceration. *Southern Economic Journal.* 2016;82(4):1062–1077. doi:10.1002/soej.12080

27. Coleman-Jensen A, Nord M. *Disability is an Important Risk Factor for Food Insecurity.* U.S. Department of Agriculture (USDA), Economic Research Service (ERS); 2013.

28. Brucker DL, Coleman-Jensen A. Food insecurity across the adult life span for persons with disabilities. *Journal of Disability Policy Studies.* 2017:1044207317710701.

29. Coleman-Jensen A, Nord M. *Food Insecurity among Households with Working-Age Adults with Disabilities.* Economic Research Service, U.S. Department of Agriculture; 2013.

30. Rose-Jacobs R, Fiore JG, de Cuba SE, et al. Children with special health care needs, supplemental security income, and food insecurity. *Journal of Developmental and Behavioral Pediatrics.* 2016;37(2):140–147.

31. Berkowitz SA, Seligman HK, Choudhry NK. Treat or eat: food insecurity, cost-related medication underuse, and unmet needs. *Am J Med.* 2014;127(4):303–310 e303.

32. Bailey ZD, Krieger N, Agénor M, Graves J, Linos N, Bassett MT. Structural racism and health inequities in the USA: evidence and interventions. *The Lancet.* 2017;389(10077):1453–1463.

33. Jones CP. Confronting institutionalized racism. *Phylon (1960-).* 2002:7–22.

34. Dunbar-Ortiz R. *An Indigenous Peoples' History of the United States.* Vol 3: Beacon Press; 2014.

35. Capps R, Koball H, Campetella A, Perreira K, Hooker S, Pedroza JM. *Implications of Immigration Enforcement Activities for the Well-Being of Children in Immigrant Families.* The Urban Institute and the Migration Policy Institute; 2015.

36. Livingston NA, Heck NC, Flentje A, Gleason H, Oost KM, Cochran BN. Sexual minority stress and suicide risk: identifying resilience through personality profile analysis. *Psychol Sex Orientat Gend Divers.* 2015;2(3):321–328.

37. Human Rights Campaign, Trans People of Color. *Addressing Anti-Transgender Violence: Exploring Realities, Challenges and Solutions for Policy Makers and Community Advocates.* 2017.

38. Purtle J. Felon disenfranchisement in the United States: a health equity perspective. *Am J Public Health.* 2013;103(4):632–637.

39. Cook JT, Frank DA, Berkowitz C, et al. Food insecurity is associated with adverse health outcomes among human infants and toddlers. *Journal of Nutrition.* 2004;134(6):1432–1438.

40. Casey PH, Szeto KL, Robbins JM, et al. Child health-related quality of life and household food security. *Arch Pediatr Adolesc Med.* 2005;159(1):51–56.

41. Skalicky A, Meyers AF, Adams WG, Yang Z, Cook JT, Frank DA. Child food insecurity and iron-deficiency anemia in low-income infants and toddlers in the United States. *Matern Child Health J.* 2006;10(2):177–185.

42. Chilton M, Chyatte M, Breaux J. The negative effects of poverty & food insecurity on child development. *Indian J Med Res.* 2007;126(4):262–272.

43. Zaslow M, Bronte-Tinkew J, Capps R, Horowitz A, Moore KA, Weinstein D. Food security during infancy: implications for attachment and mental proficiency in toddlerhood. *Matern Child Health J.* 2009;13(1):66–80.

44. Bronte-Tinkew J, Zaslow M, Capps R, Horowitz A, McNamara M. Food insecurity works through depression, parenting, and infant feeding to influence overweight and health in toddlers. *Journal of Nutrition.* 2007;137(9):2160–2165.

45. Hernandez DC, Jacknowitz A. Transient, but not persistent, adult food insecurity influences toddler development. *Journal of Nutrition.* 2009;139(8):1517–1524.

46. Heckman JJ. Skill formation and the economics of investing in disadvantaged children. *Science.* 2006;312(5782):1900–1902.

47. Shankar P, Chung R, Frank DA. Association of food insecurity with children's behavioral, emotional, and academic outcomes: a systematic review. *Journal of Developmental & Behavioral Pediatrics.* 2017;38(2):135–150.

48. Alaimo K, Olson CM, Frongillo EA, Jr. Food insufficiency and American school-aged children's cognitive, academic, and psychosocial development. *Pediatrics.* 2001;108(1):44–53.

49. Jyoti DF, Frongillo EA, Jones SJ. Food insecurity affects school children's academic performance, weight gain, and social skills. *Journal of Nutrition.* 2005;135(12):2831–2839.

50. Howard LL. Does food insecurity at home affect non-cognitive performance at school? A longitudinal analysis of elementary student classroom behavior. *Economics of Education Review.* 2011;30(1):157–176.

51. Kleinman RE, Murphy JM, Little M, et al. Hunger in children in the United States: potential behavioral and emotional correlates. *Pediatrics.* 1998;101(1):E3.

52. Weinreb L, Wehler C, Perloff J, et al. Hunger: Its impact on children's health and mental health. *Pediatrics.* 2002;110(4):e41.

53. Murphy JM, Wehler CA, Pagano ME, Little M, Kleinman RE, Jellinek MS. Relationship between hunger and psychosocial functioning in low-income American children. *J Am Acad Child Adolesc Psychiatry.* 1998;37(2):163–170.

54. Melchior M, Caspi A, Howard LM, et al. Mental health context of food insecurity: a representative cohort of families with young children. *Pediatrics.* 2009;124(4):e564–e572.

55. Bhattacharya J, Currie J, Haider S. Poverty, food insecurity, and nutritional outcomes in children and adults. *Journal of Health Economics.* 2004;23(4):839–862.

56. Gundersen C, Kreider B. Bounding the effects of food insecurity on children's health outcomes. *Journal of Health Economics.* 2009;28(5):971–983.

57. Alaimo K, Olson C.M., Frongillo EA, Jr., Briefel RR. Food insufficiency, family income, and health in U.S. preschool and school-age children. *Am J Public Health.* 2001;91:781–786.

58. Gundersen C, Garasky S, Lohman BJ. Food insecurity is not associated with childhood obesity as assessed using multiple measures of obesity. *Journal of Nutrition.* 2009;139(6):1173–1178.

59. Eisenmann JC, Gundersen C, Lohman BJ, Garasky S, Stewart SD. Is food insecurity related to overweight and obesity in children and adolescents? A summary of studies, 1995–2009. *Obesity Reviews: An Official Journal of the International Association for the Study of Obesity.* 2011;12(5):e73–e83.

60. Hamelin AM, Habicht JP, Beaudry M. Food insecurity: consequences for the household and broader social implications. *Journal of Nutrition.* 1999;129(2S Suppl):525S–528S.

61. Rose D, Oliveira V. Nutrient intakes of individuals from food-insufficient households in the United States. *Am J Public Health.* 1997;87(12):1956–1961.

62. Radimer K, Olson C, Green J, Campbell CC, Habicht JP. Understanding hunger and developing indicators to assess it in women and children. *Journal of Nutrition Education.* 1992;24:36S–44S.

63. Fram MS, Frongillo EA, Jones SJ, et al. Children are aware of food insecurity and take responsibility for managing food resources. *Journal of Nutrition.* 2011;141(6):1114–1149.

64. Braveman P, Barclay C. Health disparities beginning in childhood: A life-course perspective. *Pediatrics.* 2009;124(Suppl. 3).

65. Shonkoff JP, Boyce WT, McEwen BS. Neuroscience, molecular biology, and the childhood roots of health disparities: Building a new framework for health promotion and disease prevention. *Journal of the American Medical Association.* 2009;301(21):2252–2259.

66. Whitaker RC, Phillips SM, Orzol SM. Food insecurity and the risks of depression and anxiety in mothers and behavior problems in their preschool-aged children. *Pediatrics.* 2006;118(3):e859–e868.

67. Casey P, Goolsby S, Berkowitz C, et al. Maternal depression, changing public assistance, food security, and child health status. *Pediatrics.* 2004;113(2):298–304.

68. Huddleston-Casas C, Charnigo R, Simmons LA. Food insecurity and maternal depression in rural, low-income families: a longitudinal investigation. *Public Health Nutr.* 2009;12(8):1133–1140.

69. Laraia BA, Siega-Riz AM, Gundersen C, Dole N. Psychosocial factors and socioeconomic indicators are associated with household food insecurity among pregnant women. *Journal of Nutrition.* 2006;136(1):177–182.

70. Heflin CM, Siefert K, Williams DR. Food insufficiency and women's mental health: findings from a 3-year panel of welfare recipients. *Social Science & Medicine.* 2005;61(9):1971–1982.

71. Coleman-Jensen A. Working for peanuts: nonstandard work and food insecurity across household structure. *Journal of Family and Economic Issues.* 2011;32:84–97.

72. Davison KM, Marshall-Fabien GL, Tecson A. Association of moderate and severe food insecurity with suicidal ideation in adults: national survey data from three Canadian provinces. *Soc Psychiatry Psychiatr Epidemiol.* 2015;50(6):963–972.

73. Hernandez DC, Marshall A, Mineo C. Maternal depression mediates the association between intimate partner violence and food insecurity. *Journal of Women's Health.* 2014;23(1):29–37.

74. Montgomery BE, Rompalo A, Hughes J, et al. Violence against women in selected areas of the United States. *Am J Public Health.* 2015(0):e1–e11.

75. Hernandez DC, Marshall A, Mineo C. Maternal depression mediates the association between intimate partner violence and food insecurity. *Journal of Women's Health.* 2014;23(1):29–37.

76. Wehler C, Weinreb LF, Huntington N, et al. Risk and protective factors for adult and child hunger among low-income housed and homeless female-headed families. *Am J Public Health.* 2004;94(1):109–115.

77. Chilton MM, Rabinowich JR, Woolf NH. Very low food security in the USA is linked with exposure to violence. *Public Health Nutr.* 2014;17(1):73–82.

78. Sun J, Knowles M, Patel F, Frank D, Heeren T, Chilton M. Childhood adversity and adult reports of food insecurity among households with children. *American Journal of Preventive Medicine.* 2016;50(5):561–572.

79. Kirkpatrick SI, Tarasuk V. Food insecurity is associated with nutrient inadequacies among Canadian adults and adolescents. *Journal of Nutrition.* 2008;138(3):604–612.

80. Leung CW, Epel ES, Ritchie LD, Crawford PB, Laraia BA. Food insecurity is inversely associated with diet quality of lower-income adults. *J Acad Nutr Diet.* 2014;114(12):1943–1953. e1942.

81. Rose D. Economic determinants and dietary consequences of food insecurity in the United States. *Journal of Nutrition.* 1999;129(2S Suppl):517S–520S.

82. Seligman HK, Laraia BA, Kushel MB. Food insecurity is associated with chronic disease among low-income NHANES participants. *Journal of Nutrition.* 2010;140(2):304–310.

83. Shalowitz M, Eng J, McKinney C, et al. Food security is related to adult type 2 diabetes control over time in a United States safety net primary care clinic population. *Nutrition & Diabetes.* 2017;7(5):e277.

84. Anema A, Vogenthaler N, Frongillo EA, Kadiyala S, Weiser SD. Food insecurity and HIV/AIDS: current knowledge, gaps, and research priorities. *Curr HIV/AIDS Rep.* 2009;6(4):224–231.

85. Seligman HK, Davis TC, Schillinger D, Wolf MS. Food insecurity is associated with hypoglycemia and poor diabetes self-management in a low-income sample with diabetes. *J Health Care Poor Underserved.* 2010;21(4):1227–1233.

86. Simmons LA, Modesitt SC, Brody AC, Leggin AB. Food insecurity among cancer patients in Kentucky: a pilot study. *Journal of Oncology Practice.* 2006;2(6):274–279.

87. Olson CM, Strawderman MS. The relationship between food insecurity and obesity in rural childbearing women. *Journal of Rural Health.* 2008;24(1):60–66.

88. Jones SJ, Frongillo EA. Food insecurity and subsequent weight gain in women. *Public Health Nutr.* 2007;10(2):145–151.

89. Pan L, Sherry B, Njai R, Blanck HM. Food insecurity is associated with obesity among US adults in 12 states. *J Acad Nutr Diet.* 2012;112(9):1403–1409.

90. Dinour LM, Bergen D, Yeh MC. The food insecurity-obesity paradox: a review of the literature and the role food stamps may play. *Journal of the American Dietetic Association.* 2007;107(11):1952–1961.

91. Ziliak JP, Gundersen C. Multigenerational families and food insecurity. *Southern Economic Journal.* 2016;82(4):1147–1166.

92. Lee JS, Frongillo EA. Nutritional and health consequences are associated with food insecurity among US elderly persons. *Journal of Nutrition.* 2001;131(5):1503–1509.

93. Lee JS, Frongillo EA, Jr. Factors associated with food insecurity among U.S. elderly persons: importance of functional impairments. *J Gerontol B Psychol Sci Soc Sci.* 2001;56(2):S94–S99.

94. Kim K, Frongillo EA. Participation in food assistance programs modifies the relation of food insecurity with weight and depression in elders. *Journal of Nutrition.* 2007;137(4):1005–1010.

95. Lee JS, Frongillo E.A, Jr. Nutritional and health consequences are associated with food insecurity among U.S. elderly persons. *Journal of Nutrition.* 2001;131(5):1503–1509.

96. Cutts DB, Meyers AF, Black MM, et al. US Housing insecurity and the health of very young children. *Am J Public Health.* 2011;101(8):1508–1514.

97. Frank DA, Casey PH, Black MM, et al. Cumulative hardship and wellness of low-income, young children: multisite surveillance study. *Pediatrics.* 2010;125(5):e1115–e1123.

98. Bengle R, Sinnett S, Johnson T, Johnson MA, Brown A, Lee JS. Food insecurity is associated with cost-related medication non-adherence in community-dwelling, low-income older adults in Georgia. *J Nutr Elder.* 2010;29(2):170–191.

99. Cook JT, Frank DA, Casey PH, et al. A brief indicator of household energy security: associations with food security, child health, and child development in US infants and toddlers. *Pediatrics*. 2008;122(4).

100. Chavkin W, Wise PH. The data are in: health matters in welfare policy. *Am J Public Health*. 2002;92(9):1392–1395.

101. Romero D, Chavkin W, Wise P, Hess C, VanLandeghem K. State welfare reform policies and maternal and child health services: a national study. *Matern Child Health J*. 2001;5(3):199–206.

102. Chilton M, Rabinowich J, Breen A, Gaines-Turner T. On the fringe: how alternative financial services are related to household food insecurity. American Public Health Association, Annual Meeting, 2012; 2012.

103. Edin K, Boyd, M., Mabli, J., Ohls, J., Worthington, J., Greene, S., Redel, N., Sridharan, S. *SNAP Food Security In-Depth Interview Study*. U.S. Department of Agriculture, Food and Nutrition Service, Office of Research and Analysis; 2013.

104. Kempson K, Keenan DP, Sadani PS, Adler A. Maintaining food sufficiency: coping strategies identified by limited-resource individuals versus nutrition educators. *Journal of Nutrition Education and Behavior*. 2003;35(4):179–188.

105. Chilton M, Rabinowich J, Breen AB, Mouzon S. When the systems fail: individual and household coping strategies related to child hunger. Paper commissioned by the National Academy of Sciences Workshop on Research Gaps and Opportunities on the Causes and Consequences of Child Hunger. Committee on National Statistics, National Academy of Sciences. Food and Nutrition Board, Institute of Medicine, April 8–9, 2013.

106. Department of Health and Human Services OoDPaP. Healthy People 2020. https://www.healthypeople.gov/2020/topics-objectives/topic/nutrition-and-weight-status/objectives

107. National Commission on Hunger. *Freedom from Hunger: An Achievable Goal for the United States of America*. 2015.

108. Interagency Working Group on Food. *U.S. Action Plan on Food Security: Solutions To Hunger*. U.S. Dept. of Agriculture, Foreign Agricultural Service; 1999.

109. Bureau of Labor Statistics, U.S. Department of Labor. Household data annual averages. Table 1. Employment status of the civilian noninstitutional population, 1944 to date. n.d.; http://www.bls.gov/cps/cpsaat01.pdf. Accessed November 12, 2015.

110. Nord M, Coleman-Jensen A, Andrews M, Carlson S. *Household Food Security in the United States, 2009*. Economic Research Service; 2010.

111. Acemoglu D, Autor D, Dorn D, Hanson GH, Price B. Import competition and the great U.S. employment sag of the 2000s. 2014; http://economics.mit.edu/files/9811.

112. Autor DH, Dorn D. The growth of low-skill service jobs and the polarization of the US labor market. *Am Econ Rev*. 2013;103(5):1553–1597.

113. Romero D, Chavkin W, Wise PH, Smith LA, Wood PR. Welfare to work? Impact of maternal health on employment. *Am J Public Health*. 2002;92(9):1462–1468.

114. Hill HD. Paid sick leave and job stability. *Work Occup.* 2013;40(2).

115. Rosenbaum D. *The Relationship Between SNAP and Work Among Low-Income Households*. Center on Budget and Policy Priorities; 2013.

116. Nord M, Coleman AL. Food insecurity after leaving SNAP. *Journal of Hunger & Environmental Nutrition*. 2010;5(4):434–453.

117. Ettinger de Cuba S, Harker L, Weiss I, Scully K, Chilton MM, Coleman S. *Punishing Hard Work: The Unintended Consequences of Cutting SNAP Benefits*. Available at http://www.childrenshealthwatch.org/publication/punishing-hard-work-unintended-consequences-cutting-snap-benefits/2013.

118. Coleman-Jensen A. Working for peanuts: nonstandard work and food insecurity across household structure. *J Fam Econ Iss*. 2011;32:84–97.

119. United States Department of Agriculture. *Building a Healthy America: A Profile of the Supplemental Nutrition Assistance Program*. Food and Nutrition Service; 2012.

120. Renwick T, Fox L. *The Supplemental Poverty Measure: 2015*. U.S. Census Bureau; 2016.

121. Frank DA, Chilton M, Casey PH, et al. Nutritional-assistance programs play a critical role in reducing food insecurity. *Pediatrics*. 2010;125(5):e1267; author reply e1267–e1268.

122. Almond D, Hoynes HW, Schanzenbach DW. Inside the war on poverty: The impact of food stamps on birth outcomes. *The Review of Economics and Statistics*. 2011;93(2):387–403.

123. Ettinger de Cuba S, Weiss I, Pasquariello J, et al. *The SNAP Vaccine: Boosting Children's Health*. Children's HealthWatch; 2012.

124. Institute of Medicine, National Research Council. *Supplemental Nutrition Assistance Program: Examining the Evidence to Define Benefit Adequacy*. 2013.

125. Breen A, Cahill R, Ettinger de Cuba S, Cook J, Chilton M. *The Real Cost of a Healthy Diet: 2011*. Children's HealthWatch; 2011.

126. Metallinos-Katsaras E, Gorman K, Wilde P, Kallio J. A longitudinal study of WIC participation on household food insecurity. *Matern Child Health J*. 2011;15(5):627–633.

127. Black MM, Cutts DB, Frank DA, et al. Special Supplemental Nutrition Program for Women, Infants, and Children participation and infants' growth and health: a multisite surveillance study. *Pediatrics*. 2004;114(1):169–176.

128. Jackson MI. Early childhood WIC participation, cognitive development and academic achievement. *Social Science & Medicine*. 2015;126C:145–153.

129. U.S. Department of Agriculture FaNS. Child and Adult Care Food Program (CACFP): Adult Day Care Centers. 2017; https://www.fns.usda.gov/cacfp/adult-day-care-centers. Accessed April 14, 2017.

130. U.S. Department of Agriculture FaNS. *Engaging Special Populations*. 2016.

131. U.S. Department of Health and Human Services AfCL. *Older Americans Act Nutrition Programs*. 2016.

132. Administration for Children and Families OoCS. LIHEAP Fact Sheet. 2016; https://www.acf.hhs.gov/ocs/resource/liheap-fact-sheet-0.   Accessed   April 14, 2017.

133. Frank DA, Neault NB, Skalicky A, et al. Heat or eat: the Low Income Home Energy Assistance Program and nutritional and health risks among children less than 3 years of age. *Pediatrics.* 2006;118(5):e1293–e1302.

134. Schwartz AF. *Housing policy in the United States.* Routledge; 2014.

135. Currie JM. *The Invisible Safety Net: Protecting the Nation's Poor Children and Families.* Princeton University Press; 2006.

136. March EL, Ettinger de Cuba S, Gayman A, et al. *Rx for Hunger: Affordable Housing.* Children's HealthWatch and Medical-Legal Partnership Boston; 2009.

137. March E, Cook JT, Ettinger de Cuba S, Gayman A, Frank DA. *Healthy Families in Hard Times: Solutions for Multiple Family Hardships.* Children's HealthWatch; 2010.

138. Yarnoff B, Anater A. *Research to Support Potential Recommendations of the National Commission on Hunger to Reduce Very Low Food Security: Estimating the Potential Impact of Reductions in Very Low Food Insecurity on Medicaid and Medicare Costs.* Research Triangle Institute; 2015.

139. Harper A, Shattuck A, Holt-Giménez A, Lambrick F. Food policy councils: lessons learned. 2009; https://foodfirst.org/publication/food-policy-councils-lessons-learned/. Accessed March 11, 2017.

140. Calancie L, Allen NE, Weiner BJ, Ng SW, Ward DS, Ammerman A. Food policy council self-assessment tool: development, testing, and results. *Prev Chronic Dis.* 2017;14:E20.

141. Clayton ML, Frattaroli S, Palmer A, Pollack KM. The role of partnerships in U.S. Food Policy Council policy activities. *PLoS One.* 2015;10(4):e0122870.

142. Roncarolo F, Adam C, Bisset S, Potvin L. Traditional and alternative community food security interventions in Montreal, Quebec: different practices, different people. *J Community Health.* 2015;40(2):199–207.

143. Roncarolo F, Adam C, Bisset S, Potvin L. Food capacities and satisfaction in participants in food security community interventions in Montreal, Canada. *Health Promot Int.* 2016;31(4):879–887.

144. McCullum C, Desjardins E, Kraak VI, Ladipo P, Costello H. Evidence-based strategies to build community food security. *J Am Diet Assoc.* 2005;105(2):278–283.

145. Knowles M, Rabinowich J, Gaines-Turner T, Chilton M. Witnesses to Hunger: Methods for photovoice and participatory action research in public health. *Human Organization.* 2015;74(3).

146. Chilton M, Rabinowich J, Council C, Breaux J. Witnesses to hunger: Participation through photovoice to ensure the right to food. *Health and Human Rights.* 2009;11(1):73–86.

147. Ashbrook A, Hartline-Grafton H, Dolins J, Davis J, Watson C. *Addressing Food Insecurity: A Toolkit for Pediatricians.* American Academy of Pediatrics & Food Research and Action Council; 2017.

148. Council on Community Pediatrics Committee on Nutrition. Promoting food security for all children. *Pediatrics.* 2015;136(5):e1431–e1438.

149. Barnidge E, LaBarge G, Krupsky K, Arthur J. Screening for food insecurity in pediatric clinical settings: opportunities and barriers. *J Community Health.* 2016:1–7.

150. Adams E, Hargunani D, Hoffmann L, Blaschke G, Helm J, Koehler A. Screening for food insecurity in pediatric primary care: a clinic's positive implementation experiences. *J Health Care Poor Underserved.* 2017;28(1):24–29.

151. Hager ER, Quigg AM, Black MM, et al. Development and validity of a 2-item screen to identify families at risk for food insecurity. *Pediatrics.* 2010;126(1):e26–e32.

152. Thomas KS, Mor V. Providing more home-delivered meals is one way to keep older adults with low care needs out of nursing homes. *Health Affairs (Project Hope).* 2013;32(10):1796–1802.

153. Sahyoun NR, Vaudin A. Home-delivered meals and nutrition status among older adults. *Nutr Clin Pract.* 2014;29(4):459–465.

154. An R. Association of home-delivered meals on daily energy and nutrient intakes: findings from the National Health and Nutrition Examination Surveys. *J Nutr Gerontol Geriatr.* 2015;34(2):263–272.

155. Campbell AD, Godfryd A, Buys DR, Locher JL. Does participation in home-delivered meals programs improve outcomes for older adults? Results of a systematic review. *J Nutr Gerontol Geriatr.* 2015;34(2):124–167.

156. Cho J, Thorud JL, Marishak-Simon S, Frawley L, Stevens AB. A model home-delivered meals program to support transitions from hospital to home. *J Nutr Gerontol Geriatr.* 2015;34(2):207–217.

157. Frongillo EA, Wolfe WS. Impact of participation in home-delivered meals on nutrient intake, dietary patterns, and food insecurity of older persons in New York state. *J Nutr Elder.* 2010;29(3):293–310.

158. Tappenden KA, Quatrara B, Parkhurst ML, Malone AM, Fanjiang G, Ziegler TR. Critical role of nutrition in improving quality of care: an interdisciplinary call to action to address adult hospital malnutrition. *J Acad Nutr Diet.* 2013;113(9):1219–1237.

159. Thielking M. Does good food count as health care? New research aims to find out. *STAT News* [Newspaper]. March 24, 2017; https://www.statnews.com/2017/03/24/nutrition-food-medicine-chronic-disease/.

160. Patton-Lopez MM, Lopez-Cevallos DF, Cancel-Tirado DI, Vazquez L. Prevalence and correlates of food insecurity among students attending a midsize rural university in Oregon. *J Nutr Educ Behav.* 2014;46(3):209–214.

161. Morris LM, Smith S, Davis J, Null DB. The prevalence of food security and insecurity among Illinois university students. *J Nutr Educ Behav.* 2016;48(6):376–382 e371.

162. Mirabitur E, Peterson KE, Rathz C, Matlen S, Kasper N. Predictors of college-student food security and fruit and vegetable intake differ by housing type. *J Am Coll Health.* 2016;64(7):555–564.

163. Bruening M, Brennhofer S, van Woerden I, Todd M, Laska M. Factors related to the high rates of food insecurity among diverse, urban college freshmen. *J Acad Nutr Diet.* 2016;116(9):1450–1457.

164. Goldrick-Rab S, Richardson J, Hernandez A. *Hungry and Homeless in College: Results from a National Study of Basic Needs Insecurity in Higher Education.* University of Wisconsin–Madison; 2017.

165. Riches G. Food banks and food security: welfare reform, human rights and social policy. *Social Policy & Administration.* 2002;36(6).

166. Chilton M, Rose D. A rights-based approach to food insecurity in the United States. *Am J Public Health.* 2009;99(7):1203–1211.

8

Obesogenic Environments and Public Health Mitigation Strategies

Allison Karpyn

Chapter Highlights

- The Health Impact Pyramid
- Efforts to increase supermarket access
- Healthy Corner Store strategies
- Community Farmers Markets
- Fast food industry

Introduction

In this chapter, we will discuss the food environment that promotes the over-consumption of food high in sugar, salt, and fat, sometimes referred to as an obesogenic environment, as well as review strategies underway to reduce the presence of such environments. Although researchers do not entirely understand all of the mechanisms that drive how and why we eat what we do, our scientific understanding of the problem is growing. Today there is wider recognition that an individual's behavior is affected by multiple factors including the structure of our resources and norms at the community level, and the ways in which policy drives decisions across the food system to either promote, or detract from, health.

What We Eat Is Not a Matter of Individual Choice Alone

Today obesity is one of the most significant global health and social problems and is in part responsible for seven of the top ten causes of death, including heart disease and some cancers. In the United States, more than 80% of all healthcare dollars are spent on chronic conditions, the majority of which are exacerbated by obesity. Approximately 36% of the adult population and 17% of children (ages 2–19) are considered obese (Body Mass Index [BMI] > 30),[1] and families with lower incomes are disproportionately affected.[1]

The term **obesogenic environment** has been used to describe the manifestation of a culture that supports the overconsumption of foods high in salt, fat, and sugar. Coined approximately 25 years ago by Boyd Swinburn after his work on a Native American reservation in Arizona, the concept intended to direct attention away from the notion that obesity was brought about by an individual's lack of willpower and shift attention to the environments that encourage a sedentary lifestyle and overconsumption of unhealthy foods.[2] The term brings together the built environment and dietary decisions in a way that recognizes aspects of how the built environment contributes to obesity; what surrounds us is likely to influence our physical activity and dietary behaviors at both an individual and community level.

Obesogenic environments are particularly troubling as we recognize that obesity has a strong socioeconomic connection, wherein those who are most significantly impacted also struggle with poverty and lack of community resources generally. Together these issues contribute to a troubling scenario where the food environment, available resources, and struggling economic conditions perpetuate health inequalities and exacerbate disparities.

In 2010, the Director of the Centers for Disease Control and Prevention (CDC), Tom Frieden, published a seminal article titled, "A framework for public health action: the health impact pyramid."[3] The article introduced a five-tier pyramid that clarified the types of interventions and their potential public health impact. At the base of the pyramid lie the socioeconomic factors that are key contributors to the health of populations. The second tier from the bottom is described as "changing the context to make individuals default decisions healthy," while the next tier is focused on "long-lasting protective interventions," and the top two tiers include "clinical interventions" and "counseling and education."

Although the importance of the community to public health was already an integral component of public health, the health impact pyramid, as articulated by the CDC Director, swiftly redirected attention to the critical importance of our nation's policies, systems, and environments. It further advanced the notion that the best investment in public health was in changes that would yield broad-basedpopulation impact while at the same time limiting the amount of effort put forth by individuals themselves to achieve changes in daily behavior. By changing the default, Frieden argued, Americans would have to expend effort **not to** benefit from the public health intervention.

One example of the potential impacts of changing the default is the application of fluoride to water. Fluoride, once in the city or county supply is, by default, provided to individuals, and to avoid public health benefits would require considerable effort. Making the healthy choice the default, he postulated could and should, also be applied to cardiovascular disease risk factors such as sodium or trans-fat levels in manufactured food. If the food environment were to shift so that products did not contain trans-fats and by default had lower sodium content, the nation's health would improve.

Frieden's framework was given a sizable boost when, shortly after the publication of the paper, the Reinvestment and Recovery Act of 2010 awarded a half billion dollars in the form of Communities Putting Prevention to Work grants for state and local public health prevention efforts. Although a variety of approaches were supported, three food policies were clearly articulated as promising parts of a new national framework for action. These included altering food prices such that healthier foods are less expensive; shifting our exposure to food to increase exposure to healthier foods and decrease exposure to less healthy foods; and improving the image of healthy food to increase its attractiveness relative to less healthy food alternatives.[4]

The Food Environment and Food Deserts

In 1968, an innovative concept was born when the country gave birth to the first African American-owned shopping center, Progress Plaza. Anchored by a beautiful A&P supermarket in the heart of Philadelphia's Yorktown neighborhood, more than 10,000 residents gathered on a crisp October day to mark the opening of a much-needed retail center, which provided critical services and jobs to the community.

What is notable about this shopping center was that the project was financed entirely by the community. Residents were motivated by Reverend Leon Sullivan, leader of the nearby Zion Baptist Church, who called for members of the congregation to self-finance the project by contributing $10 a month each month for three years. The market offered an important resource to the community for many years, but, after thriving for decades, the market closed its doors in 1998. And, despite legal challenges by the community to stay in business, the store closed, leaving community members again with no choice but to travel to get affordable food. Furthermore, with the supermarket gone, the number of shoppers in the business corridor also waned, and slowly the other stores nested within the plaza also closed.

Although this story is a bit unusual given its historical significance, the account chronicles a challenge felt by many communities. In the 1980s and 1990s, there was a slow and steady change in the distribution of supermarkets across the nation, leaving many neighborhoods without a neighborhood store.[5] Today, such localities are more commonly referred to as food deserts. According to the USDA economic research service, more than 23.5 million Americans live in an area of the United States where affordable nutritious food is more than 1 mile away, for urban areas, or more than 10 miles away, for rural areas and, therefore, considered out of reach.[6]

Across the nation, over 6,529 food desert communities exist where residents face the struggles of low incomes while at the same time having insufficient access to a supermarket or large grocery store. Furthermore, food deserts exist in every state in the continental United States and in all types of communities—not just urban.

The absence of healthy affordable foods, although a challenge for anyone, presents an even greater challenge to those living in lower income neighborhoods, communities of color, and rural areas. Dr. Alfio Rausa of the Mississippi State Department of Health clearly summed up the challenge, and the definition, when he said

"There's this thing called a food desert. So out in the county you have these mom-and-pop shops and they don't have fruits and vegetables. There are several issues . . . The big 18-wheelers deliver to Walmart and Kroger and these other chains, but they don't go through the back roads . . . You know they're off the beaten path . . . They don't fit the business model maximum delivery, minimum cost. And so we're consuming what's available to us."[7]

Not unlike many parts of the world, much of the history of food shopping in America dates back to a time when local vendors sold fish locally, brought their farm product to neighborhood produce stands, and worked as butchers in spaces where they gathered alongside other vendors. Whether a large public market or a smaller mom-and-pop store, the purchase of groceries occurred vendor by vendor. By the end of World War I, however, the country began to see the emergence of larger markets and even grocery chains.

By 1930, the first modern supermarket opened in Queens, New York, which introduced the supermarket business as we know it today.[7] The modern supermarket model operates on a high volume of products with thin profit margins. Volume buying is the name of the game. The modern supermarket quickly grew, and, by the 1960s, 70% of retail food sales were transacted in supermarkets. Over time, larger stores with larger parking lots were built, many of which moved to thriving suburbia, where space was more readily available at an affordable price.

Take the example of Kenosha, Wisconsin. This is one of the communities identified as a food desert by the USDA. In 1950, the town had 126 grocery stores, but in 1970 the number declined to 60, and by 1980 only 37 were left.[7]

The change in retailer location preferences also coincided with the growth of suburban development, a result of shifts away from declining manufacturing in cities, as well as advances in technology that displaced farmworkers as agricultural production became more mechanized. Most of those moving to the suburbs were white. Later known as "white flight," the shift in population resulted in cities having disproportionately more minority residents.[8]

It stands to reason that those living in neighborhoods without good sources of healthy affordable food will have a harder time maintaining a healthy diet. Many studies support this theory, though some newer research has found the problem may be more complex than originally thought.[9] Foundational research showed that across 132 studies the preponderance of evidence supported the connection between food deserts and poor health.[7] For example, low-income zip codes have 25% fewer chain supermarkets and many more convenience stores compared with middle-income areas, though those statistics may be changing.[10] In the Mississippi Delta, for example, more than 70% of households that rely on food stamps also need to travel over 30 miles in order to use their food stamps at a local supermarket.[11]

As our understanding of food deserts continues to evolve, greater emphasis has been given to the nature and quality of supermarkets as an indicator of access to healthy food—not just whether a store is nearby. For example, a study of 226 stores across the city of Baltimore revealed that nearly half of low-income neighborhoods lacked stores with a minimally adequate healthy food selection.[12] Furthermore, nearly a quarter of the city's black residents lived in a neighborhood with low healthy-food availability, while in comparison, only 5% of white residents faced the same challenge.

In addition to their influence on the availability of a variety of food, supermarkets are also economic anchors providing 100 to 200 jobs per supermarket for area residents. As with the story of Progress Plaza, retailers generate economic activity along their local corridors, often stimulating additional investment.

In 2000, The Food Trust, a not-for-profit in Philadelphia, joined with local leadership to explore ways to reduce the number of people experiencing a food desert. Initially, a task force was formed to better understand the places where access would be most important and to examine maps where high rates of diet-related disease coincided with higher rates of poverty and lower retail access to food. At the conclusion of the three meeting process, State Representative Dwight Evans championed a recommendation to create a statewide fund to stimulate fresh-food retail development. In 2004, the state general assembly appropriated $30 million over three years to create the Fresh Food Financing Initiative. These monies were further leveraged with a 3:1 private capital match generated by the reinvestment fund. Today, the program has created 83 new or improved grocery stores across the state of Pennsylvania. From these projects, 5,000 full- or part-time jobs were created or retained, together improving access to nutritious food for 400,000 residents.[13,14]

Although the Pennsylvania Fresh Food Financing Initiative initially began as a way to address the supermarket problems across the state, the program came to offer flexible financing, which allowed funding for a variety of fresh food retail enterprises. These included corner stores, food co-operatives, and farmers markets, in addition to more traditional grocery stores.

Today, over 17 similar programs are modeled after the initial Pennsylvania program. States such as California, Illinois, New York, Louisiana, New Jersey, Colorado, Massachusetts, Texas, Ohio, and others have developed programs to provide one-time start-up funding for new food projects. Furthermore, in 2010, the federal government created the Healthy Food Financing Initiative, a funding mechanism that distributes funds to Community Development Financial Institutions (CDFI) or Community Development Corporations (CDCs) through the Department of Agriculture, the Department of the Treasury, and the Department of Health and Human Services to further promote the development of retail healthy food in and around underserved communities in America.[15]

Corner Stores

About the same time as efforts to address the gap in supermarket access were underway, so, too, was a new national healthy corner store network, which sought to share resources of programs and projects to increase healthy food access at the small-store level.

Corner stores and similar small stores such as bodegas, convenience stores, and small rural grocers face challenges in offering healthy affordable food. Yet, neighborhood residents often rely on these establishments in the absence of any nearby supermarkets. Across America, there are approximately 154,000 stores peppered throughout communities urban and rural, together constituting a $550 billion industry. Most of the stores, however, have names that you may not recognize, because over 62% of the industry is represented by family-owned stores.[16]

The National Association of Convenience Stores provides an umbrella organization for many small-store retailers, though many still face challenges achieving an adequate supply of high-quality, low-cost products to sell.[17] At the local level this translates to small stores selling soda and high-calorie junk foods alongside tobacco and alcohol. Although profit margins on fresh products are often higher than on packaged snacks and canned goods, they require a different kind of distribution and in-store operation. Because packaged foods are regularly delivered by their distributors, stores do not have to deal with the same challenging logistics in stocking these products as they do when stocking fresh or perishable foods, which have to be handled differently store to store and delivered more frequently.

Farmers Markets

In 2016, the United States Department of Agriculture recorded 8,675 farmers markets, 733 Community Supported Agriculture operations (CSAs), 1,393 on-farm markets, and 170 food hubs nationally.[18] Throughout these venues. consumers purchased $1.4 billion worth of local food directly from farmers. These types of markets have become increasingly popular over the past 20 years as demonstrated by the significant uptick in the number of sites. In fact, since 1994 the number of markets has increased by nearly 400% and the value of food sold has more than doubled.[18]

Yet, it makes sense that farmers markets are not a new concept in America. Dating back to the colonial period, public markets such as those in Philadelphia and in Faneuil Hall in Boston have, for decades, been a staple resource for communities. By the 1960s and 1970s, however, the number of recognized farmers markets in the United States began to decline.[19]

Farmers markets most often are found outdoors in parking lots, in parks, or next to public facilities, though many indoor markets also exist. Because farmers bring products directly from their fields to the customer, markets often are held just one or two days a week for a limited period of time. The product offerings at farmers markets vary widely, and some markets have been criticized for carrying more crafts than food. The majority of markets, however, sell locally grown fresh fruits and vegetables, cheese, meat, honey, jams, and prepared food.

Many believe that farmers markets are an important strategy for remedying declines in fruit and vegetable intake and for revitalizing community public spaces (Figure 8.1). Shopping at farmers markets can empower consumers to directly combat the growing packaged food industry, which can substitute cheaper ingredients and add sweeteners, salt, fats, and preservatives to lower the costs of its packaged items. Furthermore, there is evidence that prices at farmers markets are actually less than in the supermarket. Several studies have reported that because of cost savings to farmers achieved by removing the intermediary and allowing them to sell directly to the customer, prices at farmers markets are lower by 10% to 28% as compared with nearby grocery stores.[20] The impacts are likely economic, social, and health-related, and public health agencies such as the Centers for Disease Control and Prevention have recognized the development of farmers markets as an important health priority. As such, efforts to expand farmers markets and explore new ways to increase produce purchases, particularly among low-income, high-risk, or vulnerable

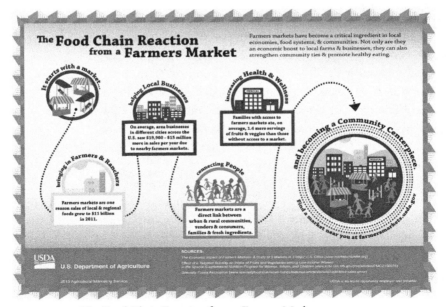

FIGURE 8.1 The Food Chain Reaction from a Farmers Market.
https://www.flickr.com/photos/usdagov/9441954041/sizes/l/in/photostream/

residents, represent one of a number of obesity prevention strategies intended to improve the food environment.[21] Buying local often means purchasing fewer processed and prepared foods while at the same time supporting local farm preservation efforts.

The majority of research studies about farmers markets have considered the characteristics of those who use farmers markets and the traits of the markets themselves, including the types of products they offer and the volume of farmers and customers participating.[22-24] Generally, findings show that women shop more than men and that markets appeal to those with higher incomes, though the number of low-income shoppers is growing.[25-27] Studies particularly focused on underserved communities and the farmers markets that serve them, find positive associations between shopping at farmers markets and fruit and vegetable consumption.[28-30] Findings on the relationship between obesity (BMI > 30) and farmers market use have been inconclusive.

Several public and private programs exist to support farmers markets and consumers with lower incomes. The Farmers Market Nutrition Program, for example, an effort developed by the United States Department of Agriculture and supported locally by states, makes available funds for individuals participating in the Women Infants and Children (WIC) program (WIC FDMNP) as well as for low-income seniors (SENIOR FMNP). These benefits are designated specifically for the purchase of fresh, locally grown fruits and vegetables at authorized farmers markets.[31,32] Although the value of the benefit varies from state to state, most offer about $20 per year to recipients.

After considering a number of options, the WIC program was expanded in 2009 to include a monthly allowance, otherwise called a cash value voucher (CVV), for participants to purchase fruits and vegetables, further advancing the purchasing power of low-to-moderate income customers at farmers markets.[33]

At the same time, electronic benefits transfer systems (EBT) have begun to take hold as a mechanism of transaction at markets allowing for even greater sales among low-income residents.[34] Farmers markets accepting EBT have grown dramatically over the past five years, creating food environments that are supportive of healthy eating for everyone, especially those who have fewer resources to purchase food.

Fast Food

The availability of fast food, the products it offers, and the way it is advertised, are often criticized as key contributing factors to the obesogenic environments across the world and the poor health of citizens. Often high in fat, salt, and calories, fast food products such as pizza, French fries, and burgers (now chicken, too) are a key factor in the growing obesity epidemic.

In 2016, fast food sales reached $237.7 billion. McDonalds continues to have the largest share of the market with 15% of all sales, though this number is declining and chicken fast food sales are increasing, with companies such as Chick-fil-A showing increases of 16% or more in sales. Table 8.1 lists the top 15 chain retailers. Some have reported, in fact, that Chick-fil-A generates more revenue per restaurant than any other fast food chain in the United States.[35]

Although many have come to the conclusion that a greater number of low-income individuals consume fast food than do middle- or upper-income people, today, in fact, more and more Americans across socioeconomic groups rely on fast food for a quick meal on the go. The issue of fast food consumption is no longer a problem just for lower income, urban areas. Recent research has begun to re-examine the assumption that those who eat fast food in America are largely low-income Americans, and findings show that it is

Table 8.1 Top 15 Chain Fast Food Companies: Percentage of World Brand Shares 2014–2016

Brand Name	2014	2015	2016
McDonald's (McDonald's Corp.)	3.2	3.1	3.1
KFC (Yum! Brands, Inc.)	0.9	0.9	0.9
Burger King (Restaurant Brands International, Inc.)	0.7	0.7	0.7
Subway (Doctor's Associates, Inc.)	0.7	0.7	0.7
7-Eleven (Seven & I Holdings Co., Ltd.)	0.6	0.6	0.7
Pizza Hut (Yum! Brands, Inc.)	0.4	0.5	0.4
Domino's Pizza (Domino's Pizza, Inc.)	0.3	0.4	0.4
Wendy's (The Wendy's Co.)	0.3	0.4	0.4
Taco Bell (Yum! Brands, Inc.)	0.3	0.3	0.3
Dunkin' Donuts (Dunkin' Brands Group, Inc.)	0.3	0.3	0.3
Chick-fil-A (CFA Properties, Inc.)	0.2	0.3	0.3
Tim Hortons (Restaurant Brands International, Inc.)	0.2	0.2	0.2
Panera Bread Co. (Panera Bread Co.)	0.2	0.2	0.2
Family Mart (FamilyMart Uny Holdings Co., Ltd.)	-	-	0.2
Sonic Drive-In (Sonic Corp.)	0.1	0.2	0.2

Source: Euromonitor International from official statistics, trade associations, trade press, company research, trade interviews, and trade sources.

becoming more and more common for middle-class Americans to purchase food on the go. Indeed, one large 2017 study found that poor people were actually less likely to eat fast food, and did so less frequently, than those with higher incomes. And, middle-class individuals were only slightly more likely than the rich to report eating fast food.[36] Overall, the wealthiest eat just one less fast food meal in a 21-day period on average than the poorest.

Research tells us that consumption of fast food is beginning to equalize across socioeconomic status subgroups, but what is unclear is what the relationship between the density of fast food establishments and the types of establishments is when it comes to impacting our health. It is possible that a Starbucks is different than a Chipotle or Burger King. Because most of the research lumps all "fast food" together, we do not know whether the type of establishment has an impact on the total contribution to diet, and how those impacts may differ between wealthier and poorer neighborhoods.

One way to regulate the growth and development of fast food in neighborhoods is with zoning policies. The CDC and others have provided information that supports changing zoning as a way to empower local governments and residents to restrict land uses or incentivize development of lands to encourage more of one kind of use and less of another.[37] Local jurisdictions can use zoning to encourage farming in urban areas, support the development of grocery stores or specialty corner markets that sell fish or produce, restrict unhealthy establishments in close proximity to schools, and reduce the density of fast food restaurants. When it comes to fast food in particular, efforts to use zoning policies to control the growth of fast food establishments at a neighborhood or community level have been in place nationally since at least the 1980s.

In 2008, for example, Los Angeles adopted a policy that created a one-year moratorium on the construction of fast food restaurants in South Los Angeles.[38] Yet the effectiveness of these policies in reducing health disparities is unclear. More recent research indicates that there are greater densities of fast food establishments in poor neighborhoods,[39,40] but that research doesn't tease out the differences by types of fast food outlets, which can vary widely.

Conclusions

In the United States and across much of the world, our food environment is defined by the social and physical surroundings that influence what we eat. Obesogenic environments can create challenges as we work to maintain a healthy diet, while healthy environments make the healthy choice the easy choice. When fast food, and a lack of affordable healthy food abound, it becomes a challenge to eat well. Instead of the default being healthy, the default is often a salty or sweet packaged food.

By understanding more about how our food environment shapes our diets, we are able to influence policy and shift our framework from one-on-one interventions to the broader systems that, in turn, impact our behaviors. Challenges are particularly abundant for those who have lower incomes, less education, and are members of ethnic or racial minority groups.

New approaches to intervene in the places where we live, work, and play, including how our neighborhoods are planned and how people are encouraged to interact with one another and with food are yet to be discovered. Furthermore, the ways in which families influence dietary choices and how they address barriers to healthy eating borne out of their food environment are still largely unexplored. How and when families and neighborhoods interact at the local level may differ from the ways in which policies and systems impact zip codes or county statistics. As we continue down the path of understanding how the food environment and public health interact, we also will begin to uncover more of the pathways through which effective interventions can operate.

Quiz Questions

1. Obesity is responsible for 7 of the top 10 causes of death in the United States. True or false?
2. Obesogenic environments include all but which of the following:
   a. Restaurant portion sizes
   b. Food marketing to children
   c. Willpower to make healthy choices
   d. Workplaces where baked goods are frequently left out for others
   e. A, B, and D above
3. The health impact pyramid has:
   a. 8 tiers
   b. 7 tiers
   c. 6 tiers
   d. 5 tiers
   e. 4 tiers
4. The health impact pyramid is important because it:
   a. Sheds light on the critical nature of socioeconomic factors in health
   b. Emphasizes the importance of educational interventions for health

    c.   Draws from successful public health approaches to shift the default

    d.   All of the above

    e.   A and C above

5. Fluorination is one example of how public health interventions can adopt clinical interventions to improve community health. True or false?

6. The Health Impact Pyramid is organized such that the closer to the top you go the more likely you are to have a population impact. True or false?

7. In the United States, food deserts:

    a.   Affect over 6,500 communities

    b.   Are in all states except two

    c.   Predominately impact urban areas

    d.   Are caused in part by suburban development

    e.   A and D above

8. The availability of a store is an adequate marker of access to healthy food. True or false?

9. The Pennsylvania Fresh Food Financing program is a model for:

    a.   Public–private partnerships

    b.   Policy to address food deserts

    c.   Addressing food deserts in urban and rural areas

    d.   All of the above

    e.   A and B above

10. The Farmers Market Nutrition Program (FMNP) provides additional funds for the purchase of locally grown produce in supermarkets across the United States. True or false?

Discussion Questions

- To what extent does the fast food or food retail environment where you live influence your daily habits?
- In what ways does the changing media environment impact how you think about your food landscape?

References

1. Condon E, Drilea S, Jowers K, et al. *Diet Quality of Americans by SNAP Participation Status: Data from the National Health and Nutrition Examination Survey, 2007–2010*. Prepared by Walter R. McDonald & Associates, Inc. and Mathematica Policy Research for the Food and Nutrition Service; 2015.

2. Swinburn B, Egger G Fau—Raza F, Raza F. Dissecting obesogenic environments: the development and application of a framework for identifying and prioritizing environmental interventions for obesity. *Prev Med.* 1999;29:563–570.

3. Frieden TR. A framework for public health action: The Health Impact Pyramid. *Am J Public Health*; 2010:100:590–595.

4. Frieden TR, Dietz W, Collins J. Reducing childhood obesity through policy change: acting now to prevent obesity. *Health Affairs.* 2010;29:357–363.

5. Karpyn A, Manon M, Treuhaft S, Giang T, Harries C, McCoubrey K. Policy solutions to the "grocery gap." *Health Affairs.* 2010;29:473–480.

6. Ver Ploeg M, Breneman V, Dutko P, et al. *Access to Affordable and Nutritious Food: Updated Estimates of Distance to Supermarkets Using 2010* Data; 2012.

7. Karpyn A, Truehaft S. *The Grocery Gap: Finding Healthy Food In America.* Public Affairs Media; 2013.

8. Lehmann Y, White A, Tucker J, Karpyn A. State-Level Interventions: Pennsylvania's Fresh Food Financing Initiative. In: Morland KB, ed. *Local Food Environments: Food Access in America.* CRC Press; 2015.

9. Dubowitz T, Zenk SN, Ghosh-Dastidar B, et al. Healthy food access for urban food desert residents: examination of the food environment, food purchasing practices, diet and BMI. *Public Health Nutr.* 2015;18:2220–2230.

10. Rundle A, Neckerman K, Freeman L, Lovasi, G., et al. Neighborhood food environment and walkability predict obesity in New York City. *Environmental Health Perspectives.* 2009;117:442.

11. Morland K, Wing S, Diez Roux A. The contextual effect of the local food environment on residents' diets: the atherosclerosis risk in communities study. *Am J Public Health.* 2002;92:1761–1767.

12. Gittelsohn J, Franceschini M, Rasooly I, et al. Understanding the food environment in a low-income urban setting: implications for food store interventions. *Journal of Hunger & Environmental Nutrition 2.* 2008;2:33–50.

13. Lehmann Y, White A, Tucker J, Karpyn A. *State level interventions: Pennsylvania's fresh food financing initiative.* In K. Morland Local Food Environments: Food Access in America, 2015; CRC Press: Boca Raton FL, 323 pages. Morland, K. (Ed.). (2014). Local Food Environments. Boca Raton: CRC Press.

14. Giang T, Karpyn, A., Laurison, H. B., Hillier, A., & Perry, R. D. Closing the grocery gap in underserved communities: the creation of the Pennsylvania Fresh Food Financing Initiative. *Journal of Public Health Management and Practice*; 2008:14:272–279.

15. The Food Trust, Policy Link. *A Healthy Food Financing Initiative: An Innovative Approach to Improve Health and Spark Economic Development.* 2009.

16. Fact Sheets: The Association for Convenience & Fuel Retailing. 2017.

17. Bentzel D, Weiss S, Bucknum M, Shore K. *Healthy Food and Small Stores: Strategies to Close the Distribution Gap.* The Food Trust; 2015.

18. United States Department of Agriculture. *Farmers Market Promotion Program 2016 Highlights.* United States Department of Agriculture; 2017.

19. Brown A. Counting farmers markets. *Geographical Review.* 2001;91:655–674.

20. Floury R. Healthy Food, Healthy Communities: PolicyLink; 2011.

21. Khan L, Sobush K, Keener D, et al. *Recommended Community Strategies and Measurements to Prevent Obesity in the United States.* Centers for Disease Control and Prevention; 2009.

22. Gao Z, Swisher M, Zhao X. A New Look at Farmers' Markets: Consumer Knowledge and Loyalty. *Hortscience.* 2012;47(8):1102–1107.

23. McGarry Wolf M, Spittler A, Ahern J. A Profile of Farmers' Market Consumers and the Perceived Advantages of Produce Sold at Farmers' Markets. *Journal of Food Distribution Research.* 2005;36(1):192–201.

24. Wood P. *National Farmers Market Manager Survey Shows Farmers Markets Continue to Grow.* USDA Agriculture Marketing Service; 2015.

25. Young CR, Aquilante JL, Solomon S, et al. Improving fruit and vegetable consumption among low-income customers at farmers markets: Philly Food Bucks, Philadelphia, Pennsylvania, 2011. *Prev Chronic Dis.* 2013;10:E166.

26. Grin BM, Gayle TL, Saravia DC, Sanders LM. Use of farmers markets by mothers of WIC recipients, Miami-Dade county, Florida, 2011. *Prev Chronic Dis.* 2013;10: E95. Published online 2013 Jun 13. doi:10.5888/pcd10.120178 PMCID: PMC3684356

27. Young C, Karpyn A, Uy N, Wich K, J Glyn. Farmer's markets in low-income communities: impact of community environment, food programs, and public policy. *Community Development.* 2011;42:208–220.

28. Pitts SBJ, Gustafson A, Wu Q, et al. Farmers' market use is associated with fruit and vegetable consumption in diverse southern rural communities. *Nutrition Journal.* 2014;13:1.

29. Jilcott Pitts SB, Wu Q, McGuirt JT, Crawford TW, Keyserling TC, Ammerman AS. Associations between access to farmers' markets and supermarkets, shopping patterns, fruit and vegetable consumption, and health indicators among women of reproductive age in eastern North Carolina. *Public Health Nutr.* 2013;16(11):1944–1952. doi:10.1017/S1368980013001389. Epub 2013 May 24.

30. Racine EF, Vaughn AS, Laditka SB. Farmers' market use among African-American women participating in the special supplemental nutrition program for women, infants, and children. *J Am Diet Assoc.* 2010;110(3):441–446. doi:10.1016/j.jada.2009.11.019.

31. United States Department of Agriculture FaNS. *Senior Farmers' Market Nutrition Program (SFMNP).* 2015.

32. United States Department of Agriculture FaNS. *WIC Farmers' Market Nutrition Program (FMNP).* 2017.

33. Consortium SIT. *Analysis of Alternatives for Implementing a Cash Value Voucher Program: United States Department of Agriculture, Food and Nutrition Service;* 2007.

34. Why Farmers Markets?: The Farmers Market Coalition; 2013.

35. Peterson H. How Chick-fil-A's restaurants sell three times as much KFC2015.

36. Zagorsky J, Smith P. *The association between socioeconomic status and adult fast-food consumption in the U.S. US National Library of Medicine National Institutes of Health.* 2017.

37. Centers for Disease Control and Prevention. *Zoning to Encourage Healthy Eating.* 2016.

38. Los Angeles City Council. Ordinance No. 1801032008.

39. Hilmers A, Hilmers D, Dave J. Neighborhood disparities in access to healthy foods and their effects on environmental justice. *Am J Public Health.* 2012;102:1644–1654.

40. Fleischhacker S, Evensong K, Rodriguez D, Ammerman A. A systematic review of fast food access studies. *Obesity Reviews.* 2011;12.

9

Food Controversies

THE HEALTHY PULSE OF A DEMOCRACY?

F. Bailey Norwood

Chapter Highlights

- How facts are accepted or rejected based on their implications
- How debates about specific issues are sometimes proxies for much more complex issues
- How policies should be evaluated partly based on the social movements surrounding them
- The difficulties that arise when debating science and policy proposals simultaneously
- The role of intuition and life-worlds in explaining different beliefs about food issues

In 2013, I began putting together an online course called Farm to Fork, where I intended to cover the science behind modern agriculture and discuss many of the controversies surrounding food. An agronomist at my university heard I would include some lectures on genetically modified organisms (GMOs), and he requested I meet with him. It turned out he was concerned that I was going to criticize GMOs, when, as a professor in an agricultural college, he felt I should be promoting them. When he realized I was not against the technology, and considered me on "his team," he began disparaging anti-GMO activists, remarking how they had not taken the time to study the science behind the technology and thus were not qualified to render criticisms.

I responded that I agreed with him regarding the *science* of GMOs, but that sometimes it seemed like GMO critics were more concerned with political issues than the physical sciences. In particular, I mentioned an Internet meme showing how more than a dozen influential people in the federal government were also previous employees of Monsanto, the leading producer of GMO seed. This revolving door between companies and their regulators make some fear that biotechnology companies have excessive influence over regulations.

Referring to the diagram I mentioned, the agronomist then asked, "Is it true?" He was unaware of this political dimension to the GMO debate, and though he had taken activists to task for not taking the time to understand the science, he had not taken the time to understand the activists. It was then that I gained a much clearer picture of how food became so controversial. We don't just have different opinions: we don't *understand* each other's opinions!

Rather than attempt to settle some of our contemporary food controversies (something I probably could not achieve, anyway) I will use this chapter to help the reader avoid the mistake made by my agronomist friend. Together, we will explore why two equally kind and intelligent people can form such radically different notions about food—and why each is adamant that he or she is in the right.

Between Fact and Conclusion

People argue about food for many reasons. Money can be a prime motivator, of course. One often encounters the remarkable coincidence that people's opinions are usually consistent with their self-interest. A company selling a product always seems to find compelling reasons why that product is safe, and interest groups whose funding derives from a stated mission of opposing those products always seem to find reasons it is unsafe. In fairness, this is partly because people find occupations where their beliefs and their wallets are in harmony. We can all identify with Upton Sinclair when he remarked, "It is difficult to get a man to understand something, when his salary depends on his not understanding it."[1]

Of course, in debates, both sides attempt to make irrelevant their biases by arguing facts. We have all heard the saying, "You are entitled to your own opinions but not your own facts," but it is rare (2016 presidential election aside) for people to make up their own facts for use in arguments. Blatant lies are too easily exposed. Instead, people choose to emphasize different facts and give them different interpretations.

Values matter also. When personal values clash there is seldom a compromise suitable to all. In the obesity debate, some stress the importance of the government caring for children, while others stress that this responsibility rightfully belongs to the parents, even if both sides agree on the facts about obesity rates and their causes. Yet part of food debates involves convincing others that your values are more noble, and that persuasion is conducted, at least in part, with facts.

If John Adams is right and facts are indeed "stubborn things," and if facts feature so prominently in food debates, then why do disagreements arise, persist, fester, and divide? Because, although we live in an age replete with facts, there is still a chasm between the facts that are known and the conclusions we wish to draw. We know facts about obesity, but what we want to know is what to do about it, and the facts aren't clear on this point. Yet we must decide *something*, and that something usually requires us to decide between allowing markets or government to reign. Given a decision must be made, and given the facts do not make clear what this decision should be, we heap into the chasm between fact and conclusion our intuitions and our perceptions—things that are not quite as stubborn as facts (at least not the type of stubbornness to which Adams alludes).

In this chasm, the food battles take place, and the issues become even more complex because any one specific issue is often about much bigger issues as well. Facts become much more than tools of discovery. They become weapons in policy debates and mantras to inspire movements. The consequence is that the interpretation of facts becomes something like cultural myths: to one group, a silly notion; to other people, the sacred core of their identity.

Not Enough Facts

Astronomers know more about the universe than ever before, but our growing knowledge only seems to present us with more questions. We have solid theories as to how the universe began, but we now struggle with invisible matter. Newton and Einstein revealed a few equations governing the stars, but others discovered spooky mysteries within the quantum world. It is like one light bulb coming on only to reveal thousands of other unlit bulbs.

The same can be said for our knowledge about food. Though we know how to prevent scurvy and the precise type of fats women should consume during pregnancy, disagreements about healthful and safe food are alive and well. Scientists today can edit genes, yet people still rely on celebrities for health advice. For all that we know, we know there is still much left to learn. Consider a few examples.

Pesticides

I once interviewed an organic farmer about how he became involved in organic food. He described a scientific study by Chensheng Lu and others (2006) in which the researchers took urine samples of children before and after they went on an organic food diet and measured the pesticide residues in the urine.[2] When children were consuming conventional foods, pesticide residues could be detected in their urine, whereas the levels fell to non-detectable levels once an organic food diet was adopted. To this farmer the results were striking and suggested to him that unless one ate organic food one would consume dangerous pesticides. The science seemed to say that feeding children conventional food was dangerous.

Yet this same study was criticized by Alex Avery of the Center for Global Food Issues (CGFI) for being misleading. Avery argued that the levels of pesticide residues in the children were far, far below the threshold determined by scientists to pose any health harm. Indeed, the Environmental Protection Agency (EPA) does regulate pesticides to ensure they are not ingested at a level that would cause health harms, and that seemed to be the case in the children. Lu (2006) responded that, though this may be true, fewer pesticide residues are always better.[3]

Who is correct? The scientists measuring the pesticide concentrations in children's urine or Avery, who belongs to what is considered a very conservative think tank? From my perspective they are both right; and this represents a controversy that could be settled by science if the science just wasn't so expensive. The EPA determines the level of threshold residues that would cause harm by exposing laboratory animals to various levels, and then requires the actual amount that shows up in food to be only a small fraction of this threshold. So, Avery cited established science when making his argument. Lu and his colleagues also cited basic science when they argued that less pesticide exposure is better because individuals can be exposed to multiple pesticides through diverse foods and reducing this total exposure should eliminate some health risks. This is a controversy about science, one that can be settled by science, and until it is, it is in our interests that such controversies continue.

The pesticide debate becomes even more complex when economics are considered. In a 2013 debate on organic food in the *Wall Street Journal*, the same Lu Chensheng[4] made the same arguments that reducing pesticide exposure by eating organic foods is always good, while an equally prestigious scientist argued that because organic food is more expensive, buying organic would reduce consumption of fruits and vegetables, and that in itself would cause health harms.[5] After all, reducing the price of fruits and vegetables by 30% is estimated to save about 200,000 lives over a 15-year period.[6]

Who is correct? One cannot say. This isn't because the question couldn't be answered through a combination of health and economics studies, but because those studies are expensive and have not been conducted. Data could settle the question, but until such data are available scientists are left to speculate based on their experience and intuition, and we should not expect them to all arrive at the same conclusions.

This is a controversy that exists for a very good reason.

Obesity

Among the top 10 public health problems identified by the Centers for Disease Control and Prevention, alongside HIV, tobacco use, and heart disease, is obesity.[7] Increasing numbers of Americans are obese, and they are suffering the health consequences of it.[8] Because obesity is seen as a preventable condition, and given that it affects over 12 million children (CDC, 2016b), considerable efforts have been devoted to determining the cause of obesity, and using that information to reverse this trend.

In one sense, this is easy. People gain weight when they consume more calories than they burn. That explanation isn't sufficient though, because the response to this calorie surplus differs among individuals. Moreover, science also must investigate why it is that some people have a calorie surplus in the first place.

Identifying the cause of obesity has been highly successful and highly futile at the same time, because everything under the sun seems to influence obesity in some way. I keep a folder titled "Causes of Obesity," and every time I come across a study suggesting or demonstrating a link between some factor and obesity rates, I place it in this folder. Browsing through it one can find the following causes: irregular eating times, genes, having harsh parents, media, exposure to chemicals, gut bacteria, insufficient sleep, sedentary lifestyles, television viewing, stress, excessive food choice, economic security, proximity to fast food outlets, sugar, having obese friends, childhood trauma, having obese parents, gut viruses, not exercising, childhood poverty, being called fat by others, inactive mothers, junk food, not being breast fed, environmental pollutants, living in cold climates, your relationship with your mother, impulsive personalities, behaviors of your mother when you were in the womb, insecticides, IQ, absence of home cooking, attention deficit disorder, having divorced parents, soda, insufficient exercise, smoking, grilling, screen time, food and clothing labels, attending day-care, mental health problems, falling cost of food, air conditioners, PBDE (polybrominated diphenyl ethers) concentrations, antidepressants, and so forth.

Name a change in lifestyle over the past 50 years, and it is probably correlated with obesity rates.

Of course, correlation is not causation. The difficulty of studying obesity is that it is difficult to conduct controlled experiments, where researchers obtain two nearly identical groups and vary only one factor for an extended period of time to observe the weight difference. If investigating the role of air conditioning, imagine the difficulty of getting one half of a large group of similar people to live without their ACs for a few years. This is an experiment that technically could be conducted but is so difficult that it will likely remain a hypothetical scenario.

Instead, you observe people who already happen to not have an AC, along with their weight, and then you observe people who already have AC and consider their weight. The people without ACs are very different people though, mostly likely living on smaller incomes, probably eating a poorer diet, and possibly consisting of more smokers. So, what actually caused one group to weigh more than the other? The AC factor, the income factor, the diet factor, or the smoking factor—or all of them?

If the issue of what causes obesity is ever settled, it won't be for many years. In the meantime, society speculates on the main causes, and this speculation results in controversy.

Some point to soda, producing documentaries like *Sugar Coated* and passing soda taxes, and though some studies show reducing sugar consumption can reduce weight,[9] other studies show that underweight people consume more soda and sweet snacks than those who are overweight.[10]

Farm subsidies are often blamed, as in the documentary *Fed Up*. The idea is that farm subsidies are given to producers of crops like corn, and one of the many uses of corn is corn syrup (sugar). Fruit and vegetable farmers receive far fewer subsidies, so it seems the government is encouraging unhealthful diets. Such an argument conveys the truth about large subsidies given to crop producers, but they ignore the fact that some government policies, like sugar import quotas, work to increase the price of unhealthful foods. Indeed, agricultural economists estimate that removing all of these government programs would have only a very small impact on calories consumed.[11] Still, farm subsidies continue to receive blame and probably always will, and if someone like me points to the studies showing they are insignificant factors, because I am an agricultural economist, I will probably be labeled as biased.

Gluten

Gluten sensitivity is another controversy that could be settled by science, if the science were conducted. A person with gluten sensitivity does not have Celiac disease but nevertheless experiences intestinal discomfort when consuming gluten (gluten is a mixture of proteins found in wheat, barley, and rye—and sometimes oats). In 2013, about 30% of the American adult population said they were reducing gluten in their diet, and more people said they are trying to be gluten-free than said they are dieting.[12]

Is there such a thing as gluten sensitivity? Science can answer this question, but the verdict so far is nuanced. Some studies have found that gluten can cause intestinal discomfort,[13,14] but later studies found that the problem might be due to a specific class of carbohydrates and not the gluten.[15] Although these studies are conducted well, the samples are small, sometimes with fewer than 40 individuals. Without more studies with larger samples, the true health impact of gluten remains unclear, leaving ample room for controversy.

The marketplace has made a decision about gluten, though, and that decision is to replace many sales of gluten products with gluten-free varieties. For example, sales of products labeled "gluten-free" rose from $11.5 billion in 2009 to $23 billion in 2013.[16] Many of these products never contained gluten in the first place, but the label is still necessary because of considerable confusion about gluten.

People wrongly associate gluten with unambiguously more healthful foods,[17] and people have difficulty identifying which grains contain gluten.[18] This confusion has been made the source of humor in Jimmy Kimmel's YouTube video *Pedestrian Question—What is Gluten?* (viewed over 4 million times) and movies such as *This is the End*. This means people who fear gluten need the label indicating whether it is present in the food, because they don't know what it is. Some of my own research shows that many people consider a gluten-free diet to be a valid weight-loss strategy, when there is no obvious reason this would be the case.

Perhaps surprisingly, some of this confusion may lead to desirable outcomes. If people seek to avoid gluten by shunning a broad array of conventional grains, they may begin consuming unusual grains such as Teff and Quinoa, which are generally consumed in whole grain form, and whole grains are more nutritious than their refined grain counterparts. Or, they may consume more vegetables. Either of these choices might lead to a more healthful diet, and as people feel better, they may attribute their improved health not just to better foods but to reducing their gluten consumption. In this sense, even people without Celiac disease or gluten sensitivity may find the gluten-free diet improves their health.

The gluten controversy is about much more than just gluten, then; it is about the overall diet of a people. The same is true for the pesticide and GMO controversy. Two sides may be debating food safety, but that is just one food battle in a much larger war.

A Single Controversy Can Be a Proxy War

It doesn't get any more controversial than food made with genetically modified organisms (GMOs), and the debate seems unresolvable partly because it is unclear what the debate is even about. At first it might seem obvious that the debate concerns whether foods made with GMOs are safe, but most of the world's prestigious scientific organizations have stated that GM foods are as safe as non-GM foods, and these endorsements have done little to settle the issue. This suggests that the GMO debate may be about more than food safety.

I have interviewed a number of anti-GMO activists and have come to believe that some of these activists feel that most foods produced from GMOs are indeed safe to eat. One of them was a young lady who abstains from GM foods, yet she is also a type 1 diabetic, which means she relies on the insulin produced by genetically modified bacteria to live. No one better understands the benefits reaped from genetic modification, yet she embraces it for medicine and rejects it for food. Others have expressed to me that they do believe the foods are probably safe and can provide some benefits, but the corporate world in which GMOs are developed introduces a number of other dangers, and it is these other dangers that motivate their opposition to the technology.

This isn't to say that all GMO opponents see GM foods as safe, but I find that the higher their educational level and understanding of the science, the more likely they are to oppose such foods based on reasons other than food safety.

The debate about GMOs is less about food safety and more a proxy war concerning the role of large corporations, ownership of genetics, and food sovereignty. Transgenic crops such as Round Up Ready Soybeans (transgenic means genes from one organism are inserted into the genome of a different organism) just happen to provide a platform where this proxy war can take place.

Biotechnology requires enormous amounts of financial investment, and so GMOs typically are developed only by very large corporations. One of these corporations is Monsanto, and many food activists have an intense dislike for the company. As the Bayer corporation sought to purchase Monsanto in 2016, the *Wall Street Journal* ran an article with the title, *If Monsanto Loses Its Name, What Will Opponents Oppose?* Crafted in humor, the title suggests that GM activists are so focused on opposing Monsanto that it has become their *raison d'etre.*

The Monsanto corporation is called out by Wise Intelligent in his hip-hop song *Illuminati*, protesting the control of a small minority over much of the world's wealth and power (Arnold, 2011). The lyrics state:

> Before they collapse the market, they're criminalizing farming
> They're silencing you for talking, while turning us all into peasants
> Agricultural patents, ConAgra created the famines
> Monsanto's seeds that terminate the natural birthing action
> Controlling the food supply, choosing who should live or die
> Confusion rules you choose the lie, illusion illuminates your mind
> —*Illuminati* by Wise Intelligent

The rap connects Monsanto's dominance in the market for crop seeds with enslavement of blacks and British colonization. The corporation isn't just being scolded by African Americans. Neil Young recently released an album titled *The Monsanto Years*, which *Rolling Stone* described as, "... a jeremiad against the agrochemical behemoth of the title and what he sees as American farming's Frankenstein future" (Dolan, 2015). The publication *Modern Farmer* even ran a 2014 article titled, "Why Does Everyone Hate Monsanto?"

Monsanto is not the only producer of genetically modified seed, but it seems to receive all the animosity, perhaps because it was the first corporation to really be successful marketing transgenic seeds. In their haste to acquire first-mover's advantage in the market they were aggressive in their marketing and in their lobbying, and to some it appeared as if they were not so much working with government regulators but controlling them.[19]

As GM seed began to be marketed in developing countries it was interpreted as a form of quasi-colonialism. When DNA sequences from genetic corn were found to have infiltrated the DNA of traditional corn in Oaxaca, Mexico, it was viewed as a threat to traditional culture and the preferred food

system. Feeling like they were losing control of their cherished corn varieties, they protested the use of GMOs in the region. Others, such as residents
of the country of Colombia, did likewise, and as the movement solidified,
the term *food sovereignty* was coined, referring to the ability of a people to
control their own food production, distribution, and trade. In Fitting's
interviews with scientists associated with the food sovereignty movement in
Mexico, the scientists remarked that they were not opposed to biotechnology
itself, but to the raising of transgenic corn in Mexico.[20] In 2014, researchers
at Iowa State University attempted to conduct a study where they would pay
people to consume a genetically modified banana. The experiment wasn't to
determine whether the banana was safe (the gene inserted already exists in
other bananas) but to determine the rate at which the banana would increase
Vitamin A levels in people. The GM banana was produced with funding from
the Bill and Melinda Gates Foundation to help reduce Vitamin A deficiencies
in countries such as Uganda.

The experiment hasn't yet been conducted due to protests from a small
group of Iowa State University graduate students. These were not radical
activists who understand little about biology or food. Most of these students
studied food systems and one was even an agronomy student. They started
a petition that made headlines and stymied the university's progress. Why
would any group pose obstacles to the Gates' philanthropic efforts? For many
reasons other than fears about the safety of the banana. Because they believe
efforts to enhance Vitamin A in Africa are best achieved not through tinker-
ing with the genetics of existing bananas but by helping Africa diversify its
food supply—by raising amaranth, for instance.

Most genetically modified crops are specifically designed to be used in an
industrial agricultural system, which relies heavily on chemical fertilizers, synthetic pesticides, and extensive use of monocultures. For individuals dream-
ing of a food supply without these three elements, GMOs have no allure. Yet,
it is difficult to just protest industrial agriculture in general—where do you go
with your protest signs? You can, however, protest an active member of the industrial agricultural world, a member like Monsanto. So when the Monsanto
chief technology officer visited Iowa State University to speak, a group of students attended, and at one point in the speech donned gas masks and a protest sign reading, *conventional ag = chemical ag*.

The battle regarding GMOs is not just about GMOs, and it isn't just about
food safety. Yet, because transgenic crops are a relatively new technology,
can sound scary at first, require a new approach to regulation, and have the

potential to make industrial agriculture more appealing to farmers, controversy over GMOs has become the battleground over a host of food issues. It is a proxy war, where the spread of GMOs is seen as victory for industrial agriculture, and its hindrance seen as a victory for organic food, food sovereignty, and the like.

It Is Easy to Conflate Specific Policies and Social Movements

Belloc Hilaire wrote the poem "On Food" to describe the varieties of food tastes around the world, and included the lines:

The French are fond of slugs and frogs,
The Siamese eat puppy dogs.
...
And all the world is torn and rent
By varying views on nutriment.
And yet upon the other hand,
De gustibus non disputand umest

—Hilaire, Belloc. 1930. "On Food." Published in *Lapham's Quarterly,* Vol. IV, No. 3, page 140.

The last line can be interpreted as, "there's no disputing taste." Some people like mangos and some don't, but there is little point in two people arguing whether they taste good or not. Likewise, we did not need Hilaire's poem to tell us that culture has a profound effect on people's tastes. Just compare the type of food consumed in China and the type of food sold in the United States as "Chinese food" (hint: the latter has much more sugar!).

Culture can change considerably even in the same region and over a relatively short period, especially when there are social movements afoot. Fifty years ago, many Americans thought a cigarette the ideal way to end a meal. Today most cannot even stand the smell or sight of smoking around food. The recent unpopularity of smoking was not just a random alteration of tastes, but the result of decades of battles between health advocates and tobacco companies. Similar movements occur around food, and understanding their power is essential to understanding food controversies.

The Movement Against Soda

The combination of our food problems and desire to rectify them has led to a plethora of policy initiatives to encourage more healthful eating. Taxes on foods with a high fat, sugar, and/or calorie content are highly favored among some, as are mandatory calorie labels in restaurants and restrictions on the size of soft drinks. The country of Mexico enacted a 10% tax on all sugary drinks, and in 2016 the U.S. city of Berkeley, California passed a similar measure. Do such taxes work? A study found the Berkeley tax did reduce soda consumption four months later, but will the reduction be sustained? Mexico also saw its soda consumption numbers fall after the tax, only to see them rise again later.[21]

When evaluating these ideas scientists typically focus on the impacts of one individual policy, and their findings are mixed. Yes, taxing certain unhealthful foods such as soda would curb its use (taxes tend to do that), but it is not clear that any one of these policies have a remarkable impact on health. One cannot just judge a soda tax by its impact on soda consumption. It must also be determined whether those calories from soda are replaced with calories in another form, and if they are, whether the soda sugar is replaced with healthful foods such as fruits and vegetables or unhealthful foods such as French fries. For example, one study has found that people who drink diet beverages often replace those sugar calories with other foods that are high in sugar and fat.[22] Requiring restaurants to post calorie counts associated with their items is helpful for those wanting lower calorie meals, but most research finds the impacts of such information to be either small or undetectable.[23]

The obesity problem can be described as a problem with manifold causes and no obvious policy solution. So, if the direct impacts of any one policy are negligible, does that mean the policy has no value? No, because policy experiments are part of the *movement* to curb obesity, and a movement is greater than the sum of its parts.

Proposals to tax sodas, and other proposed soda restrictions, such as limiting the amount of soda one can purchase at a time, are controversial—both because their impacts are uncertain and because they are seen to encroach on individual freedom. Yet, as these policies are debated, the public becomes increasingly aware of the role of sugar in obesity. Most Americans are not ravenous consumers of health news, but millions watched the *Parks and Recreation* episode making fun of soda restrictions, which drew attention to the enormous soda sizes available at gas stations. In their Netflix queue, people saw documentaries, such as *Fed Up,* linking sugar with obesity. The limit proposed by New York City Mayor Michael Bloomberg on soda drink sizes was discussed on every major news outlet and many talk shows. Oprah Winfrey is arguably the most respected person in America, and her endorsement of Dr. Oz crowned him the king of health advice for many of her viewers, so when he says to avoid sodas (and he has), people listen.

When people pay attention to the news, they often hear health officials stigmatizing sugar and urging the Food and Drug Administration to limit soda's sugar content. They hear of schools banning sales of soda, and they see products such as Coca-Cola and Pepsi referred to disparagingly as "Big Soda," which is surely an allusion to "Big Tobacco."

This is what a movement against soda in the United States looks like, and it worked. Sales of high calorie sodas have fallen by more than 25% in the last two decades, and these sales aren't being replaced by diet soda, but mostly by water.[24,25] I teach a course on measuring consumer preferences for foods, where we often conduct taste-tests of foods. Once, when introducing a soda taste-test I asked students which brand of soda they preferred. Out of 22 students, only a few even claimed to drink soda regularly (my generation was very different at this age). What they did bring to class, though, were personalized water containers and coffee. This is not the result of smart policy, new scientific findings, or good journalism alone. It is the outcome of a social movement against soda whose overall impact is larger than its individual components.

This is important to understanding food controversies because it helps us understand exactly what we are arguing about, and usually we are arguing about different things. In a debate over soda taxes, fat taxes, food restrictions, and the like, one side might cite research showing that any one of these policies has only small effects, while the other side may not seem to care about that research and argue, "we need to do something" anyway. Both sides can be correct. The direct impact of any one policy may be small, but as discussions of that policy circulate in society, and the goals of the policy become integrated into a social movement, its indirect effects may be considerable.

It would be nice if we could separate policy discussions from social movements, but doing so is difficult. Evaluating one piece of individual policy is hard enough, but measuring its overall impact as part of a social movement is nearly impossible. Perhaps food would be less controversial if we could have food movements without the need for policy. After all, stigmatizing a food can be done without policy. But that is not how democracies tend to work. Social movements tend to pursue both policy changes and cultural changes simultaneously.

The Local Foods Movement

The local foods movement is another issue where controversies emerge from a blurry distinction between policy and movements. I have written on local foods, and in my first writings I failed to notice that it is indeed a movement that is difficult to analyze using traditional economics. My first writing on the issue was coauthored at the Library of Economics and Liberty[26] and critiqued the local foods movement on several grounds. My coauthor and I argued that local does not necessarily mean more healthful, better for the environment, or better for the local economy. It *could* be all those things, but simply being local doesn't guarantee that it is. Because of this, we did not agree with proposals to require organizations such as schools to acquire a certain percentage of their food from local sources.

Many people resented the article. They felt as if I had attacked something sacred, because in a way, I had.

Negative reactions to the article taught me two things. First, people have very fond feelings for local foods. That first lesson taught me a second one: These fond feelings are creating a new food movement wherein people are taking a greater interest in what they eat—and that is a good thing. Carrots at the local farmers market may or may not be more healthful than carrots at the grocery store, but if going to a farmers market makes someone more likely to eat carrots and less likely to eat junk food, then this local food may promote healthful eating. Becoming a supporter of Community Supported Agriculture (CSA), in which customers buy a share of whatever the farm harvests, might expose people to new types of vegetables they otherwise might not try.

Concomitant with the local food movement are a variety of social justice issues, such as efforts to bring fresh food into food deserts and low-income areas. The local food movement is also associated with education, because many schools are using school gardens to teach children about how food is produced and to help them develop a taste for healthful foods early in life. Locavores get more than just food from farmers markets and other nearby food sources; they acquire social goods related to community.[27]

Being an economist, I only recently gained an appreciation for everything involved in a social movement. One can't just pick apart a movement and analyze all its elements separately, and one can't just view a movement as a mechanism through which consumers are attempting to get certain goods. That is, people aren't just shopping at farmers markets, CSAs, and dining at underground restaurants to acquire certain types of foods. They are expressing their values, as well as discontents with the existing food system. They are searching for something more meaningful than a market transaction.[28,29]

That first article I coauthored on local foods was not meant to discourage people from buying local food, but to discourage policies that would force people to buy local, and to caution policymakers to be careful before subsidizing it. I still hold these views, but now when I write about the topic I am careful to acknowledge that local food is a *movement* with many potential benefits. Only if I praise the movement will my critiques regarding policy be taken seriously. Because of this, my writings are less controversial than they once were.

It Is Difficult to Debate Science and Policy Simultaneously

It is reasonable to want to first designate what science can tell us about important social issues, and then to discuss the best policies (including no policy at all) to address it. Gathering facts before forming strategies just makes sense. This may be the preferred mode-of-operation for scientists and business consultants, but not necessarily for politicians and interest groups. The reason is that policy is the result of negotiations, and every admission made in the fact-gathering stage impacts a person's negotiating power in the policy stage.

Consider when Senator Jim Inhofe (Republican from Oklahoma) threw a snowball on the U.S. Senate floor as an argument against the idea of climate change. Inhofe has the reputation of being the staunchest climate denier in Congress. It could be that the Senator does not believe the science showing that carbon absorbs long-wave electromagnetic radiation bouncing from the earth's surface. Chances are, if he had real reason to believe this science wrong he could assert these reasons and soon accept his Nobel Prize. It is also unlikely that Inhofe believes that we are not emitting more carbon than we are sequestering.

He gladly accepts the role of foremost climate denier in Congress because he is doing everything he can to prevent government action to mitigate climate change. Hobbling the ability of the federal government to confront problems is what has made him popular among his constituents. By asserting that climate change is a hoax, he sends a clear message to his constituents that he will not even consider a government policy intended to curb emissions. It is a negotiating tactic, like telling a potential buyer of your used car that you paid $6,000 for it last year when in fact you paid $4,000.

Of course, the snowball was probably more than just a negotiating tactic. It was a publicity stunt also, one that he knew would be covered by media and circulated on social media. Moreover, discussing this stunt drew attention away from the real debate on climate change.

And so it goes with food. Organic food is generally purchased by political liberals (i.e., in the United States, Democrats), yet both Republicans and Democrats have similar beliefs about the health benefits of organic foods. If you told me that you prefer foods that don't have genetically modified ingredients, and then asked me to guess your political affiliation, I would guess a Democrat (if you were an American). Most others would also. Yet the percent of Republicans and Democrats who believe GM foods are unhealthful is nearly identical.[30] Despite these agreements on GM foods, when California voted on whether to require labels for genetically modified foods in 2012, Democrats were much more likely to vote for the requirement while Republicans were much more likely to vote against it.[31]

The explanation for this difference is simple. Although citizens of both political parties possess the same perceptions regarding the potential dangers of GM foods, they disagree on the ability of government regulation to do any good. Polls show that Democrats have a more negative opinion of big business (e.g., those producing GM foods). Republicans have a more negative opinion of government, which would regulate those businesses.[32] So when Republicans and Democrats trade arguments over labeling of GM foods, though they generally agree on potential dangers from GM foods, Republicans have the incentive to claim there are no dangers in order to help them negotiate for no regulations, while Democrats have the incentive to exaggerate dangers to bolster their claims for why regulations are necessary.

The Power of Intuition

Most of us have seen established science undergo a correction, and though this is the natural course of intellectual progress, it can understandably cause one to be skeptical of scientific claims. A recent Pew poll found that Americans frequently encounter news stories regarding food and health that seem to conflict with earlier studies, and 37% of respondents say that such research cannot be trusted because it is contradictory. These individuals may find the consistent message of food celebritiessuch as William Davis (who argues that all wheat products are dangerous because its genes have changed in the last century), reassuring despite a lack of scientific credibility. This lack of scientific credibility may not matter for many, given that only 19% of

Americans believe scientists understand the health effects of GM foods "very well" anyway.[30]

Most people born in the 1970s or earlier have witnessed a scientific reversal regarding the role of fat in a healthful diet. During the 1980s most of the health advice boiled down to one tip: avoid fat. The American Heart Association was even advising us to drink soft drinks to avoid it. Many Americans heeded this advice, yet health problems in the United States didn't improve; in fact, they only worsened. Eventually, we discovered that the "science" did not really document a link between fat consumption and health, at least not the type of link we were led to believe.

Now fat is no longer a public enemy (that role seems to have been given to sugar, at least for now). Based on the best types of health research (randomized controlled trials), scientists now say that the fat guidelines introduced in the United States and the United Kingdom in decades past should never have been introduced.[33] When investigative journalists such as Gary Taubes and Nina Teicholz described what went wrong, their accounts did not sound like normal science correcting itself based on new information. This was not Einstein standing on the shoulders of Newton and leading us into science revolution. Health researchers had concluded from poorly designed studies that fat was bad for health, and then when the findings from other—often better—studies contradicted that notion, they simply assumed those new findings were flawed. Believing those new studies to be flawed, even the authors sometimes did not submit them for publication, or if they did, reviewers rejected the articles because the results contradicted their beliefs.[34,35] This was not how science was supposed to work, so why should anyone trust what is deemed to be "established science"?

However much we like to think of science being receptive to new ideas and willing to set old theories aside for new ones when the evidence demands, there is a reason Max Plank (a member of science's pantheon) remarked, "A new scientific truth does not triumph by convincing its opponents and making them see the light, but rather because its opponents eventually die, and a new generation grows up that is familiar with it."[36] Only those familiar with the history of science would be unsurprised at the length of time it took to correct this mistaken notion about fat and health. Although scientists may see the correction as vindication of scientific institutions, its belatedness must have made many skeptical of any new scientific claims.

As this reversal on fat unfolded, some must have recalled a fellow with rather odd views named Dr. Atkins. In 1972, he published a book advocating a diet where you avoid all carbohydrates but eat as much fat as you like.

This must have seemed crazy in the 1980s, when cookies were deemed healthful as long as they didn't contain fat; but in 2016, the odd Dr. Atkins might seem more knowledgeable than the entire health profession to some. It is not all that surprising, then, when some give up all wheat after reading William Davis's *Wheat Belly* and take their nutrient recommendations from Dr. Oz.

The reversal on fat also might have led people to begin placing greater trust in their intuitions than in science. On July 6, 2015, Susannah Mushatt Jones was the oldest human at 116 years, and she gave partial credit for her longevity to the four strips of bacon she ate every morning.[37] Born in 1899, Susannah continued to eat an old-fashioned diet—the diet of our grandparents. Maybe, some people suspected, there is more wisdom in traditional eating than there is in the most advanced scientific institutions?

There was a time when cattle were fed the rendered carcasses of sheep. However unnatural it may seem to the ordinary person, scientists considered it perfectly safe, and even advantageous given that it allowed us to extract greater value from every sheep slaughtered. If you expressed skepticism of its safety in the 1970s, most scientists would calmly explain the process to you, and make you believe your skepticism was the result of ignorance, not wise intuition.

Yet it would be your intuition that would be vindicated. In the last two decades of the 20th century the phenomenon of "mad cow" disease (bovine spongiform encephalopathy) emerged, where prions destroyed the brains of cattle—and the brains of humans, if they ate the diseased beef. The current consensus is that these prions originated in the sheep, were transferred to the cattle in feed, and then transferred to humans in beef. Between 1996 and 2014, this disease killed 177 people in the United Kingdom, where feeding of sheep to cattle was most prevalent, and 27 deaths occurred in France.[38]

Only four deaths occurred in the United States, and this might explain why Europeans are more fearful of livestock production technologies such as synthetic growth hormones. Although growth hormones are considered safe by most scientists who study the issue, it is understandable that the British and French might prefer to avoid them, trusting their intuition that because the hormones are "unnatural" they might eventually be proven dangerous. For over 20 years, the European Union has prohibited imports of beef from the United States that were administered synthetic growth hormones (Johnson, 2015), despite all scientific evidence finding their use safe. In the United States, the majority of beef is produced using synthetic growth hormones. It is hard to say exactly why Europeans and Americans have such different views, but it does seem that their intuitions regarding the hormones differ, and these intuitions are formed by multiple factors. There is no reason to believe these intuitions will begin to resemble each other soon, and thus no reason to believe the hormone controversy will not continue.

This also could explain some of the controversy regarding local foods, minimal ingredient foods, and organic foods. It is not clear whether local foods would be safer or more healthful than their non-local counterparts, but some people do believe they would be,[39] and there is no science to prove them wrong (or right). For many there is a strong intuition that local foods are more healthful, and that intuition has some logic to it. After all, intuition is a feeling of knowing based on thoughts that occur below the realm of consciousness.

It is difficult for a local food producer to produce highly processed foods because that requires expensive equipment and often poses high regulatory burdens. If less processed foods are then more healthful, perhaps local foods are as well? Yet, someone else could argue that importing foods allows people to expand their field of choices and find more healthful foods than they could acquire locally. It would be unwise for Swedes, for example, to try to acquire all their fruits within 20 miles of their homes. With no clear science to reconcile conflicting intuitions, controversies continue, including the extent to which local schools should pay higher food prices to incorporate locally produced foods.

Highly processed foods only use ingredients demonstrated to be safe for consumption, and food ingredients are usually in the Food and Drug Administration's "Generally Recognized as Safe" category. In 2014, many Americans heard from news reports that the Subway restaurant chain was being petitioned to remove a chemical from their breads that is also used in yoga mats. This chemical is called (cue the scary music) azodicarbonamide—the name is enough to make bread seem dangerous to eat. The public may not have known about this chemical, but scientists did. The Food and Drug Administration (FDA) has studied it and found that it is safe in bread dough so long as its concentration is 45 parts per million or less.[40] Not everyone, however, is willing to mute their intuition and just assume that what the FDA says is correct.

Each Person Is a Life-World

For a research project, I once had to learn a mathematical optimization technique called artificial neural networks, which is a mathematical procedure that attempts to mimic the neural networks of the brain. In the process

I gained some insights into how humans think that forever changed my understanding of food controversies.

What follows is my attempt to explain neural networks in the simplest way possible, using an analogy. Suppose Jim calls a meeting for anyone interested in protesting the use of transgenic genetic modification in food production. Jim decides that if at least 20 people show up, that suffices for starting a protest in his town. With his own money he funds advertisements for the meeting on Facebook. Of the thousands of people in his town who see the advertisement, 26 decide to attend.

Five of those are local gardeners who have spent their lives gathering seed from their gardens and trading it with others to preserve heirloom varieties of vegetables. They had read that farmers planting transgenic soybean seed are prohibited by law from planting any of the seed they harvest. In the past, many soybean farmers would reserve a portion of their harvest and use it to plant next year's crop, but because corporations "own" the genetics of the seed they can prevent farmers from doing so. This strikes those five gardeners as not only unethical, but a violation of a sacred practice. Mostly for this reason, those five gardeners attend Jim's meeting.

Another five attendees are activists who protest any form of corporate power. They attended the 1999 anti-globalization protests in Seattle and the 2011 Occupy Wall Street movement. They are concerned that, as more and more seed is owned and sold by large corporations like Monsanto, the world's food supply will be held hostage by organizations with only their own interests in mind. One of the activists watched his mother's retirement fund vanish with the Enron scandal, another saw a documentary on the catastrophic chemical spill in Bhopal, India, and the others were exposed to a variety of music, art, and literature that depicted the private sector as evil and the corporate world as a danger to society.

Ten attendees are concerned parents, some of whom have children with food allergies, one with an unexplained autoimmune disease, and others who feel as though they no longer have any control over what their children eat. They stare at the list of ingredients in a standard bread loaf and grow fearful about the words they do not understand. Recalling that their grandmothers once made bread with only flour, water, salt, and yeast, they suspect these other ingredients are meant to save the companies money at the expense of their children's health. When they hear that scientists have taken a gene from a bacterium and inserted it into the plants that comprise some of their food supply, they see this as a step too far. Their deep attachment to their children and fear of the unknown, along with the refusal of any regulatory agency to respond to their concerns (government agencies only like to communicate through vetted press releases), makes them resent the current food system and eager to strike back in any way.

Three attendees are actually in favor of genetic modification in agriculture, but they believe that regulation is excessively permissive, and that the genetic makeup of crops is changing too fast to really understand the dangers. Though not opposed to GMOs, they want to slow the practice down, but because there is no "slow-down" movement, their conscience tells them that, for now, the opposition is on the right side of history. One of these three is actually a botanist, and so understands the genetic modification process better than the vast majority of people.

One of the attendees does not really understand GMOs, but he is looking for something meaningful to do in his life. The idea of fighting power appeals to him, but he is neither a member of a minority group nor poor and so cannot portray himself as a victim. Perhaps being a consumer of conventional foods his whole life is his victimhood? Of the two remaining attendees, one is an undercover spy for a seed corporation, and another is a reporter.

What I describe above is a reasonable story, but it is also a metaphor for how one person's neural network might work. Though a brain is more complex than this, suppose that your "decision" to sneeze is determined by one neuron in the brain. A neuron receives signals from other neurons, and a neuron can—in a way—count. It counts the number of signals it receives from other neurons, just as Jim counted the number of attendees, and if that number exceeds a threshold, the neuron itself sends a signal. As this neuron considers whether to sneeze, it receives a signal from neurons that receive signals from other neurons indicating that a cat hair has been detected in the nose. It also receives signals from other neurons that draw on memory to evaluate whether the cat hair is an allergen. Indeed, the cat hair is in the nose, and the brain long ago decided cat hair is an allergen, and so a sufficient number of signals reach our neuron of interest, and it itself releases its own signal that causes the body to sneeze.

After begging forgiveness from neurologists for this crude metaphor, I hope you can see the analogy. Jim is the neuron of interest, and the attendees are the signals sent from other neurons. The important thing to grasp about neural networks, and this metaphor, is the complexity of signals. Even more important to see is the impossibility of ever describing clearly why the GMO protest movement is taking place in Jim's hometown (or why you sneeze).

Yes, you sneeze because a cat hair entered your nose and you are allergic to cats, but why are you allergic to cats in the first place? Yes, the five gardeners oppose transgenic seed because they believe the farmer should own any seed she harvests, but exactly why do they hold this belief, when they also know that companies are more likely to develop better genetics if they own those genetics. After all, these gardeners do not oppose patents on tractor engines, or the software running their computers.

Your body decided cat hair was an allergen due to a complex interaction of many environmental stimuli and thousands more interactions between the 100 billion neurons in the human brain. The same could be said for the gardeners. They grew up saving and planting their own seed, and they have seen how that system improves genetics without patents. They also have fond memories of seed preservation, and it evokes memories of home and even spiritual stirrings. Their decision to protest GMOs is the product of billions of neurons exchanging signals, neurons evolving different connections to one another, and other changes to the brain that could never be documented fully.

If we consider that Jim is but one neuron in a *real* person named Abbie, and the five gardeners, five activists, ten parents, and the six others are metaphors for neurons connected to the Jim-neuron inside Abbie's mind, we can imagine the real, subconscious dialectics a person undergoes before deciding to oppose GMOs. Although Abbie is not a gardener, her mother was an avid collector of heirloom seed varieties. She has no actual history in activism, but a part of her believes that she should become more active on social issues—to leave her mark on the world, and ensure her life means something. Though her two children are healthy, about half of her close friends have children who are not, and she frequently hears them wonder whether modern food is the cause of their problems. Although she has encountered convincing information and people who express confidence in GMOs, the bulk of her world biases her against them, and these biases come to her in such manifold, complex, and often subtle ways that it is difficult to determine which of these influences has the largest impact on her views. She isn't completely aware of all these influences, but she "knows" GMOs are bad.

What if we ask Abbie, why? She will draw upon a wealth of arguments, some of them resonating with her real influences, some contrived at the moment to justify her beliefs. She will seem, and indeed is, very informed, and at the same time not completely cognizant of how her beliefs are constructed. Moreover, should some of her arguments be countered with facts, Abbie still has a number of other arguments from which to continue her opposition.

In fact, attempts to prove her wrong with facts may very well only solidify her original position. This isn't because she is ill-informed, unintelligent, or stubborn—it is because she is human. Referred to as a backfire effect, it is related to cognitive dissonance and the need for people to perceive that their beliefs are consistent with one another. If Abbie *knows* GMOs are a food safety threat, but all scientific organizations say they do not cause food allergies, she may very well accuse these organizations of being biased—and in her search for evidence of this bias, she will eventually discover some.

Ironically, as I was writing this paragraph, the *Food and Water Watch* and *The New York Times* published an investigative piece regarding the conflicts of interest at the National Academies of Science (NAS) regarding its panel on Sciences, Engineering, and Medicine. There is no more authoritative scientific body than the NAS, yet many of its panel members apparently profit from biotechnology ventures.[41,42] Although I still hold the NAS in great esteem, if I were looking for a reason not to, one was delivered right into my Facebook feed.

Understanding the sources of controversies requires insights into the psychology of knowing, of being certain. In his remarkable book *On Being Certain*, the neurologist Robert Burton writes, "Despite how certainty feels, it is neither a conscious choice nor even a thought process. Certainty and similar states of 'knowing what we know' arise out of involuntary brain mechanisms that, like love or anger, function independently of reason."[43] This doesn't mean that people form beliefs independent of facts, logic, or life experiences. Rather, what is believed to be true, what is deemed to be a fact, what is considered logical, and recollections of life experiences are all determined jointly by the byzantine networks of the human mind. Yet, when we debate food issues, we are compelled to present our beliefs as if they are the direct and uncontested consequence of fact and logic. And so, in our haste to win the debate we contradict ourselves, alter our priorities, reveal ourselves as hypocrites, and double down on discredited assumptions—all the while expressing amazement that anyone could come to an alternative conclusion.

Most people are probably sympathetic to this depiction of the human mind, but none more so than sociologists and anthropologists as evidenced by their frequent use of the term *lifeworld*. Though it goes by many definitions, my favorite is given by Kraus as, "Lifeworld means a person's subjective construction of reality, which he or she forms."[44] Humans do not just process information like the ones and zeros of computers. Information is colored by context, shaped by previous life experiences, illuminated or suppressed based on social pressure, and manipulated to be consistent with prior beliefs.

Science works well because the scientific method calls for experiments whose outcomes should not be influenced by the researcher's lifeworld. Every other question that cannot be answered with science, will, however, receive different answers based on people's lifeworlds. As such, one should not expect the calm introduction of new facts to reconcile all or even most disagreements.

So when interacting in a food controversy with people who disagree with you, I offer a few thoughts to keep in mind.

- However odd their beliefs may be, they possess good reasons for holding them—reasons that matter to them, if not to you.
- Their ability to process information is probably equal to yours, they are just starting from a different set of assumptions and are striving toward a different goal.
- Instead of just asking them "where they get their information," ask them about their life experiences and personal relationships that may have helped form their views. Do not appear to be psychoanalyzing them, but make a sincere effort to understand them better, and make this sincerity evident.
- Admit the gaps in your understanding and the questions you still ask. Showing that you still have much to learn will allow them to make the same admission.
- Find common ground by trying to identify the type of scientific experiments that would satisfy you both.
- Remember that you may place different levels of trust in certain authorities, like regulatory agencies and scientists. Avoid making personal attacks on these authorities, for they will be compelled to defend them regardless.
- Remember that you are one element in the other person's lifeworld. You can have an impact on the person's beliefs, but your impact is more likely to be more subtle than revolutionary.

Parting Thought

Controversy can be an obstacle to progress, but it can also be a friend. However entrenched two sides of a debate may become, they can help a society pursue the "golden mean" of sensible food policy. Without activist groups seeking to end pesticide use, the lack of social monitoring in pesticide regulations may give companies excessive influence over which pesticides are approved. Yet without lobbying on the part of these companies, the research they fund, and groups favoring conventional agriculture, regulation might become so aggressive that the price of fruits soars, making it more difficult for households to acquire adequate nutrition.

Controversy serves as a parallel enforcement mechanism to protect food safety. If some of us were not skeptical of companies' willingness to keep dangerous foods out of the food supply, we might not have learned that Saudis are eating foods with genetically modified maize, which is not supposed to be available for human consumption, due to the potential for food allergens.[45]

As debate opponents battle in the public arena they reveal information about each other that the spectators deserve to know. Many people oppose modern food technologies because they fear the organizations that sell them: corporations, whose major goal is to earn profits. Yet these same people deserve to know that the icon of the anti-GMO movement, Vandana Shiva, makes around $40,000 for every speech she gives denouncing GMOs.[46] This fact doesn't mean that Shiva would necessarily skew the truth to receive more speaking invitations, but neither are all corporations willing to peddle lies for a monetary return.

Perhaps controversy is the healthy pulse of a democracy? Perhaps we should always seek at least a modicum of controversy? There was an ancient Jewish law that said no one could be convicted of a capital offense if the verdict was unanimous. One interpretation of the law is that a unanimous verdict is a sign that the court itself was not being diligent if it could not find at least some evidence to acquit the suspect. When all beliefs aligned, it was a sign that those beliefs stemmed from something other than the facts on the ground. Indeed, a group of scientists has shown that when different pieces of evidence are not collected independently, when the amount of evidence is large, and when all the evidence supports one clear answer, there is good reason to suspect that answer. A systematic failure has occurred in how the evidence is collected that suggests real measurement error that should be considered before a final verdict is reached.[47]

With this perspective in mind, we can reinterpret food controversies to be a sign that we are on the right track—that the truth is being sought, that policies are reasonable, and that our food is more healthful and safer than if there were no food controversies at all.

Quiz Questions

1. Even if organic food has fewer pesticide residues on a per calorie basis, how might consuming non-organic fruits and vegetables actually lead to a more healthful diet?
   a. Pesticide residues cannot be expressed on a per calorie basis.

b. Non-organic food is less expensive, allowing persons to consume more fruits and vegetables.

c. Pesticide residues can act like an immunization, helping to protect the body from residues consumed in other foods.

d. Although pesticides themselves can be dangerous, pesticide residues are actually beneficial.

2. How do U.S. government subsidies given to farmers impact U.S. calorie consumption?

a. They greatly increase calorie consumption.

b. They lead to a small increase in calorie consumption.

c. They greatly decrease calorie consumption.

d. They lead to a small decrease in calorie consumption.

3. Which seed and pesticide corporation receives the most attention from anti-GMO activists?

a. Monsanto

b. Syngenta

c. Dow Chemical

d. Dupont

4. Sales of high-calorie sodas in the United States in the last two decades have

a. Fallen

b. Risen

c. Remained the same

5. In the United States, both Republicans and Democrats have similar beliefs about the health benefits of organic foods, though they differ on policy.

a. True

b. False

6. In the 1970s and 1980s, the livestock industry continued to feed cattle the rendered carcasses of sheep, despite loud protests by the scientific community.

a. True

b. False

7. Subway was recently caught adding azodicarbonamide to their bread, a chemical that is dangerous at any level consumed.

a. True

b. False

8. What term refers to a person's subjective construction of reality, formed from their genetics, environment, and life experiences?
    a. life construction
    b. life augment
    c. life world
    d. life manifestation
9. In most cases, it is impossible for someone to know the exact reasons why they believe something is true.
    a. True
    b. False
10. There are reasons to be skeptical of a claim if it is believed by everyone.
    a. True
    b. False

Discussion Questions

1. Suppose pesticide residues are detected in meals at elementary school cafeterias. Discuss why someone might argue the food is nevertheless safe.
2. Suppose pesticide residues are detected in meals at elementary school cafeterias, but at levels the government has deemed to be safe. Discuss why someone might argue the food is nevertheless unsafe.
3. Suppose a study finds that individuals consuming a high-sugar diet tend to suffer from fatigue. Describe one or two other factors that are correlated with sugar consumption that might also cause the fatigue, making it difficult to label sugar as the cause of fatigue.
4. Describe why some people oppose food made with genetically modified organisms, even if they think the food is safe to eat.
5. Describe the similarities and the differences between the anti-tobacco and anti-soda movements.
6. Describe how a farmers market can be much more than a place to buy food.
7. Name some reasons why well-informed people might be skeptical about claims made by the scientific community.
8. Consider two identical twins raised in the same household, but each goes to a different college to pursue a different major. Describe the events that might occur in each twin's college experience that would cause them to sharply disagree on whether genetically modified organisms are good for the world.

References

1. Sinclair UI. *Candidate for Governor: And How I Got Licked.* Vol 109. University of California Press; 1994.
2. Lu C, Toepel K, Rene I, Fenske R, Barr D, Bravo R. Organic diets significantly lower children's dietary exposure to organophosphorus pesticides. *Environmental Health Perspectives.* 2006;114:260–263.
3. Lu C. Organic Diets: Lu et al. respond. *Environmental Health Perspectives.* 2006;114(4):A211.
4. Lu C. Yes: It's common sense to try to avoid pesticide exposure. *Wall Street Journal.* June 17, 2013;R3.
5. Silverstein JH. No: There is little evidence organic food is worth the cost; *Wall Street Journal.* June 17, 2013;R3.
6. Leschin-Hoar C. Slice the Price of Fruits and Veggies, Save 200,000 Lives? National Public Radio. 2016.
7. Centers for Disease Control and Prevention. *Adult Obesity Facts.* September 1, 2016.
8. Centers for Disease Control and Prevention. *Childhood Obesity Facts.* November 17, 2016b.
9. Morenga LT, Mallard S, Mann J. Dietary sugars and body weight: systematic review and meta-analyses of randomised controlled trials and cohort studies. *BMJ.* 2013;346:e7492.
10. Just D, Wansink B. Fast food, soft drink and candy intake is unrelated to body mass index for 95% of American adults. *Obesity Science and Practice.* 2015;1:126–130.
11. Okrent AM, Alston JM. The effects of farm commodity and retail food policies on obesity and economic welfare in the United States. *American Journal of Agricultural Economics.* 2012;94(3):611–646.
12. Schute N. Gluten Goodbye: One-Third of Americans Say They're Trying to Shun It. National Public Radio. 2013.
13. Di Sabatino A, Volta U, et al. Small amounts of gluten in subjects with suspected nonceliac gluten sensitivity: a randomized, double-blind, placebo-controlled, cross-over trial. *Clinical Gastroenterology and Hepatology.* 2015;13:1604–1612.
14. Biesiekierski JR, Newnham ED, et al. Gluten causes gastrointestinal symptoms in subjects without celiac disease: a double-blind randomized placebo-controlled trial. *American Journal of Gastroenterology.* 2011;106:508–514.
15. Biesiekierski JR, Peters SL, et al. No effects of gluten in patients with self-reported non-celiac gluten sensitivity after dietary reduction of fermentable, poorly absorbed, short-chain carbohydrates. *American Journal of Gastroenterology.* 2013;145:320–328.
16. Jargon J. The gluten-free craze: is it healthy? *Wall Street Journal.* July 23, 2014.
17. University of Florida Institute of Food and Agricultural Sciences. When it comes to gluten-free diets, unfounded beliefs abound: *ScienceDaily.* July 29, 2014.

18. Whole Grains Council. Whole Grain Statistics. 2016.

19. Schurman R, Munro WA. *Fighting for the Future of Food*. University of Minnesota Press; 2010.

20. Fitting E. *Food Activism*. Cultures of Corn and Anti-GMO Activism in Mexico and Columbia. Edited by Carole Counihan and Valeria Siniscalchi. 2014;175–192.

21. Guthrie A, Esterl M. Despite tax, Mexico soda sales pop. *Wall Street Journal*. May 4, 2016.

22. Reopeng A. Beverage consumption in relation to discretionary food intake and diet quality among US adults, 2003 to 2012. *Journal of the Academy of Nutrition and Dietetics*. 2016;116: 28–37.

23. Mayne S, Auchincloss A, Michael Y. Impact of policy and built environment changes on obesity-related outcomes: a systematic review of naturally occurring experiments. *Obesity Reviews*. 2015;16:362–375.

24. Esterl M. Diet soda's glass looks half empty. *Wall Street Journal*. December 9, 2013.

25. Sanger-Katz M. The decline of "Big Soda." *New York Times*. 2015.

26. Lusk JL, Norwood B. The locavore's dilemma: why pineapples shouldn't be grown in North Dakota. Library of Economics and Liberty; 2011.

27. Diedrich S. Food is community. *Iowa Now*. 2015.

28. Starr A. Local food: a social movement? *Cultural Studies—Critical Methodologies*. 2010;10:479–490.

29. Hvitsand C. Community supported agriculture (CSA) as a transformational act—distinct values and multiple motivations among farmers and consumers. *Agroecology and Sustainable Food Systems*. 2016;49:333–351.

30. Funk C, Kennedy B. *The New Food Fights: U.S. Public Divides Over Food Science*. Pew Research Center; 2016.

31. Bovay J, Alston JM. GM labeling regulation by plebiscite: Analysis of voting on Proposition 37 in California. *Journal of Agricultural and Resource Economics*. 2016;41:161–188.

32. Newport F. Democrats, Republicans Diverge on Capitalism, Federal Gov't. GALLUP Politics; 2012.

33. Harcombe Z, Baker JS, et al. Evidence from randomised controlled trials did not support the introduction of dietary fat guidelines in 1977 and 1983: a systematic review and meta-analysis. *Open Heart*. 2015;2.

34. Taubes G. *Good Calories, Bad Calories*. Alfred A. Knopf; 2008.

35. Teicholz N. *The Big Fat Surprise*. Simon & Schuster; 2014.

36. Planck M. *Scientific Autobiography and Other Papers*. Philosophical Library; 1949.

37. Whitford E. Oldest human turns 116 in Brooklyn, credits longevity to sleep and bacon. Gothamist.com; 2015.

38. CNN. Mad Cow Disease Fast Facts. 2016.

39. Onozaka Y, Nurse G, McFadden DT. Local food consumers: how motivations and perceptions translate to buying behavior. Choices. 2010;25.

40. Aubrey A. Almost 500 foods contain the "yoga mat" compound. Should we care? *The Salt*. March 6, 2014.

41. Schwab T. New York Times confirms GMO industry ties at National Academies of Sciences. *Food and Water Watch*. 2016.

42. Strom S. National biotechnology panel faces new conflict of interest questions. *New York Times*. 2016.

43. Burton R. *On Being Certain*. St. Martin's Press; 2008.

44. Kraus B. The life we live and the life we experience: introducing the epistemological difference between "Lifeworld" (Lebenswelt) and "Life Conditions" (Lebenslage). *Social Work & Society*. 2015;13:4.

45. Elsanhoty RM, Al-Turki AL, Ramadan MF. Prevalence of genetically modified rice, maize, and soy in Saudi food products. *Applied Biochemistry and Biotechnology*. 2013;171:883–899.

46. Miller H. Anti-GMO activist Vandana Shiva earns $40,000 per speech advocating policies harming poor. Genetic Literacy Project; 2014.

47. Gunn JL, Chapeau-Blondeau F, et al. Too good to be true: when overwhelming evidence fails to convince. *Proceedings of the Royal Society A*. 2016:472.

10

The Obesity Pandemic and Food Insecurity in Developing Countries

A CASE STUDY FROM THE CARIBBEAN

Kristen Lowitt, Katherine Gray-Donald, Gordon M. Hickey,
Arlette Saint Ville, Isabella Francis-Granderson,
Chandra A. Madramootoo, and Leroy E. Phillip

Chapter Highlights

- Provides an overview of global trends in obesity and malnutrition
- Describes diverse policy responses to obesity
- Discusses the need for a food systems response to obesity
- Presents a case study from the Caribbean that sought to address obesity and food insecurity among school children

Global Trends in Obesity and Food Insecurity

Obesity is a significant public health concern affecting over half a billion people globally.[1] Once considered a problem limited to high-income countries, obesity has now become a problem for all countries at all incomes levels. As global economies continue to expand, many middle- and low-income countries are following the now well-worn path from undernutrition to obesity.[2] More people in the world today are overweight and obese than undernourished.[3]

Most simply, "overweight" and "obesity" are terms used to describe having too much body fat. Overweight and obesity are major public health concerns, because excess weight gain is a key risk factor for non-communicable diseases (NCDs) such as cardiovascular diseases, diabetes, cancers, and chronic respiratory diseases.[4] Overweight and obesity are commonly measured using body mass index (BMI), a basic index of weight-for-height (kg/m^2). BMI offers the most useful population-level measure of overweight and obesity because it is the same for both sexes and for all ages of adults;[1] however, for children, age also needs to be considered when using BMI.[1]

According to the World Health Organization[1], the prevalence of obesity worldwide has doubled since 1980. In 2014, more than 1.9 billion adults were overweight; of these, over 600 million were obese. It is of particular concern that obesity rates also have been steadily rising among children and adolescents. In 2010, 43 million preschool children were assessed as being overweight or obese, a 60% increase since 1990, and the number continues to rise.[5] If recent trends continue, it is estimated that by 2030 nearly 58% of the world's adult population could be overweight or obese, with developing regions experiencing the largest proportional increase in the prevalence of obesity.[6]

Although a range of factors contribute to obesity, increased intake of energy-dense foods (foods high in fat and sugar) and a decline in physical activity, have been recognized as paramount.[1] The term "nutrition transition" is used to refer to the combination of changes in access to food and decreased physical activity, and it was first observed in developed countries in the 1970s. The nutrition transition is characterized by a shift toward increased reliance upon processed foods, more eating away from home, larger portion sizes, and greater use of edible oils and sugar-sweetened beverages.[3] This is accompanied by a decline in physical activity due to the increasingly sedentary nature of many forms of work. During the early 1990s these changes began to appear in developing countries, spurred largely by economic globalization. Freer flow of trade propelled by the World Trade Organization, along with global investments in agriculture, produced large shifts in relative food prices that favored animal-source foods, edible oils, and other global commodities, including sugar.[3] Thus, the nutrition transition is deeply rooted in processes of globalization, particularly as these forces have altered the nature of global agri-food systems and thereby the quantity, type, cost, and desirability of foods available for human consumption.[7]

The nutrition transition in many developing countries has resulted in a "double burden of malnutrition."[1] This means that while some countries are still dealing with the problem of undernutrition, they also are experiencing rapid increases in the prevalence of NCDs for which obesity is a major risk factor.[1] Undernutrition and over-nutrition (energy overconsumption) also have been referred to as the "two faces" of malnutrition.[8] It is possible for this double burden of malnutrition to exist at the individual, household, and population levels. For example, an overweight or obese individual may be deficient in one or more vitamins and minerals; at the household level, a mother may be overweight and a grandparent or child underweight; and at the population level, both undernutrition and overweight can be seen in the same community, region, or nation.[9]

As this double burden of malnutrition has become better understood, it is now recognized that food insecurity (one of the main causes of undernutrition in terms of insufficient access to nutritious food) and obesity can go in hand in hand. This does not mean, however, that food insecurity and obesity are causally related; indeed, the particular association between the two is a subject of ongoing research. Nonetheless, both are increasingly viewed as consequences of social and economic disadvantage.[10] Obesity in developing countries originally was associated with those at higher-income levels but recent research suggests this trend is changing, with rising obesity rates among even the poor in the developing world.[3] Therefore, in developing countries, obesity is affecting people at all income levels. In developed countries, by contrast, studies suggest those at lower socioeconomic levels show disproportionately higher rates of obesity compared with those with higher incomes.[5] This is due, in part, to the fact that food insecure households with limited income tend to spend a larger proportion of their income on cheaper, energy-dense foods, which are satiating but have minimal nutritional benefit. In fact, studies in both developed and developing country contexts indicate that fresh fruits and vegetables tend to be the most expensive food items in terms of cost per calorie,[11,12] and it is known that limited intake of fruits and vegetables is associated with obesity.[13] In addition to household income, studies in the United States have indicated that those with lower levels of education, as well as some minority populations, have a higher prevalence of overweight and obesity.[5]

There are global trends in obesity and food insecurity that need to be understood within regional contexts. For example, undernutrition rather than over-nutrition still tends to be the dominant malnutrition problem in some parts of sub-Saharan Africa and Asia.[1] Sociocultural factors, such as norms around body size, physical activity, or a fondness for certain types of foods that may be unique to different regions of the world also can play a compounding role in determining the prevalence of obesity.[14] Overall, and especially in developing country contexts, there is a need for enhanced monitoring data on the prevalence of obesity and its key risk indicators in order to better contextualize the global obesity trends and devise strategies and interventions to curb the pandemic.

Solutions and Approaches
Policy Approaches to Obesity

To sustainably address the complex obesity pandemic facing society, diverse action is required by governments and other institutions.[15] According to Sacks, Swinburn, and Lawrence,[16] the various public health approaches to addressing obesity generally include: (1) *Upstream policies*, designed to affect broad social or economic conditions of a society, such as food systems and physical activity environments; (2) *Midstream policies,* designed to directly influence population behaviors; and (3) *Downstream policies,* designed to support clinical interventions and community health services. Each of these approaches necessarily involves different policy perspectives, actors, targets, monitoring programs, and outcome measures.

Because many countries lack sufficient population monitoring data on obesity prevalence and associated risk indicators, and because the efficacy of obesity-related interventions and potential solutions are often contested, the challenge of obesity prevention can seem overwhelming.[15] Nevertheless, governments do have a wide range of policy instruments available to achieve their policy objectives related to obesity prevention. These include government spending (grants, loans, purchasing contracts, etc.), subsidies and taxation, education, information and advocacy, direct service delivery, laws and regulations, and engaging in partnerships. The key is to recognize that no single intervention or approach will be sufficient to reduce or reverse the obesity epidemic; instead, doing so requires a mix of instruments carefully designed to facilitate mutual learning and adjustment through multifaceted, integrative, participatory, and transdisciplinary approaches across the human life course.[15]

Through this wide range of policy options, the food system has emerged as a key locus of action. There are growing calls in public health for a full food systems response in which all parts of the system—production, storage, transport and trade, processing, retail, and consumption—contribute in an integrated way to making high-quality diets more available, affordable, and appealing.[2] A food systems response is based on the fundamental recognition that global food systems are currently not well aligned with the world's dietary and healthy eating needs, and that structural changes are required to allow them to do so.[17] Governments can better use the full range of policy instruments described above to stimulate a food systems response to obesity (see Table 10.1). For example, in "upstream policies", realigning production subsidies away from commodities that get processed into cheap, high-calorie food, and toward the fruits and vegetables that are lacking in most people's diets could assist in making healthy foods more affordable. In "midstream policies", campaigns and programs on healthy eating along with institutional food procurement guidelines that prioritize nutrition could play important roles in shifting eating patterns. Lastly, "downstream policies" may include initiatives such as providing the services of a nutritionist/dietitian to those communities experiencing increased health risks related to overweight and obesity.

"Farm to School" Feeding Programs

"Farm to school," also referred to as "farm to table" or "farm to fork" programs, have emerged as a promising food systems response to help reduce obesity prevalence and improve population health. These programs, through institutionalized procurement of healthy and local foods, generally seek to stimulate a food systems response to obesity by establishing renewed relationships between farmers, schools, and wider communities.[19] They have emerged from calls for nutritional reform of the much longer-standing "school feeding programs" (SFPs) that were historically established to address childhood undernutrition, but have been slow to adapt to the newer challenge of childhood obesity and overnutrition.[20] Through research to prevent NCDs, it has become clear that once a child is overweight, it is difficult to reverse the trend; hence, early interventions to encourage healthy eating among children can be an effective approach to addressing the risk of obesity and NCDs later in life.[21]

School feeding programs first emerged after World War II as western countries grappled with childhood undernutrition. In 1946, the United States passed the Richard R. Russell National School Lunch Act, establishing the first federal school food program, which mandated the United States Department of Agriculture to administer lunch programs, provide free or reduced-price meals to low-income students, and meet minimum nutritional standards.[22] Not long after, the U.S. food system was transformed through the green revolution, which led to major increases in agricultural productivity

Table 10.1 Examples of Policy Approaches that May Stimulate a Food Systems Response to Obesity

Upstream Policies

Sector:

Primary production	• Land use policies that support local food systems • Community gardens • Nutrition-sensitive agriculture supported by subsidies and taxes
Food processing	• Product composition standards (e.g., maximum levels of sugar, fat, salt) • Food safety standards
Distribution	• Import restrictions
Marketing	• Nutrient content disclosures • Restrictions on marketing of unhealthy food; promotion of healthy food • Taxes and subsidies (e.g., taxing targeted unhealthy foods and providing financial incentives for healthier options)
Retail	• Minimizing food deserts through accessible placement of retail outlets with healthy foods • Product placement in stores to promote healthy foods

Midstream Policies

Setting:

Early childcare	• Campaigns and programs to promote healthy eating • Nutritious food policies • Nutrition education for caregivers
Education (schools, universities)	• Campaigns and programs to promote healthy eating • School food policies and institutional procurement that support healthy and local foods
Workplaces	• Campaigns and programs to promote healthy eating • Health and nutrition targets • Financial incentives to participate in health and nutrition activities
Households	• Campaigns and programs to promote healthy eating • Mass media promotion of healthy foods
Other government facilities (hospitals, military, prisons)	• Institutional procurement policies that focus on sourcing healthy and local foods

Downstream Policies

Sector:

Primary care	• Healthy living and nutrition counseling • Primary care partnerships for community health
Secondary care	• Services of nutritionists/dieticians

Adapted from Sacks, Swinburn, & Lawrence[16] and Hawkes et al.[18].

and availability of food staples, and increased vertical integration and corporate control of food systems.[23] This globally reorganized agriculture brought about dietary transformations as processed foods became increasingly more available in schools. This was compounded by declines in federal funding of SFPs during the 1980s and 1990s, which led to corporate interests assuming a more prominent role in supplying school meals through privatized SFPs.[23]

As multinational companies took over more school meals services, access to high-fat and high-sugar foods in U.S. school diets increased. With public health concerns about childhood obesity mounting, however, the spotlight on the nutritional quality of school meals sparked reform.[20] The Healthy, Hunger-Free Kids Act (HHFKA) of 2010 responded to these concerns by updating nutritional guidelines for meals and requiring more servings and a greater variety of fruits and vegetables.[22] At this time, researchers flagged the potential for "farm to school" programs to help meet the nutritional objective of increasing fruit and vegetable consumption.[19] Farm to school programs can be understood as a more localized food system approach, which, through institutional food procurement, seeks to build connections between schools, producers, and wider communities, and also may stimulate local food production through the provision of reliable markets and supportive technologies.

Developing nations also have been implementing SFPs that continue to evolve. In the late 1990s, Brazil, for example, implemented SFPs with multi-sectoral objectives such as poverty reduction, the establishment of social safety nets for low-income households, addressing undernutrition, and improving educational attendance (particularly among primary school children).[24] In 2003, Brazil's SFPs were significantly restructured in order to align better with the national multi-sectoral food and nutrition security strategy and family farm promotion.[25] The School Feeding Law adopted in 2009 was regarded as a milestone that expanded the right to a free school meal for all public school students from day care/kindergarten to high school levels.[25] The program required 30% of funds spent on school meals be purchased from foods produced by family farms. Food procurement for schools is overseen by elected local-level coordinating bodies called School Nutrition Councils, which serve as mechanisms for engaging local-level civil society in food and agriculture activities. Despite this effort, concerns persist in Brazil about an ongoing increase in the prevalence of overweight and obesity among children due to consumption of energy-dense foods within the wider society and food environments beyond schools.[25]

In low-income countries of sub-Saharan Africa, national school feeding programs have been implemented to varying degrees and have been supported by the World Food Program (WFP) since the late 1970s. Starting in the early 2000s, however, there has been a concerted effort to transform these SFPs in Africa into "home grown school feeding programs" (HGSFPs) in order to more explicitly link the dual objectives of stimulating local markets and economies and addressing nutrition needs.[26] In so doing, these programs link agricultural growth with short- and long-term objectives related to hunger alleviation for low-income households, increased school enrollment, improved nutritional status and school attendance of children, cognitive development, and the retention of schoolchildren.[24] In 2003, African governments provided policy support for such programs by including school feeding programs that source food locally from smallholders in the Comprehensive Africa Agriculture Development Programme.[26] Here, the government aims to play a supportive role by providing complementary services to farmers such as training, credit, and access to technology.[27] Related food procurement strategies are diverse and include weekly cash purchases of food items by school cooks at local markets; public tendering of food items by school districts at minimum set prices, with items delivered monthly for cooking at schools; and national level procurement for tenders to supply, prepare, and distribute cooked food.[27] Despite some progress, concerns have arisen around the need for strengthened national nutritional standards for school meals and ongoing inconsistencies in the availability of some local fruits and vegetables.[27]

Case Study: The Caribbean Region

The remainder of this chapter focuses on the food insecurity and obesity challenges in the Caribbean context, and presents the lessons learned through implementing a "farm to fork" school feeding project that was piloted in St. Kitts-Nevis.

Food Insecurity and Obesity in the Caribbean Community and Common Market (CARICOM)

The CARICOM is an economic grouping of 15 developing and predominantly small island developing states (SIDS) with a combined population of nearly 18 million. The populations of CARICOM have been experiencing increasing rates of NCDs related to obesity.[28] Between the 1970s and 1990s, the prevalence of overweight and obesity among adult populations increased dramatically from 20% to 60%, with higher prevalence among women than men.[29] Since then, rates of obesity and overweight continued to increase, reaching nearly 70% in some countries by 2010.[30] The prevalence of childhood obesity in some CARICOM countries is also greater than the global average, more than doubling from 7% in 2000 to 15% in 2012.[30]

These trends in overweight and obesity have been associated with an increasing consumer preference and regional dependence on energy-dense foods, low consumption of fresh vegetables and fruits, and sedentary lifestyles.[28] This is compounded by the fact that, until very recently, the agricultural systems of CARICOM countries were focused mainly on producing plantation-based export commodities (such as sugar, cocoa, and bananas) with little emphasis on local food production to meet domestic needs. Consequently, CARICOM countries have accumulated large and escalating food import bills, totaling approximately USD 4.25 billion in 2012; and much of these imports comprise energy-dense foods.[31] According to the former Caribbean Food and Nutrition Institute (CFNI) the intake of fats and calories by CARICOM populations is, respectively, 78% and 36% above the recommended population goals (RPG) but the intake of vegetables and fruits is 29% below RPG's.[32]

Food insecurity, obesity, and non-communicable diseases (NCDs) are significant problems that threaten the human and economic development of CARICOM nations, with economic cost of NCDs estimated to range from 1.4% to 8% of the region's gross domestic product (GDP).[33] Some CARICOM countries are also suffering from the double burden of malnutrition, with, for example, undernourishment rates reaching nearly 14% in Antigua and Barbuda and the prevalence of low birth weight infants at approximately 19% in Guyana.[30] Haiti is an exception in CARICOM with extremely high levels of undernourishment at 50% of the population.[30]

Addressing both food insecurity and obesity has become a major public health priority for the region. In 2005, the CARICOM Heads of Government endorsed a proposal, known as the "Jagdeo Initiative." The proposal, titled "Strengthening Agriculture for Sustainable Development,"[34] identifies food security as a regional priority. It outlines nine key constraints to CARICOM's ability to achieve agricultural productivity and suggests interventions to help achieve food and nutrition security objectives in the region. In 2006, mandated by the CARICOM Heads of Government, the Caribbean Commission on Health and Development issued its report on the relationships among economic development, human capital, and population health.[29] Among its conclusions, the report notes that governments must "face squarely, the problem of obesity with its co-morbidities of non-communicable diseases" (p. xviii). The report further argues that addressing the problem of obesity and NCD's "turns not only on the burden of morbidity and mortality but, also on the huge economic costs society will have to bear" (p. 98). In 2007, the CARICOM leaders signed the "Port of Spain Declaration" aimed at uniting to stop the epidemic of NCDs; this declaration recognized that the burden of NCDs needs to be addressed through comprehensive and integrated intervention strategies at various levels from the individual through to the region. Further, it specifically identified schools, including provision of healthy school meals, and consumer education about healthy eating, as an important area of intervention.[35]

Implementation of a "Farm to Fork" School Feeding Project in St. Kitts-Nevis

St. Kitts-Nevis is a twin-island state in the Eastern Caribbean with a population of approximately 55,000 people. Through the publicly owned School Meals Centre (SMC), the Government of St. Kitts-Nevis offers a free hot lunch daily to approximately 3,300 primary schoolchildren in 18 schools St. Kitts. Imported food is used widely in the school lunch program, and sugar-sweetened beverages are offered on most days; fruits and vegetables are offered rarely or offered in small quantities. For the first time in St. Kitts-Nevis, working in collaboration with the local Ministries of Agriculture, of Health, and of Education, a McGill University–University of West Indies (UWI) project sought to transform the existing school feeding program into a viable market opportunity for local smallholder farmers while also serving as a vehicle for improving nutrition outcomes and contributing to obesity prevention in children. The project was funded through Canada's International Development Research Centre (IDRC).

This "farm to fork project" centered around three core pillars of the local food system that functioned, with community and institutional support, to deliver healthy lunch meals to children. These three pillars represented: *agricultural productivity and diversity; procurement of locally grown produce* from smallholder farmers; and *children's consumption of nutritious school lunch meals* based on improved menus that were redesigned to include the locally farmed produce, especially vegetables and fruits. Agricultural, nutritional, and social science research was conducted in each of these areas to establish an evidence base for the project (see Figure 10.1).

In terms of agricultural production, extensive on-farm participatory research and training were undertaken with selected smallholder farmers (the "project farmers") in order to facilitate the adoption of environmentally

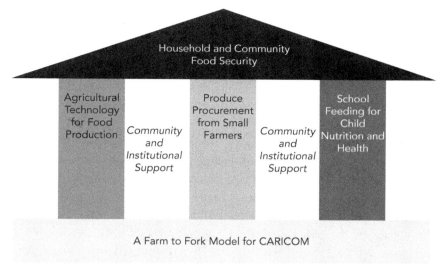

FIGURE 10.1   Farm to fork model for CARICOM.

sustainable technologies that could increase agricultural productivity and diversity, ensure food safety, and reduce post-harvest losses. Because seasonal variation in water availability is a key constraint to agricultural productivity in St. Kitts-Nevis, the project also developed and introduced a drip irrigation technology, management, and training package for project farmers. Regular monitoring of farmers' plots was undertaken to evaluate the impact of drip irrigation on food production. Recognizing that post-harvest losses (i.e., losses that take place between harvesting and consumption) are also a significant problem in St. Kitts-Nevis, the project sought to quantify these losses and train farmers in methods (including the use of plastic wrapping and the use of umbrellas to protect produce from direct sunlight and high temperatures) to improve crop handling, reduce their losses, and improve food safety.[36]

The second key pillar of the farm to fork model was the procurement of local produce for the school lunch program. Due to the historical dominance of export-oriented agriculture in the Caribbean, domestic markets for smallholder farmers in St. Kitts-Nevis are relatively undeveloped.[37,38] Given that institutions in St. Kitts-Nevis are trying to realign themselves away from export-oriented structures and toward structures better able to support diversified domestic products and markets, the farm to fork project initiated mechanisms for coordinated purchasing of produce from smallholders for school meals in order to establish a precedent for institutional local food procurement. Project funding was provided for the recruitment of a designated

Procurement Coordinator who worked at the Schools Meals Centre. This individual communicated with the farmers about the produce needs of the schools and arranged for regular pick up of produce from farmers for delivery to the Schools Meals Centre. Produce procurement data were collected weekly on the weight of the fruits and vegetables delivered by the farmers in order to measure the increase in local produce procured by the school feeding program.

The third key pillar was children's consumption of nutritious foods. A nutrition intervention in the school feeding program was facilitated through collaboration with the Ministry of Education and the Ministry of Health. Seven schools participated in the study; four schools were randomly allocated to a new 10-day cycle lunch menu ("intervention schools") that focused principally on the addition of local fruits and vegetables. Three schools represented "control schools" with no change in the normal menu, which contained virtually no fruits or vegetables (see "Example in Practice" for more details). To assess the impact of the intervention, baseline and endpoint data were collected on dietary intake, anthropometric measurements, and socioeconomic status of the children (5 to 12 years old) and their caregivers in both intervention and control schools. Height and weight were measured by community nurses at school, and household interviews were conducted with the caregiver and the child to obtain 24-hour food recall data. The U.S. Department of Agriculture (USDA) Household Food Security Survey Module was used to assess household food security status and caregiver anthropometry was also measured. Complete data at endpoint was available for 167 children and their caregivers. Foods offered to the children also were recorded and food acceptance was measured to assess children's willingness to consume new foods.

Example in Practice: Menu Modification in the Farm to Fork School Feeding Project

Table 10.2 provides a comparison of the old and new 10-day menus implemented in St. Kitts-Nevis; local fruits and vegetables were added to the new menu, which also included a fish sandwich and greater variety in meat items.

A sugar-sweetened drink was offered each day in both control and intervention schools because attempts to offer water on some days when fruit was offered in intervention schools was not seen as an acceptable change.

Table 10.2 Comparison of Control and Intervention Menus in St. Kitts-Nevis Schools

Day	Control	Intervention (Menu Change)
1	Spaghetti in browning with corned beef	Oven baked chicken in light gravy Seasoned baked sweet potato Sautéed string beans and carrots
2	Stewed turkey wings in tomato sauce Rice and pink beans	Stewed turkey wings in tomato sauce Rice and pink beans Watermelon slices
3	Stewed turkey wings and lentils Rice	Spaghetti with stewed turkey wings (in a chunky tomato sauce with cubed pumpkin and string beans)
4	Hot dogs with bread (tomato ketchup and onions as condiments)	Hot dog (in Creole Sauce) with bread
5	"Cook up" (lentils, chicken, rice, onions and seasoning)	Stewed chicken Stewed pink beans in tomato sauce with cubed pumpkin Rice Sliced Tomato
6	Spaghetti with stewed chicken	Baked chicken in light gravy Seasoned mashed sweet potato Sautéed cubed pumpkin and string beans
7	Rice and beans in tomato sauce	Baked fish sandwich Hot slaw (seasoned carrot, cabbage, and sweet pepper)
8	Split pea soup (sweet potato, white potato, pumpkin, and dumplings)	Split pea soup (sweet potato, white potato, pumpkin, and dumplings)
9	Cheese sandwich	Hamburger (in a Creole Sauce) Hamburger bun Cucumber slices Watermelon slices
10	"Cook up" (lentils, chicken, rice, onions, and seasoning and browning)	Stewed turkey wings Stewed pink beans in tomato sauce with cubed carrots Rice

Key Outcomes of the Farm to Fork School Feeding Project in St. Kitts-Nevis

Agricultural Production and Diversity

Research with vegetable and fruit crops (including tomato, pumpkin, string beans, and watermelon) among project farmers showed that adoption of drip irrigation and mulching technologies boosted overall crop productivity (see Figure 10.2) as well as increased water use efficiency by up to 20%. For example, prior to the intervention in St. Kitts-Nevis, the average national yield of pumpkin under local and rain-fed agriculture was estimated at about 17,000 kg/ha; however, with the introduction of drip irrigation by the project in 2012, the average yield of pumpkin at the irrigated sites was approximately 25,000 kg/ha, representing a 48% increase in the local productivity and annual output of pumpkin. Increases in productivity were also observed for string beans and tomatoes, with watermelon responding the least to drip irrigation. Improvements also occurred in crop diversity because with drip irrigation and water harvesting farmers can now grow crops (e.g., cucumber, squash, zucchini, and sweet pepper) that they could not cultivate before due to the lack of rain during the dry season. Not surprisingly, higher crop productivity and diversity was also shown to have the potential to increase farmer income. The project farmers were, however, all subsidized by the project for additional equipment, fertilizer, and other input costs associated with their participation in the research.

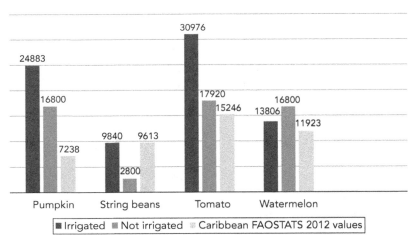

FIGURE 10.2 Comparative crop yields (kg/ha).

Produce Procurement

As a result of coordination and cooperation from 28 local smallholder farmers (including 10 "non-project" farmers), the school lunch program in St. Kitts-Nevis was able to procure, over a 15-month period (January 2013 to March 2014), 20,000 kg of 11 different locally grown fruits and vegetables, including tomatoes, sweet potatoes, carrots, string beans, cabbage, cucumber, and watermelon for use in a new lunch menu for 800 children in the four intervention schools. This new inflow of produce to the school lunch program provided market opportunities for the local farmers and represented a significant addition of fresh fruits and vegetables to the school meal lunches in the intervention schools.

Despite coordinated efforts in produce procurement, however, the local smallholder farmers were not able to supply the full needs of the school meal programs. Specifically, records kept throughout the project indicated they were able to supply less than one third of the total amount of vegetables and fruits required for the four schools participating in the nutrition intervention (see Figure 10.3). Constraints to production included challenges with crop planting schedules, water scarcity to sustain the rain-fed wells for drip irrigation, and low baseline levels of management capacity. In order to supply all 18 primary schools on the island, fruit and vegetable production would need

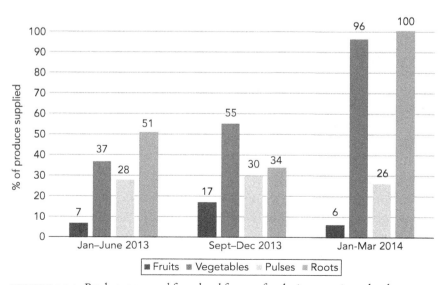

FIGURE 10.3 Produce procured from local farmers for the intervention schools.

to be very substantially increased with many more farmers involved to spread risk and improve the reliability of supply.

Children's Food Consumption

FOOD ACCEPTANCE

Results indicated that there was a progressive increase in the children's acceptance of the new food items introduced into the improved school lunch menus in St. Kitts-Nevis. Overall, vegetables were less accepted than fruits. The proportion of children accepting vegetables and fruits ranged from 51% for carrots (cooked) to 85% for watermelon.

NUTRIENT INTAKE

The 121 children who ate the school lunch on the day of the 24-hour recall at endpoint were compared for their nutrient intake through lunch meals in intervention versus control schools. The two groups did not differ in energy intake, but intervention school participants reported eating a higher amount of protein, fat, vitamin A, potassium, and vegetables in their lunch meal than those in the control schools (see Table 10.3). Overall, children in the intervention schools consumed 76% more vegetables daily in their lunch meal than those in the control schools. Fruit consumption was similar between the children in the control and intervention schools. This was likely due to fruit consumption being extremely low in both groups because of the limited supply of fruits from local farmers.

In order to assess whether the differences in the lunch meals translated into better overall intake for a whole day for each child, the 24-hour recalls for total daily intake were examined (see Table 10.4). These results indicate the children in the intervention schools consumed significantly more vegetables over the entire day, but in terms of nutrients only their potassium levels were higher. The macronutrient breakdown of the children was good overall with adequate intake of protein but low calcium intake.

OVERWEIGHT AND OBESITY

Despite increases in vegetable consumption by school children over the 15-month period, the prevalence of childhood obesity was not affected by the nutrition intervention. Over the course of the study, the rates of overweight and obesity among children increased from about 20% at baseline to 26% at endpoint. Importantly, the schools continued to offer a sugary drink to the

Table 10.3   Nutrient Intake and Food Group Portions at Lunch
for Control and Menu Change Groups of 6- to 12-year-old Children
in St. Kitts-Nevis at Endpoint

Nutrient/Food group	Children Who Consumed the School Lunch ($N = 121$)	
	Control ($n = 50$)	Menu Change ($n = 71$)
Energy, *kilocalories*	603 ± 375	529 ± 225
Percent energy as protein, %	13.8 ± 4.74	19.3 ± 10.4[**]
Percent energy as fat, %	18.3 ± 11.1	21.9 ± 9.41[*]
Percent energy as carbohydrate, %	66.8 ± 13.5	58.3 ± 15.4[**]
Fiber, *g*	3.21 ± 3.40	3.07 ± 2.56
Calcium, *mg*	141 ± 106	131 ± 88.4
Iron, *mg*	2.72 ± 2.39	2.59 ± 1.36
Potassium, *mg*	403 ± 330	481 ± 310[*]
Vitamin A, *RAE*	126 ± 300	215 ± 242[**]
Vitamin C, *mg*	66.6 ± 54.2	86.1 ± 75.5
Fruits, *portions*	0.17 ± 0.54	0.20 ± 0.65
Vegetables, *portions*	0.11 ± 0.27	0.24 ± 0.32[**]
Staple vegetables,[1] *portions*	0.06 ± 0.35	0.07 ± 0.21

Mean ± SD. [*] $p < 0.05$ [**] $p < 0.01$.

T-tests for normally distributed variables and non-parametric Wilcoxon test for those with non-normal distributions.

[1]Because staples in the Caribbean Food Guide include grain products and vegetables, the staple vegetables are reported separately.

children each day and access to sugary and high-fat snacks sold within and around the school were not changed over the study period.

OBESITY AND HOUSEHOLD FOOD SECURITY

The project also investigated household food security and its link to obesity. Among the households studied in St. Kitts-Nevis, 35% reported being food insecure and 20% reported child-specific food insecurity. There was no significant difference in weight status between those in food secure and food insecure households.

Based on WHO standards, only 1% of children were stunted (height for age) and about 4% were underweight for height (< -2 SD from median BMI

Table 10.4 Total Daily Nutrient Intake and Food Group Portions from 24-hour Recalls for Control and Menu Change Groups of 6- to 12-year-old Children in St. Kitts-Nevis at Endpoint

Nutrient/Food Group	All Children ($n = 167$)	
	Control ($n = 76$)	Menu Change ($n = 91$)
Energy, *kilocalories*	1754 ± 895	1647 ± 653
Percent energy as protein, %	14.1 ± 4.60	15.3 ± 6.71
Percent energy as fat, %	28.1 ± 9.27	27.5 ± 7.48
Percent energy as carbohydrate, %	57.5 ± 12.3	57.7 ± 9.67
Fiber, *g*	9.60 ± 6.64	10.15 ± 6.32
Calcium, *mg*	474 ± 303	478 ± 308
Iron, *mg*	11.0 ± 5.82	11.8 ± 5.44
Potassium, *mg*	1327 ± 832	1461 ± 670[*]
Vitamin A, *RAE*	880 ± 1468	570 ± 733
Vitamin C, *mg*	157 ± 132	179 ± 131
Fruits, *portions*	0.88 ± 1.41	0.57 ± 1.13
Vegetables, *portions*	0.34 ± 0.65	0.60 ± 1.13[**]
Staple vegetables,[1] *portions*	0.23 ± 0.72	0.41 ± 0.81

Mean ± SD. [*] $p < 0.05$ [**] $p < 0.01$.

T-tests for normally distributed variables and non-parametric Wilcoxon test for those with non-normal distributions.

[1]Because staples in the Caribbean Food Guide include grain products and vegetables, the staple vegetables are reported separately.

by age and sex). These findings support earlier reports that the prevalence of stunting and underweight among children in CARICOM is declining.[31] The dietary and anthropometric data collected in this project indicate that the problem of undernutrition has given way to a growing problem of overweight and obesity among children and adults in St. Kitts-Nevis.

COST OF THE IMPROVED SCHOOL LUNCH MEAL

The cost of improving the lunch menu in St. Kitts-Nevis increased because fruits and vegetables were considered an addition to the menu and not a substitute for other foods. The school lunch program offered meat most days in all the schools and menu improvements included adding fish and better-quality meats, which increased the costs. Although fruits and vegetables were the main target of the intervention, improved choice or quality meats also were seen as ways of improving the meals offered. Decreasing the consumption of certain foods which are well liked presented a challenge (e.g., the imported fruit drink and very low use of meat alternatives). Clearly, improving the quality of the lunch menus entails "trade-offs," which would have both economic and health policy implications for the adoption of the farm to fork model. On-site nutritional expertise to adapt meal offerings to local food availability and ensure the nutritional value of each day's meal to meet the daily food needs of children in a given environment would be valuable.

Conclusions and Lessons Learned

The "farm to fork" case study in St. Kitts-Nevis indicates that while bringing about dietary and behavior change to improve health outcomes is a significant challenge, such change is possible through improvements in existing food systems and institutional commitment. Children receiving the improved school lunch meal in St. Kitts-Nevis consumed more fruits and vegetables while smallholder farmers likewise benefited from access to new markets.

Reflecting on this case study offers some insights into ways forward for farm to school programs to support a food systems response to obesity. First, farm to school programs need to be part of a multifaceted food systems response that involves a combination of upstream, midstream, and downstream policies for greatest public health impact. Although the farm to fork project in St. Kitts-Nevis contributed to improvements in nutrition among children in intervention schools, rates of overweight and obesity among the children nonetheless continued to rise. Although this may be due in part to the short time frame over which overweight and obesity rates were monitored, it also demonstrates the importance of influences beyond school meals in shaping consumption. There is ample evidence of the role played by the food environment and food policy[18] in shaping food preferences, eating habits, and obesity. To address obesity and food insecurity better, improved school feeding programs need to be part of a multifaceted approach that involves not only schools but also other institutions, households, and workplaces. In St. Kitts-Nevis, limiting children's access to sugar-sweetened beverages and unhealthy snacks, enhancing nutrition education of the broader population, and extending the farm to fork model to include local foods procurement in other institutions (such as hospitals) are all specific policy actions that may assist in stabilizing the escalation of childhood obesity.

A second key insight offered by the farm to fork case study in St. Kitts-Nevis makes clear that although agricultural technologies, improved food procurement, and dietary practices in school feeding are core pillars of the model, these need to be supported by a strong "community of practice"—including school teachers and principals, parents, farmers, school meals staff, dietitians, and government decision-makers across different sectors—that can collaborate and coordinate toward the goal of improved school feeding.[39] Such a community of practice needs to be deliberately cultivated from the start of the project by involving all actors in goal setting and providing networking opportunities that help build trust and rapport among actors. Collaborative relationships were central to the outcomes of the farm to fork project in St. Kitts-Nevis; hence, ensuring that collaborative and coordinated relationships are in place will be important to supporting the long-term sustainability of local farm to school projects, particularly after project funding ends.

Integrated policymaking is also crucial to the long-term success of local farm to school feeding programs.[16] One of the main challenges to supportive policy for these types of programs is coordinating efforts across the various mandates and jurisdictions responsible for different facets of food and public health-related policy, including trade, education, health, agriculture, and environment.[40] The most successful farm to school programs are those supported by appropriate policy and legislative frameworks, with the Brazil school feeding program being a key example.[25] In St. Kitts-Nevis and the CARICOM specifically, research has shown that policymaking on food security is fragmented among a number of different regional bodies and national governments;[41] thus, ongoing efforts to improve policy coherence will be important to the long-term functioning of an improved school feeding program. For example, in St. Kitts-Nevis, building on the initial relationships established through the project, there is an opportunity for ongoing collaboration between the Ministry of Agriculture (to encourage the production of local foods suitable for school feeding), the Ministry of Health (to define and monitor healthy and safe food offerings to children), and the Ministry of Education (to oversee food production, offer education in food literacy, and set standards for other foods offered in schools). Clearly, more integrated policymaking that considers the interplay of food and health factors may also help encourage investment in improved school meals by recognizing that this can contribute to beneficial public health outcomes and reduced healthcare costs in the longer term.[42]

Finally, there is a need for ongoing research and evaluation of farm to school programs to inform best practices. Research and evaluation from the farm to fork school feeding project in St. Kitts-Nevis points to some operational challenges that would need to be further considered in future initiatives, particularly in developing area contexts. For example, ensuring healthy substitutions and menu flexibility requires the skills of a trained nutritionist; adding more fruits and vegetables to a menu can require additional cleaning, peeling, and chopping of vegetables, which creates more work for kitchen staff; adding new foods may be easier than taking away popular foods despite nutritional guidelines (such as the example of sugar-sweetened beverages in the case study). In addition, inconsistencies in local production can impact the desired menu and nutritional changes and thus any agricultural production barriers need to be addressed through appropriate investments in infrastructure, technology, and farmers' information needs.

Discussion Questions

1. What skills do you think a professional dietitian/nutritionist would need to successfully implement a farm to school program like the one described in this chapter?
2. What types of public policies do you think could help support more effective farm to school feeding programs?

Quiz Questions

Multiple choice: (answers are in bold)
1. The "nutrition transition" refers to which of the following: (a) a decline in physical activity; **(b) a decline in physical activity and increased consumption of energy-dense foods**; (c) increased consumption of energy-dense foods; (d) the erosion of traditional diets; (e) consuming too many calories
2. The "double burden of malnutrition" refers to which of the following: (a) the coexistence of diabetes and heart disease; (b) the coexistence of obesity and overweight; **(c) the coexistence of undernutrition and overnutrition**; (d) the coexistence of undernutrition and underweight; (e) the coexistence of food insecurity and underweight
3. Body mass index (BMI) is a basic index of weight-for-height (kg/m^2) used to measure overweight and obesity. When using BMI for children the

following variable must also be considered: **(a) age;** (b) rate of growth; (c) level of nutrition; (d) level of undernutrition; (e) stunting

4. Farm to school programs can best be described as which of the following: (a) building school farms; (b) bringing farmers into the classroom; **(c) schools sourcing local and healthy food to improve children's nutrition;** (d) including education about agriculture in the classroom; (e) bringing more fruits and vegetables into schools

5. Overweight and obesity are key risk factors for which of the following: (a) food insecurity; **(b) non-communicable diseases (NCDs);** (c) overnutrition; (d) stunting; (e) underweight

6. Which of the following best describes projected trends in global overweight and obesity in the coming decades: **(a) rising;** (b) declining; (c) remaining steady; (d) declining rapidly; (e) declining, then leveling off

7. All of the following are benefits of a Farm to School program *except*: (a) create or promote economic development; (b) increase fruit and vegetable consumption; (c) enhance overall academic achievements; **(d) increase food waste of local foods;** (e) increase parental engagement in early childhood educational opportunities

8. Two causes of obesity in humans are: (a) set-point theory and BMI; **(b) genetics and physical activity;** (c) genetics and low-carbohydrate diets; (d) mineral imbalances and fat-cell imbalance; (e) high-carbohydrate diets and BMI

Short-Answer Questions

1. Briefly compare and contrast trends in overweight and obesity in developed and developing country contexts.
2. Describe what is meant by a food systems response to obesity.
3. Identify and describe three types of policy instruments governments can use to address obesity.
4. Describe how farm to school programs seek to promote a food systems response to obesity.
5. Describe two upstream aspects that one would expect to help reduce obesity.

References

1. World Health Organization. Overweight and obesity. http://www.who.int/mediacentre/factsheets/fs311/en/ Published 2016. Retrieved June 20, 2017.
2. Haddad L et al. A new global research agenda for food. *Nature.* 2016; 540: 30–32.

3. Popkin BM, Adair LS, Ng SW. Now and then: The global nutrition transition: The pandemic of obesity in developing countries. *Nutrition Reviews.* 2012;70(1):3–21.

4. World Health Organization. Non-communicable diseases. http://www.who.int/gho/ncd/en/ Retrieved June 20, 2017.

5. Harvard School of Public Health. Obesity trends. https://www.hsph.harvard.edu/obesity-prevention-source/obesity-trends/#ref1 Published 2017. Retrieved June 20, 2017.

6. Kelly T, Yang W, Chen CS, Reynolds K, He J. Global burden of obesity in 2005 and projections to 2030. *International Journal of Obesity.* 2008;32:1431–1437.

7. Hawkes C. Uneven dietary development: Linking the policies and processes of globalization with the nutrition transition, obesity and diet-related chronic diseases. *Globalization and Health.* 2006;2(4).

8. Eckholm E, Record F. *The Two Faces of Malnutrition.* Worldwatch Institute; 1976.

9. World Health Organization. Nutrition. http://www.who.int/nutrition/double-burden-malnutrition/en/ Published 2017. Retrieved June 20, 2017.

10. Frongillo E, Bernal J. Understanding the coexistence of food insecurity and obesity. *Current Pediatrics Reports.* 2014;2(4):a284–a290.

11. Prentice A. The emerging epidemic of obesity in developing countries. *International Journal of Epidemiology.* 2006;35(1):93–99.

12. Bhurosy T, Jeewon R. Overweight and obesity epidemic in developing countries: A problem with diet, physical activity, or socioeconomic status? *The Scientific World Journal.* 2014.

13. World Health Organization. Diet, nutrition and the prevention of chronic diseases: Report of the joint WHO/FAO expert consultation. WHO Technical Report Series 916. 2003.

14. Kanter R, Caballero B. Global gender disparities in obesity: A review. *Advances in Nutrition: An International Review Journal.* 2012;3:491–498.

15. Gortmaker SL, Swinburn BA, Levy D, et al. Changing the future of obesity: Science, policy, and action. *The Lancet.* 2011;378(9793):838–847.

16. Sacks G, Swinburn B, Lawrence M. Obesity Policy Action framework and analysis grids for a comprehensive policy approach to reducing obesity. *Obesity Reviews.* 2009;10(1):76–86.

17. Stuckler D, Nestle M. Big food, food systems, and global health. *PLoS Med.* 2012;9(6).

18. Hawkes C, Smith T, Jewell J, et al. Smart food policies for obesity prevention. *The Lancet.* 2015;385(9985):2410–2421.

19. Nicholson L, Turner L, Schneider L, Chriqui J, Chaloupka F. State farm to school laws influence the availability of fruits and vegetables in school lunches at US public elementary schools. *Journal of School Health.* 2014;84(5):310–316.

20. Lyson HC. National policy and state dynamics: A state-level analysis of the factors influencing the prevalence of farm to school programs in the United States. *Food Policy.* 2016;63:23–35.

21. Brotman L, Dawson-McClure S, Huang KY, et al. Early childhood family intervention and long-term obesity prevention among high-risk minority youth. *Pediatrics*. 2012;129(3):e621–e628.

22. Yoder AB, Liebhart JL, McCarty DJ. Farm to elementary school programming increases access to fruits and vegetables and increases their consumption among those with low intake. *Journal of Nutrition Education and Behavior*. 2014;46(5):341–349.

23. Schafft K, Hinrichs C, Bloom J. Pennsylvania farm-to-school programs and the articulation of local context. *Journal of Hunger & Environmental Nutrition*. 2010;5(1):23–40.

24. Aliyar R, Gelli A, Hamdani S. A review of nutritional guidelines and menu compositions for school feeding programs in 12 countries. *Frontiers in Public Health*. 2015;3.

25. Sidaner E, Balaban D, Burlandy L. The Brazilian school feeding programme: An example of an integrated programme in support of food and nutrition security. *Public Health Nutrition*. 2013;16(06):989–994.

26. World Food Programme. Home grown school feeding resource framework. http://documents.wfp.org/stellent/groups/public/documents/resources/wfp290721.pdf Published 2017. Retrieved June 20, 2017.

27. Sumberg J, Sabates-Wheeler R. Linking agricultural development to school feeding in sub-Saharan Africa: Theoretical perspectives. *Food Policy*. 2011;36(3):341–349.

28. Saint Ville A, Hickey G, Locher U, Phillip L. Exploring the role of social capital in influencing knowledge flows and innovation in smallholder farming communities in the Caribbean. *Food Security*. 2016;8(3):535–549.

29. Report of the Caribbean Commission on Health and Development. Pan American Health Organization (PAHO) and the Caribbean Community Secretariat. Ian Randle Publishers; 2006.

30. Food and Agriculture Organization (FAO). State of food insecurity in the CARICOM Caribbean. http://www.fao.org/3/a-i5131e.pdf Published 2015. Retrieved June 20, 2017.

31. Food and Agriculture Organization (FAO). CARICOM food import bill, food security and nutrition. http://www.fao.org/fsnforum/caribbean/sites/caribbean/files/files/Briefs/Food%20Import%20brief%20.pdf Published 2013. Retrieved June 20, 2017.

32. FAO/CARICOM/CARIFORUM Food Security Project Report. The Caribbean Food and Nutrition Institute (CFNI). Published August 2007.

33. Theodore K, Lalta S, Althea La Foucade A, Cumberbatch A, Laptiste C. Responding to NCDs under severe economic constraints: The links with universal health care in the Caribbean. In Legetic B, Medici A, Hernández-Avila M, Alleyne G, Hennis A, eds. *Economic Dimensions of Noncommunicable Diseases in Latin America and the Caribbean*. Pan American Health Organization and the University of Washington; 2016.

34. Private Sector Commission. The jagdeo initiative. Technical Information Bulletin No. 8. Georgetown, Guyana: The Private Sector Commission of Guyana, Ltd; 2007.

35. Caribbean Community. Declaration of Port-of-Spain: Uniting to stop the epidemic of chronic NCDs. http://caricom.org/media-center/communications/statements-from-caricom-meetings/declaration-of-port-of-spain-uniting-to-stop-the-epidemic-of-chronic-ncds Published 2007 Retrieved June 28, 2017.

36. Cortbaoui P, Ngadi M. Characterization of postharvest practices and losses of fresh produce along the Caribbean supply chain: Guyana and St. Kitts-Nevis. *Journal of Post-Harvest Technology.* 2016;4(1):6–15.

37. Saint Ville AS, Hickey GM, Phillips LE. Institutional analysis of food and agriculture policy in the Caribbean: The case of Saint Lucia. *Journal of Rural Studies.* 2017;51:198–210.

38. Saint Ville A, Hickey GM, Phillip LE. Addressing food and nutrition insecurity in the Caribbean through domestic smallholder farming system innovation. *Regional Environmental Change.* 2015;15(7):1325–1339.

39. Lowitt K, Hickey G, Ganpat W, Phillip L. Linking communities of practice with value chain development in smallholder farming systems. *World Development.* 2015;74:363–373.

40. McRae R. A joined-up food policy for Canada. *Journal of Hunger and Environmental Nutrition.* 2011;6(4):424–457.

41. Lowitt K, Saint Ville A, Hickey G, Phillip L. Challenges and opportunities for more integrated regional food security policy in the Caribbean Community. *Regional Studies, Regional Science.* 2016;3(1):368–378.

42. United Nations System Standing Committee on Nutrition. Investments for healthy food systems. https://www.unscn.org/uploads/web/news/document/EN-final-Investments-for-Healthy-Food-Systems-UNSCN.pdf Published 2016. Retrieved June 20, 2017.

11

Intersections of Food and Culture

CASE STUDIES OF SUGAR AND MEAT FROM
AUSTRALIA, JAPAN, THAILAND, AND NIGERIA

*Wakako Takeda, Cathy Banwell, Kelebogile T. Setiloane,
and Melissa K. Melby*

Chapter Highlights

- Culture is a primary determinant of food preferences.
- Culture has been ignored to a large extent in public health.
- Four case studies demonstrate how culture influences food preferences.
- Better approaches are needed to incorporate cultural understandings into community and policy responses to food issues.

Introduction

"What makes people eat the food they do? If you want one answer it is culture. People eat the food of their culture. In particular, it is availability and cost that are part of culture. And they eat what they like, based on sensory properties, the context and the meaning. This is a dominant motivation of what people eat. Convenience and health are also important but what they like is more important."

Paul Rozin, December 2015[1]

Paul Rozin trained as a biologist and psychologist and, often in collaboration with food sociologist Claude Fischler, spent many years working to understand the role that culture plays in deciding what and how we eat. Although there are various definitions of culture across academic disciplines, Rozin considers culture as a full range of values, behaviors, and systems embedded in the society that underline food choices and preferences of people. This chapter starts with his premise that culture is a major determinant of food preference and consumption.

Culture and Food Preferences

Through much of our history, humans have foraged for their food. The domestication of food production began in roughly 10,000 BCE, relatively recently on an evolutionary time scale. Most humans have learned what is adequate and appropriate to eat, not only from what is grown around them, but through the norms and cultures of their community.[2] Cultural transmission of knowledge carries social, moral, and religious meanings or logic that influence people's beliefs about which food is adequate, appropriate, and desirable to eat. Symbolic aspects of food can be observed through food practices ranging from restriction of certain foods, to cooking styles and manners associated with sharing food. Environments, including availability and affordability of food and drink, play an important role in shaping food practices and preferences of individuals, as well as collective ones shared among groups of people. Thus, meanings of food and food practices have evolved to function as more than just a source of nutrients to be powerful influences over food choices and dietary behavior.

Until a few hundred years ago, most societies and cultures were separated by geographical and ecological barriers as well as resistance to interacting with others, which left them relatively isolated from global influences.[3] Today, the global nature of our economy and communication networks have resulted in profound cultural changes. A useful framework for considering the potential range of impacts is shown in Figure 11.1, which summarizes how cultural influences can impact food choice, ranging from individual food preferences, to differential access within households, to availability and affordability of households within a community, to a larger local system that may involve ecological influences on food production and availability, and economic influences on affordability, to the global system with historical, political, economic, environmental, and cultural influences.

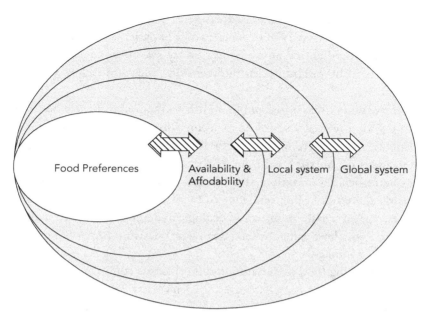

FIGURE 11.1 Interactions between levels of culture as they relate to food preferences.

Interactions between Culture and Public Health

Despite a strong focus on food choices and behaviors, public health has had a poor history of incorporating the notion of culture in its intervention "tool box." Historically, the theoretical foundation of modern public health was based on a biomedical focus on determinants of disease, laboratory-based diagnosis,[4] and epidemiology, which focus on the quantification of prevalence and distribution of diseases. This orientation often has obscured the role of more subtle and complex cultural factors and led to a struggle to operationalize the interconnectedness of individuals, communities, and their cultures. Although culture is important in disease prevention, it may be even more critical to understanding effective strategies for health promotion.

The common biomedical and public health views of disease causation are often vector focused and fail to incorporate the multifactorial etiology of culture or people's ways of life, which are often intangible and difficult to measure. For example, the biomedical public health intervention of antiretrovirals (ARVs) in the AIDS epidemic in Mozambique contributes to dramatic recoveries and longer lives. The ARV treatment, however, also increases hunger and leads to competition for limited food resources and conflicts among people.[5] This occurred because the intervention focused on increasing access to treatment, but paid little attention to hunger and food security or to social justice of patients and their communities, thus highlighting how complex impacts of culture have frequently been ignored by public health interventions and approaches, with dire consequences.

At the same time, initial public health work around dietary best practices led food-related research to focus on calories and macro- and micronutrients,[6,7] which are measurable. Public health mandates on nutrition often focus on nutrient deficiencies that lead to disease, or increasingly on obesity-related chronic disease caused by excess caloric intake. Until recently there has been a tendency to focus on what people put in their bodies, rather than on broader ecological determinants and cultural practices—the how, when, where, who, why questions providing the context of food intake.

In examining food preferences and diets across countries, regions, and different groups of people, however, it is clear that culture is enormously influential in determining what people eat, as Rozin observed. Recently, there have been efforts to advocate comprehensive approaches in public health interventions. The idea of "cultural competence," the ability to understand social and cultural diversity, has emerged as a key strategy to reduce health disparities across populations.[8] Leaders such as Risa Lavizzo-Mourey of the Robert Wood Johnson Foundation have recognized the importance of a *Culture of Health,* which emphasizes multifaceted approaches to improve the health of people across geographic, demographic, and sociocultural backgrounds.[9] As outlined in her 2014 speech, Lavizzo-Mourey emphasizes the interconnectedness of health care, work, family, and community life alongside the importance of economic opportunity, employment, and education. Following this emerging trend in contemporary public health, we examine case studies of sugar and animal proteins and demonstrate how the multifaceted nature of culture complicates patterns of consumption and preference in certain populations and societies. These two food items have been valued as commodities that not only provide substantial energy, but also are initially considered luxuries and cultural status symbols.[10,11] At the same time, changes in consumption patterns of these foods are considered key indicators of the global transition from undernutrition to overnutrition as well as the global pandemic of obesity and non-communicable diseases (NCDs).[12]

Overview of Case Studies Exploring the Intersection of Food and Culture: Focus on Sugar and Animal Protein

With economic growth, urbanization, modernization, and globalization, many countries and populations have experienced dramatic dietary changes. In particular, many societies have seen increased consumption of sugar and animal products, both of which have been linked to obesity and NCDs. The rise of hyper-processed foods with saturated fats and refined sugars is a key determinant of rapid increases in overweight and obesity in high-income countries as well as low- and middle-income countries.[13] A closer examination of changes in diets in various societies, however, reveals cross-cultural variations in patterns of consumption and health profiles in societies. In this chapter, we examine case studies of sugar and animal proteins from four countries (Australia, Japan, Thailand, and Nigeria) with different health profiles, socioeconomic conditions, food production, and consumption environments and cultures. Table 11.1 shows demographic and economic profiles, as well as supply of sugar and meat, of the four countries in comparison to the United States, the world, and low-income, lower- and upper-middle income, and high-income countries.

Australia is an English-speaking western country with a high-income economy, and of the four case studies has the highest food production index, an indicator of edible food crops with nutritive values (i.e., although coffee and tea are edible they have no nutritive value and are not included). Fostered by industrialized agriculture and food processing as well as geographic proximity to consumers in the Asia-Pacific region,[14] Australia is now a major producer and exporter of many agricultural products, including meat, wheat, alcoholic beverages, fruits and vegetables.[15] Japan, also a high-income economy, differs from Australia in that its domestic food production industry is small and has the lowest food production index among the four case-study countries. Thailand provides an example of a newly industrialized country whose economy has grown considerably in recent years. Now the second largest economy in Southeast Asia, the nation rapidly transitioned to achieve a gross domestic product (GDP) of an upper middle-income country by 2011.[16] These three countries have seen increases in NCDs along with their economic development, and now NCDs are their major causes of death. Although most of contemporary public health focuses on obesity and overconsumption,

Table 11.1 Demographic and Economic Profiles and Supply of Sugars and Meats of Selected Countries

Country	Population (1,000s)[a]	Urban Population (%)[b]	GDP[1] Per Capita PPP[2,c]	Life Expectancy (yrs)[d]	Death by NCDs[e] (%)	Food Production Index[3,f]	Supply of Raw Sugar Per Capita (kg/yr)[g]	Supply of Meat Per Capita (kg/yr)[g]
Australia	23,789.75	89	46,270.80	82	90	119.5	36.46	116.23
Japan	126,958.47	93	40,763.40	84	82	97.9	16.17	49.45
Thailand	67,959.36	50	16,340	75	71	128.5	37.69	29.33
Nigeria	182,201.96	48	6,003.90	53	26	114.9	10.11	9.2
United States	321,418.82	82	56,115.70	79	88	113.2	31.71	115.13
World	7,346,705.90	54	15690.6	72	70	123	20.53	43.22
Low-income	638,286.29	31	1635.9	62	37	133.4		
Lower-middle income	2,927,468.84	39	6443.1	68	59	130.7		
Upper-middle income	2,593,857.85	64	15935.9	75	82	128		
High-income	1,187,092.92	81	45,648	81	88	107.7		

[1]Gross domestic product; [2]Purchasing power parity; [3]Food Production Index is an indicator of edible food crops that contain nutrition values, Food and Agricultural Organization of the United Nations (FAO) electric files and websites; [a]World Bank. "Population, total" 2015, http://data.worldbank.org/indicator/SP.POP.TOTL; [b]World Bank. "Urban population, % of total" 2015, http://data.worldbank.org/indicator/SP.URB.TOTL.IN.ZS?view = chart; [c]World Bank. "GDP per capita, PPP (current international $)" 2015, http://data.worldbank.org/indicator/NY.GDP.PCAP.PP.CD?view = chart; [d] World Bank. "Life expectancy at birth, total (years)" 2015, http://data.worldbank.org/indicator/SP.DYN.LE00.IN?view = chart; [e] World Bank. "Cause of death, by non-communicable diseases (% of total)." 2015, http://data.worldbank.org/indicator/SH.DTH.NCOM.ZS?view = chart; [f]World Bank. "Food production index (2004-2006=100)." 2013, http://data.worldbank.org/indicator/AG.PRD.FOOD.XD?view=chart; [g]FAO. "Food Balance Sheet, food supply quantity (capita/kg/year)." 2013, http://www.fao.org/faostat/en/#data/FBS.

much of the world's population still struggles with hunger, undernutrition, and food insecurity. Elimination of hunger and food insecurity are key priorities in the United Nations' sustainable development goals for 2030.[17] The final case-study country, Nigeria, is a nation located on the coast of West Africa with the largest population in Africa. Compared to the other three case-study countries, overnutrition, NCDs, and consumption of processed sugars are not major problems in Nigeria. Yet the population's overall diet has inadequate protein, particularly given its infectious disease load. In the Yoruba community in Nigeria, meat is a prestige food that often is withheld from children. Similarly, sugar was also a commodity that was historically only accessible by the wealthy, until mechanization led to decreased prices. In Thailand, sugar has become a symbol of modernity and urbanism, and for Australians it is part of a lifestyle valuing convenience and is used to reward and motivate children. In Japan, for complex political, economic, historical, and cultural reasons, sugar is less a symbol of modernity—at least in the form of beverages, while sweets are often consumed with tea. Taken together these four case studies allow comparisons between developed and developing countries, Western, Eastern, and African cultures, and complex historical, political, and economic factors, including colonialism, colonization, immigration, and globalization, as well as accessibility and food preferences.

Australia

Our first case study focuses on an economically advanced country, Australia, where concern has been growing over the last few decades about the prevalence of NCDs such as type 2 diabetes (2.5%), cardiovascular disease (5.2%), and hypertension (11.3%) associated with overweight and obesity (63.4%).[18] Recently, attention has turned to sugar as a major contributor to these health problems. Australians consume almost double the World Health Organization (WHO) recommendation of six teaspoons a day, while children in Australia consume even larger quantities than adults.[19] Sugar has long played an important part in the Australian diet and is embedded in the country's colonial and post-colonial culture as an economically valued agricultural product (Figure 11.2).[14]

The Growth of the Australian Sugar Industry

Sugar cane was domesticated in New Guinea, situated about 150 kilometers north of Australia. Despite its proximity to Australia, sugar cane was transported around the world to become commercially established in many other

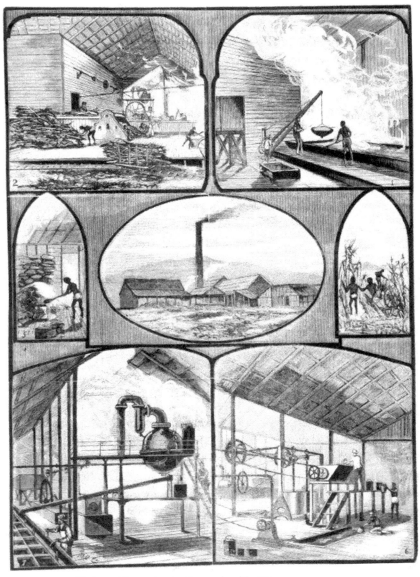

FIGURE 11.2 "A Sugar Plantation in Queensland," 1886.
Courtesy of The State Library of Victoria.

countries before it arrived on Australian shores. The area around Sydney, Australia was established as a penal colony by the British in 1788. Because the British already had developed a taste for sugar over the course of the 18th century, they brought it to their new colony. After several failed attempts to grow sugar cane around Sydney, its cultivation became established in tropical coastal areas of Queensland from 1862 onward.[20] Following the example of sugar plantations in the New World, Queensland plantation owners sought cheap, non-European labor. Approximately 62,000 laborers were brought from Melanesia to work on these rapidly growing plantations. Many were indentured, some forcibly kidnapped, and others were coerced or tricked into relocating. Figure 11.2 shows that the more laborious and unpleasant tasks associated with a sugar plantation were given to Pacific Islanders and Asians, indicating Australian colonial views of race and division of labor.

The development of the sugar industry in the 19th century was linked to other emblematic colonial business enterprises, which received support from the government and investment from local and international business entities. In 1901, the Federal Government of Australia legislated a stop to the import of Pacific Islands cane workers, and many were deported in the following years.[21] The plantations that had relied heavily on cheap labor were replaced by small-scale farms supplying centralized mills.[20] Migrants from Italy and other European countries worked in the cane fields in the early 20th century with some eventually becoming wealthy enough to buy their own farms. During the first half of the 20th century, much of the process of sugar production became mechanized, reducing the demand for labor.

Currently, according to the Australian Sugar Milling Council, there are "4400 cane farming entities growing sugar cane on a total of 380,000 hectares annually, supplying 24 mills, owned by 7 separate milling companies."[22] The sugarcane industry is ranked ninth among Australia's agricultural export earners. It is Queensland's largest agricultural industry and produces 4.5 million tons of raw sugar per annum. Eighty-five percent of raw sugar is sold overseas, earning 1,500 million AUD, and the rest supplies the Australian sugar market.[22] In other words, this is an important source of export earnings for the Australian government. Australia currently ranks as one of the top 10 major sugar exporters in the world market.[23]

A Taste for Sugar

From Australia's early colonial days, sugar was consumed in large quantities. It was supplied in rations to convicts and workers and from the late 1850s onward it was cheap and affordable. In a country with high summer temperatures and primitive transport, it had the advantages of being portable, non-perishable, and unaffected by heat. In the 18th and 19th centuries, people often subsisted mainly on tea, sugar, and bread. Large quantities of sugar also were contained within the prodigious amounts of beer consumed.[24] Sugar consumption was strongly connected to that of tea, which was also cheap, portable, and storable. Indeed, for many years Australians consumed more tea and more sugar than any other nationality.

By the 1930s, in Queensland it was common for people to drink four lumps of sugar in every cup of tea.[25] For most of the 20th century, Australians had the highest per capita apparent sugar consumption in the world (based on quantities sold, rather than self-reported consumption), averaging around 50 to 55 kilograms per annum. Consumption dipped slightly during the Depression (1926 to 1935) but rose again rapidly to 60.5 kilograms from 1936 to 1940.[25(144)] Due to rationing during the Second World War consumption dropped again. From the 1950s to the mid-1960s, it declined to about 52 kilograms, although it was still higher than in many countries. It continued to decline slowly; by the 1990s, it was down to 46.5 kilograms. Griggs attributes this partially to the large influx of European immigrants, who had a much lower sugar consumption,[25] thereby reducing the per capita average.

Through interviews with Australians born in the 1920s and 1930s, and their children and grandchildren, Banwell and colleagues[26] discussed these trends through accounts of common food practices. They described family meals over the first half of the 20th century consisting of a main course and a dessert, sweet, or pudding. The latter were made at home and were stewed fruit or jelly during summer and baked or steamed puddings, rice puddings, and custards during winter. Homemade scones and cakes were usually served to visitors and were sent to school and work in lunchboxes. These baked goods were relatively inexpensive ways to fill hungry stomachs and women used them to display their domestic skills. Furthermore, over the same period, women made jams, pickles, and chutneys at home to preserve produce when refrigeration was not readily available. Although commercially prepared replacements could be bought, interviewees generally described making their own. Cookbooks in the first half of the 20th century devote many more pages to recipes for cakes, desserts, and pastries than for vegetables, suggesting that these types of products were held in higher regard. Indeed, accounts from the period emphasize that only a limited range of vegetables were eaten, and these were often so overcooked that they were nearly inedible.[26]

Until the 1940s, Australian Bureau of Statistics (ABS) data did not differentiate among refined sugar added to foods, sugar consumed in processed products, and other sugar products such as treacle, golden syrup, and honey. Once the ABS began collecting these data, however, the figures from the 1950s to the 1990s show a drop in consumption of added sugar and an increase in sugar consumed in manufactured products.[25] Once again personal accounts illustrate this trend. By the 1970s, Australian women were beginning to enter the workforce. They reported during interviews that they had less time for domestic activities. To manage this time shortage, they stopped making desserts and cakes, although they continued to prepare the evening meal, consisting of a main course of meat and vegetables.[26] This aligns with the trend commencing in the mid-1960s of increasing amounts of sugar consumed in manufactured products rather than added to foods. By the early 1970s, almost 60% of sugar was consumed this way and this has continued to grow. This shift demonstrates Australians' continued devotion to sweet foods, although in a different form. It is supported by other socioeconomic trends, such as the development of supermarkets selling manufactured goods; the growth in car use, allowing Australians to purchase their food from supermarkets in a weekly shopping expedition; and the purchase of home refrigerators.[26] One of the most obvious dietary changes that illustrates these trends is the replacement of homemade desserts, sweets, and cakes with ice cream, which is likely to contain more sugar and calories on average than the homemade desserts it has replaced. In Australia in the 1990s, ice cream, among all the frozen foods, was sold in the highest quantities, surpassing vegetables, poultry, frozen desserts, and convenience meals.[27] Rather than a novelty or high status food, ice cream has become an everyday food in many households.

Sugar Wars: Sweetness or Health

The extraordinary consumption of sugar over the 19th and 20th centuries was driven by strong domestic support for Australia's sugar industry by politicians, while consumers were encouraged to view sugar as a benign substance. Over the 20th century, a subtle war was conducted over the healthfulness of sugar. In the early 1940s, the Commonwealth Department of Health advocated sugar as "a useful addition to a diet, especially for active people."[25(147)] In contrast, Australian dentists began issuing warnings in the 1930s about the association between sugar consumption and dental cavities.[25] In the late 1960s and 1970s, sugar began to be associated with obesity, diabetes, and other NCDs. A corresponding decline in consumption encouraged the sugar industry to mount vigorous advertising campaigns promoting the wholesomeness and naturalness of sugar and its importance to the Australian economy; in addition, the industry began to sponsor sporting activities as a way to address rising rates of obesity. Despite these efforts, Australian consumers have not markedly increased their consumption of sugar. Since the 1990s, however, the Australian sugar industry has managed to achieve overseas expansion.[25]

Since the mid-19th century, sugar has been affordable and available and low prestige enough to be given to children. Sweet foods and lollies were used to socialize them and as rewards for desirable behavior. Desserts were offered to children as an incentive to eat the more nutritious and less desirable meat and vegetable portions of meals. As the Australian diet has become industrialized over the last 50 years or so, much of children's sugar consumption has taken the form of highly processed foods that are explicitly marketed to them. In 2011–2012 over half (52%) of the free sugar in the Australian diet was consumed in beverages, such as soft drinks (or sodas), electrolyte and energy drinks (19%), fruit and vegetable juices and drinks (13%), and cordials (4.9%). Confectionary and cakes/muffins each contributed 8.7%. Teenaged boys were the biggest sugar consumers.[28] Over the same period, Australian children have gained weight. In 2014–2015, some 27.4% of Australian children were overweight or obese.[18] Concern now focuses on children, particularly those from poorer families, who are consuming quantities of inexpensive sweetened foods and not enough fruit, vegetables, or other healthful foods. Australian public health campaigners are now attempting to undo the culturally embedded association between sugar and reward, and the use of convenient, highly processed foods. An additional difficulty is that it is likely that Australians are unaware of just how much sugar they are eating, and indeed, experts are not sure either. Some experts, using self-reports of sugar consumption and sales data, argue that sugar consumption has declined, even as obesity rates have increased,[29,30] leading to discussions on whether sugar should be targeted in obesity reduction efforts. In an attempt to address the broader *obesogenic* food environment, calls have gone out for taxes on sugar-sweetened beverages, along with other public health measures to reduce sugar consumption, but these have been brushed aside by government and strongly resisted by industry groups.

Japan

The second case study is from Japan. Like Australia, Japan is a country with a high-income economy.[16] However, after post-World War II economic development and declines in rural agriculture, many food products consumed in Japan are no longer produced domestically but rather are imported from overseas. About 60% of sugar consumed in Japan is imported, and domestic sugar production is limited to three prefectures in the South (Kagoshima and Okinawa) and North (Hokkaido).[31] From a macro-economic perspective, Japan is a sugar deficit country where domestic demands for sugar exceed domestic production, and it must rely on imports to feed Japanese consumers. This Japanese case study examines the history of sugary products in Japan and shows how the Japanese food system and food culture influence sugar consumption in contemporary Japan.

Development of Sugary Products in the Meiji and Taisho Periods

Similar to the Australian case study, sugar consumption in Japan is an indicator of modernity and industrialization in the late 19th and the early 20th centuries (the Meiji and Taisho periods). Japanese adoption of sugar, however, cannot be solely explained by the development of international trade and adoption of "western" eating practices. Kushner[32] suggested that consumption was fostered by a combination of changes in consumer practices, the expansion of market culture, and imperial colonial policies in the Meiji and Taisho periods. In particular, the 1895 military acquisition of Taiwan, a producer of sugarcane, helped expand the imperial economy and increased sugar availability in Japan. When the government introduced school lunch programs to build a healthy nation in the 1920s, sugar was considered a nutritious food to provide calories, not as an item to be avoided.[32] This idea was also reflected in advertisement and packages of new sugary products like caramels and chocolates, which emphasized the nutritional values of sugar. Figure 11-3 is an advertisement of Morinaga confectionary company in 1919. The advertisement describes how their confectionery products are developed to support people's health (*"morinaga no seihin ha hoken ni rikkyaku suru"*), together with its good taste and nutrition (*"bimi to jiyō towo kanete"*).[33]

In terms of changes in consumer practices, the rise of the tea break,[32] treating guests with sweets,[34] and increasing consumption of tea fostered consumption of a range of sweets eaten with tea among a wider population. These consecutive socioeconomic and cultural changes during this period enabled Japanese businesses to expand the market for sweet products which accompany tea breaks.

The association between sugar consumption and tea drinking is not unique to Japan. Mintz[35] showed that sugar consumption in Great Britain increased together with the consumption of items, such as tea and jam, which use sugar. The Australian case study also discussed how sweetened tea became an economical and convenient source of energy. In Japan, although sugar is sometimes consumed with British-style black tea, it is rarely consumed with

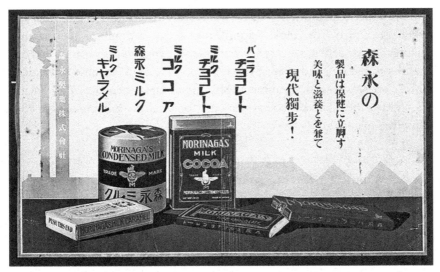

FIGURE 11.3 "Daihyōtekina morinaga 5 seihin (five major products of Morinaga)," 1919. Courtesy of Morinaga & Company, Ltd. Taichiro Morinaga.

green tea. Green tea's bitter taste distinguishes it from sweet "foreign" products introduced during the modern era. Originating from Chinese Buddhist and Taoist notions of health and healing, appreciation of the bitter taste of tea was inherited through Zen Buddhism in Japan.[36] In the pre-modern period, tea drinking was an aesthetic practice only for elite men such as aristocrats, *samurai* warriors, and businessmen. At tea ceremonies (*sadō*) and gatherings (*chakai*), sweets (*kashi*) were prepared to be presented and served along with tea. The Japanese word *kashi* means fruits and the *kashi* did not necessarily contain added sugars. Sugary sweets became popular at the end of the 17th century when domestic and imported sugars became available.[37] However, some *kashi*, such as *senbei* (rice crackers), do not contain sugars or other sweeteners even today. During the Meiji and Taisho modernization periods, tea drinking practices changed dramatically. Fostered by imperial policies to promote nationalism, green tea became a tool to characterize the essence of national culture and was promoted to the non-elite population, especially middle-class housewives.[38] Mass production of tea leaves also assisted in changing tea drinking from an aesthetic to a daily practice for the masses. Green tea became a national beverage for the Japanese people. Thus, consumption of bitter green tea developed almost simultaneously with the development of sweets in Japan. Appreciation of bitterness and sweetness became key features of modern tea culture in Japan.

Japanese Sugar Market and Tea Drinking in the 21st Century

After World War II, colonial sugar production was replaced by international trade, which enabled Japan to access cheap sugar from overseas. To protect domestic sugar production, however, the government imposed high tariffs on imported sugar and set the domestic sugar price very high. In 2014, the average price of refined white sugar in Tokyo (JPY 185.50/kg or USD 1542/ton)[39] was about five times higher than the world price of raw sugar (USD 295.85/ton).[40] In contrast to increasing demands for sugar in the rest of the world, the sugar market in contemporary Japan is shrinking. Although sugar supply and consumption rapidly increased between the 1960s and the early 1970s, both exhibited declines beginning in the mid-1970s (Figure 11.4).

In contrast to direct consumption of sugar, the market for "ready-to-drink (RTD)" non-alcoholic beverages (*seiryō inryō*) has grown rapidly since the 1960s. The total production was 1.18 million kiloliters[41] in 1964 and increased tenfold (10.74 million kiloliters)[41] by 1990 and twentyfold (20.47 million kiloliters)[42] by 2015. In the 1960s, sugary drinks, including carbonated drinks and fruit drinks, were the most popular RTD non-alcoholic beverages.[41] From the 1990s, however, production of RTD tea, especially unsweetened tea (i.e., green tea, barley tea, and blend tea) rapidly increased (Figure 11.5) and now comprise the largest share (28% in 2015) of the RTD market in Japan.[42]

The rise in unsweetened tea consumption is not simply because more Japanese consumers have begun drinking non-sugar-sweetened tea for health

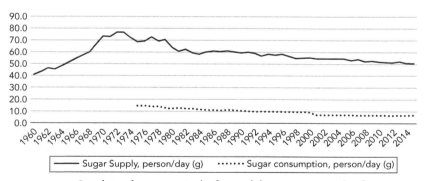

FIGURE 11.4 Supply[a] and consumption[b] of sugar (g) per person per day from 1960 to 2015. [a] Includes both domestically produced and imported sugars available; [b] Consumption of raw sugar at the household from 1975 to 2015.

Created based on *Shokuryo jyukyū hyō* (Chart of food supply and demand time series data) from 1960 to 2015, Ministry of Agriculture, Forestry and Fisheries; and *Kokumin Kenkō Eiyō Chōsa* (National Health and Nutrition Surveys) from 1975 to 2015, Ministry of Health, Labor and Welfare.

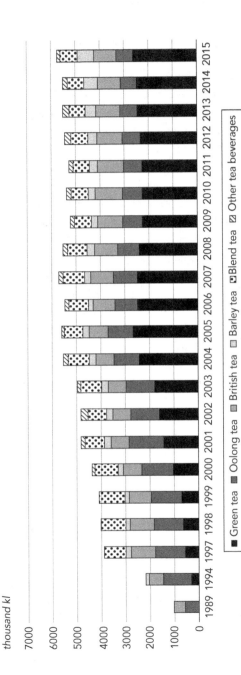

FIGURE 11.5 Production of "ready-to-drink" (RTD) tea beverages in Japan from 1989 to 2015.

Created based on *Seiryō inryō sui kankei toukei shiryō* (documents related to non-alcoholic beverages) 2016, Japan Soft Drink Association.

reasons, but also because more Japanese consumers are buying RTD tea instead of making tea from leaves at home and in the workplace. In fact, household expenditures on green tea leaves dropped 40% while expenditures on RTD tea increased 67% between 2000 and 2015.[43] Thus, in addition to Japanese consumers' preferences for drinking green tea without sugar, industrialization of tea and a culture valuing convenience also contribute to tea drinking culture in contemporary Japanese society.

Recent Trends and Emerging Public Health Issues

Sugar supply and consumption are expected to continue declining in Japan.[40] This is not only because of increasing awareness of the health risks in consuming excessive sugar, but also because of competition from sweeteners such as high-fructose corn syrup (HFCS). The use of HFCS is more prevalent among countries with higher sugar prices, such as Japan, Korea, and the United States, because the low production cost of HFCS provides more profits compared with sugar. The HFCS market in Japan is growing and profitable due to domestically produced HFCS made from corn imported from the United States with zero tariffs, combined with domestic starch.[44] The cost-savings, however, benefit only the HFCS producers, because Japanese consumers still pay high prices for both sugar and HFCS.

Government regulation focuses on protecting domestic sugar production and stabilizing sugar prices. Beginning in 1982, surcharges on HFCS were imposed and this income generates subsidies for domestic sugar producers.[45] The government considers domestically produced sugar to be key to contributing to the nation's food and caloric self-sufficiency, and its contribution is crucial especially in emergencies such as natural disasters.[46] Nonetheless, health concerns about HFCS have not yet been explicitly communicated to consumers, and the Ministry of Health, Labor and Welfare, the ministry which oversees the health risks of food additives, has been quiet on this issue.

The Japanese experience shows how the import-influenced food system and tea drinking culture affect sugar consumption in contemporary Japanese society. Unlike in other developed nations, consumption of sugary drinks is not a major public health issue due to the popularity of unsweetened tea. Along with high sugar prices and absence of regulation by the public health sector, however, the consumption of HFCS is growing and replacing domestic demands for sugar.

Thailand

Located in mainland Southeast Asia, Thailand is a major producer and exporter of a range of food products including rice, cassava, seafood, and sugar.[47]
Rice has been a main food product and an export item, iand a majority of the
population has engaged in its production and consumption since the 19th
century.[48] Although rice is still the top food product produced in Thailand,[47]
today the country has become a major producer of a range of raw, frozen,
canned, and processed food.[49] In 2015, the Thai food industry contributed
about 23% to the nation's GDP.[50] Increased domestic food production and
income improvement have contributed to a rapid reduction in stunting and
poverty as well as to a transformation of the Thai food system and consumption culture. Among foods produced in Thailand, cane sugar is a key player in
the changing food production and consumption culture in this newly industrialized society.

From Local Palm to Global Cane Sugar

Sweetness (*waan*) is an important element in Thai cuisine. "Proper" Thai
meals normally consist of three to five dishes varied in flavor, color, ingredients, and type of cooking techniques.[51] Sweetness is one of the essential flavors
along with spiciness (*phet*), bitterness (*kom*), sourness (*preaw*), and saltiness
(*kem*). In traditional dishes and sweets, sweetness comes from palm sugar,
the sucrose-rich sap of the palmyra palms found in the region. Sugarcane was
grown in Thailand as early as the 13th century,[52] and cane and palm sugars
were produced on a small scale by part-time workers.[53] Refined cane sugar
imported from Indonesia and the Philippines was consumed only by the
wealthy.

The Thai sugar industry changed dramatically in the mid- to late-20th
century when the government began mass production of cane sugar for export by establishing modern sugar mills, imposing tariffs on imported sugar,
and introducing the revenue sharing system among the planter and millers.
With this support, the sugarcane producers' associations have emerged to become one of the most powerful interest groups influencing domestic policies.
Ramsay[52] suggested that the emergence of well-organized sugarcane producers' associations was crucial for the rapid expansion of the sugarcane industry
in Thailand in contrast to other politically weak, rural farmers. This state involvement changed Thailand from a net importer in the late 1950s to one
of the largest cane sugar exporters in the world by the 1980s. Furthermore,
the growth of the domestic sugarcane industry and the support from the

government also changed palm sugar production, which was controlled by the local elites, and enabled the producers to earn a more stable and higher income than rice production, which had remained under control of the local elites.[54]

Cane sugar became not only a major export product generating substantial income for the country, but also an accessible item enhancing the domestic population's caloric intake. The Food and Agricultural Organization (FAO) food balance sheet estimates that in Thailand only 3.91 kilograms per person per year of raw sugar was available in 1961, but availability increased almost tenfold to 37.69 kilograms in 2013.[55] The change in sugar availability, however, is not explicitly reflected in the consumption of raw sugar reported in national surveys, but rather appears in the consumption of beverages. Table 11.2 shows the average consumption of sugar and beverages in Thailand reported in five national surveys.

Average amounts of sugar consumption (all forms combined) increased from 1960 to 1995, but slightly decreased in the latest survey (2016). Consumption of palm sugar was listed under the vegetable section as well as included as jaggery under the sugar section in 1986[56] and 1995,[57] but it was not reported in later surveys.[58-60] The consumption of beverages increased most dramatically between 1986 and 2016. Although Coca Cola was the most consumed beverage in 2016, tea showed the highest increase between 1986 and 2016 followed by fruit juice. Unlike the United States and other countries where carbonated drinks are the most consumed sugar-sweetened beverages,[61] in Thailand, non-carbonated sweetened beverages such as sweet tea and fruit juices are consumed more frequently. The latest national survey on consumption frequency showed that only 5.9% of people drink carbonated drinks (i.e., soda) every day, while about one third of people drink other sugar-sweetened beverages including sweetened tea, coffee, and fruit juices daily.[62]

Sweetened Tea Market in Contemporary Thailand

In contrast to Japan (see Japan section), most ready-to-drink (RTD) green tea beverages in Thailand are sweetened. In 2003, the Thai brand *Oishi* launched its first RTD sweetened green tea and quickly attained the highest share in the market within a few years. Since the mid-2000s, Japanese beverage companies (i.e., *Kirin, Itoen*, and *Pokka*) have attempted to sell Japanese-style unsweetened green tea in the Thai market, but have not successfully broken into the market dominated by sweetened green tea.[63] The total share of Japanese companies' green tea sales in Thailand is less than 10% of the RTD tea market.[64] The market competition is not just a matter of different taste preferences

Table 11.2 Average Amounts of Sugar (g) and Beverage (g/ml)[a]
Consumption Per Capita Per Day in 1960, 1975, 1986, 1995, and 2016

	1960	1975	1986	1995	2016	Increase Between 1986 and 2016
Sugar (combined)	0.2	7.0	10.5	13.6	12.2	16%
White sugar			8.4	11.4		
Brown sugar			0.0	0.3		
Jaggery[b]			1.3	1.8		
Sugarcane juices			0.9	0.1		
Others				0.0		
Palm sugar (young)			2.2	0.5		
Beverage (combined)			8.2	14.0	270.7	3206%
Coffee			0.3	0.1	10.8	3067%
Juices			0.1	0.1	38.8	48419%
Coca Cola			3.6	3.6	78.8	2119%
Carbonated sweet drink			2.0	2.0	26.8	1242%
Milo, Ovaltine			0.3	0.3	10.1	3255%
Tea			0.0	0.0	56.8	246764%
Cocoa			0.0	0.0	0.0	473%
Soy milk			1.9	8.0	37.1	1864%
Mineral water					11.5	

Created based on the first to the fourth national nutrition surveys in 1960, 1975, 1986, and 1995, and food consumption data of Thailand in 2016.

[a] Surveys in 1986 and 1995 reported all beverages in grams and the survey in 2016 reported beverages sold in powder form in grams and beverages sold in liquid form in milliliters.

[b] Traditional non-centrifugal sugar made from evaporation and concentration of sugarcane, date, or palm sap.

between Thai and Japanese consumers. Amornpetchkul[65] suggested that the Thai green tea market grew rapidly due to price competition among several brands (i.e., *Oishi, Yenyen,* and *Ichitan*) investing heavily in aggressive marketing such as "lucky draw" campaigns, giving away prizes worth hundreds of millions of Thai *baht*. The lucky draw campaign was effective in attracting low-income consumers to buy green tea beverages for the draw rather than for the taste of green tea. The price of these green tea beverages begins at 10 baht (about $0.30 USD)[66] and is cheaper than some bottled mineral waters and most of the available carbonated sweet drinks.

Another factor contributing to the low price of sweetened RTD tea is the current taxation system. Since 1984, the Thai government has imposed tax on some non-alcoholic beverages based on price or volume. In the current system,[67] tax is levied on 25% of ex-factory value (or 0.77 baht per 440 ml) for soda water and 20% (or 0.37 baht per 440 ml) for carbonated soft drinks and some fruit and vegetable juices. Yet, RTD tea and coffee are exempt from the tax. Jou and Tachakehakij[68] suggested that the price-based tax rate is higher than that in the United States and ineffective for reducing obesity in Thailand, where consumption of these taxed beverages (i.e., carbonated drinks) is relatively low. This system enables RTD tea and coffee to set lower prices than carbonated sweetened drinks.

Would a Sugary Drink Tax Work in Thailand?

Recently, the Thai government started preparing to introduce a new tax on beverages that contain certain amounts of sugar.[69] This move is driven by public health concerns for Thailand's relatively high prevalence within Southeast Asia of individuals who are overweight, obese,[70] and have diabetes.[71] Skeptics argue, however, that the sugary drink tax may not be the best solution for preventing obesity and diabetes in Thailand.[72-74] Firstly, increased prices of sugary drinks may affect consumption among low-income households only and may not influence consumption among high-income households, which are the major consumers of sugary drinks in Thailand.[72,73] Secondly, the sugary drink tax will be imposed on beverages with nutrition labels sold at convenience stores and supermarkets, and the sugary drinks sold at cafés and street vendors will not be taxed.[74] Sugar added to dishes and sweets is not subject to the tax. Although modern retailers such as supermarkets and convenience stores dominate half of food sales in Thailand, traditional fresh markets and street vendors not only provide affordable food to poor Thais but also support local food culture and social networks for many Thais.[75] Thus, the introduction of the new tax may affect sales of RTD beverages at modern retailers, but not the consumption of sugar from local markets and vendors.

From the Privileged to the New Urban Consumers

In addition to the industrialization of the Thai sugar system and the rise of sugar-sweetened beverages, there is a shift in the definition of sugar and sweetness. A Thai writer, Kham Paka,[76] noted that although refined white sugar was a product for the privileged few in the past, it has now become a symbol of new urban consumers. For urbanites, refined sugar is believed to be clean and its quality standardized, compared with "local" sugar, such as palm and coconut sugar, which varies in quality and hygienic standards. She concluded that this attitude is reflected in the practice of adding sugar to most dishes people consume. From the consumption surveys employing 24-hour dietary recalls, or the semi-quantitative Food Frequency Questionnaire (FFQ) and self-report household data, it is hard to estimate how much sugar is added to dishes prepared outside of the household,[77] and to what extent urbanites consume more refined sugars than traditional sugars outside of the household. Eating out is a common practice in urban Thailand,[78] however, and food away from the household tends to be high in calories, fat, and sugar compared with home-cooked food.[79] More importantly, as discussed earlier in the Australian section, most of the sugar intake in contemporary societies is from processed food and drinks, with little from traditional methods of sweetening food and drinks using palm and coconut sugars. Appreciation of sweetness within the complex mix of flavors in Thai culinary culture has gradually been replaced by the mass production of cane sugar and the symbol of busy urban consumers, and sugar has become a health threat as rates of obesity and diabetes increase.

Sweetness is an important element of Thai meals. The complex mix of flavors created by local ingredients is now replaced by mass-produced cane sugars and manufactured syrups. Public health concerns about obesity and diabetes have encouraged the government to regulate prices of sugar-sweetened beverages. The expected impacts are limited, however, because taxation focuses only on sugar in beverages and ignores social mechanisms and cultural meanings of sugar consumption.

Nigeria

Nigeria is situated on the shores of the Gulf of Guinea along the coast of West Africa. Nigeria is the most populous country in Africa, having an estimated population in 2015 of 182.2 million people.[80] Well over half of the population of West Africa and between one fifth and one sixth of that of Africa as a whole live in Nigeria. The Yoruba ethnic group of southwest Nigeria make up about 20% of the Nigerian population. The food production growth rate is well below the population growth rate,[81] leading to a heavy reliance on the import of food items to supplement domestic production. This food supply situation is now even more serious because of the increasing difficulties in meeting import bills due to the decline in foreign exchange earnings. As in many developing countries, there is a marked inequality in income distribution and a steep gradient in nutrient consumption from the poorest to the wealthiest, with the result that a high proportion of the population has an intake of nutrients below requirements.[82]

Nutritional Status of Children

In many low-income African communities, including those in Nigeria, growth failure or stunting of young children continues to be a problem. This is due not only to the high burden of infection and parasites, low energy intake, and a deficit in overall food intake, but also to inadequate intake of high-quality protein and micronutrients.[83] Animal source foods (ASF) supply not only high-quality and readily digested protein and energy, but are also a compact and efficient source of readily available micronutrients.[84] Researchers have become increasingly aware that access to ASF, even in relatively small amounts, can lead to improvements in the health and nutrition of young children,[85,86] and that consumption of ASF is significantly correlated with child growth when access to food is not limited.[84]

Nigeria continues to have a significant portion of the burden of undernutrition in the world: Worldwide, over 5% of all children under five years of age who are stunted live in Nigeria, and the country is the second largest contributor to the global prevalence of stunting, ranking just below India.[87] Also, in southwestern Nigeria, where the Yoruba predominate, 31% of children under five years of age had moderate-to-severe stunting.[88] Furthermore, the prevalence of micronutrient deficiencies in Nigeria is quite high, with recent national estimates reporting the prevalence of vitamin A, zinc, iron, and iodine deficiencies in children five years of age and under to be 29.5%, 20.0%, 27.5%, and 27.5% respectively.[89]

Beliefs and Animal Source Foods

Animal protein foods are therefore especially important in this part of the world. Proteins provide important nutrients for the healthy development of children and their mothers in a place where diarrhea, measles, and malaria often compromise health and have an impact on young children at an age when cultural restriction of animal protein foods is most severe.[83,90] Infection increases the protein requirements of young children,[83] and cassava and similar starchy foods that many rely on for a large part of their diets are deficient in protein.

Eating snail, grass-cutter (marsh cane-rat or ground hog) meat, and eggs for example can provide needed protein in Southwestern Nigeria, yet food taboos and cultural traditions may advise against it. Cultural traditions have held for generations that starting children on eggs early in life can predispose them to stealing later in life, that snail consumption can make a child sluggish, and that grass-cutter meat may make labor difficult.[91] As a result, food beliefs that restrict protein foods for young children have been cited as an especially important determinant of the low nutritional status and increased mortality seen in young children.

Food habits, including beliefs and practices that prohibit certain foods, do not exist in a cultural vacuum; they are interwoven with a people's entire way of life.[92,93] As shown in the United Nations International Children's Emergency Fund (UNICEF) framework of undernutrition,[94] for effective interventions, especially in developing countries, it is important to understand that food beliefs and practices continue to be a strong force in the life of society. Often these societies are changing from rural traditions to more modern, urban lifestyles, and food traditions help to maintain cultural identity and familiar traditional values. Importantly, food beliefs and practices also are influenced by the environmental resources of the people, especially in simple low-technology societies where humans have developed a sensitive and intimate relationship with nature. The fauna and flora of an indigenous environment considerably influences what foods will be produced and cultivated generation after generation.

Vegetation Zones and Nutritional Deficiencies

The distribution of nutritional deficiencies in Nigeria follows the four broad vegetation zones of the country and the agricultural activities in each of these regions. Generally, the northern and coastal parts of the country do not have as great a protein deficiency problem as the inland southern areas, because the environment allows for the rearing of animal products in the form of cattle in the north, and seafood in the coastal zone. The forest zone, which stretches from the southwestern to the eastern part of the country does not have as much animal protein, because the thick forest and presence of the tsetse fly inhibit raising of livestock. As far back as 1949, Bascom[95] observed that in southwestern Nigeria, where the Yoruba predominate, meat was a food for ceremonies and special occasions, and only chiefs and the wealthy could afford to buy it regularly in the market or to kill a domestic animal simply for food. Meat, therefore, was considered a rare and luxurious food in the Yoruba community. It remains difficult and expensive to obtain and is often restricted and reserved for important occasions and important people. According to Bascom,[95] British foreign influence has helped to increase the amount of meat in the average Yoruba diet, even though meat is still considered a food of the well to do. Because meat and other animal protein are considered prestige foods to be relished by special people, and because their use is influenced by cultural beliefs and practices, they are given only sparingly to children or withheld from them completely.

Beliefs and Restriction of Animal Source Foods

Earlier studies in Nigeria indicated that meat and eggs were restricted in the diets of preschool children due to beliefs that too much of these led to the child's moral degradation by causing them to steal and become "spoilt."[96–98] More recent studies continue to document such beliefs in both urban and rural areas of southwestern Nigeria,[99] as well as in other parts of west Africa.[100]

The rationale for this belief is an example of the age-old practice, found in many parts of the world, of using food in the socialization of children. In this particular example, meat and other similarly scarce or prestigious foods serve not only as food but also as educational material for teaching children the culturally accepted rules for behavior within the social group. Specifically, parents restrict animal source foods to young children to teach them concepts of self-denial and deferred gratification. Because of the thick forest vegetation in southwestern Nigeria, animal source foods are difficult to rear and are therefore scarce and expensive. Parents rationalize that if children become used to eating such expensive foods on a regular basis, they will develop a preference for them even when the food ceases to be available. According to this rationale, they will steal from others in order to satiate the craving for the food. Also, parents fear that children (once grown) will not be able to save money for those things that signify good social standing, such as buying a home or being prepared for expensive ceremonial rituals, because all their money will go toward buying expensive meat. Parents fear that giving children too much meat will spoil them and eventually lead them to steal, and thus parents act in a preventive manner in restricting animal source foods to young children.

Discussion: Lessons Learned from Cross-Cultural Comparisons of Four Case Studies

Human biology and genetics may have some influence on food preferences and eating behaviors. However, innate desires for certain tastes and foods are not the absolute determinant of food practices. Our case studies from Australia, Japan, Thailand, and Nigeria illustrate that culture, including economic, social, and environmental factors can embed a preference for certain foods into the population's everyday food practices. These four case studies highlight Paul Rozin's statement, "What makes people eat the food they do?... [C]ulture." Yet not only does culture influence food preferences, but food practices, particularly as taught to children, are used to instill and reinforce cultural beliefs. As we see in the example from Australia, where sugar and sweets have been used as rewards and motivation for children's behavior, and in the example from Nigeria where restricting meat and other prestige foods prevents "spoiling" children and letting them "develop a liking (sweet tooth)" for foods their families cannot afford to give them, adults use food to enculturate the next generation and transmit cultural values.

Although practices and functions may overlap between cultures, a closer examination highlights how cross-cultural generalizations may come up short, and how one size or pattern "does not fit all." For example, taxation of sugar-sweetened beverages is a popular policy intervention for preventing obesity, and several countries and states have introduced such taxes.[101,102] Yet, the case study of Thailand highlights how a sugar tax may not have the same effects in the Thai context. Historical, political, and economic contexts are clearly important for understanding how preferences for the same food, such as sugar, may vary widely. Cultural comparisons also raise questions about the appropriate metrics and questions. For example, although sweetened beverage consumption has increased in many countries, including Thailand, most Japanese prefer to drink unsweetened tea. Yet tea often is consumed with sweets, but these are increasingly processed foods containing added sugar or HFCS. Thus, to what extent does tea consumption in Japan and Thailand directly and indirectly contribute to increased sugar consumption? Answers to these questions are needed for public health policy and interventions that aim to reduce sugar consumption and associated chronic disease. Yet focusing exclusively on calories, or reducing food to its biochemical components, leads to a limited understanding of the role of food in human life and health.

Food preferences may vary among individuals, but to some extent can be considered properties or characteristics of groups, and these preferences travel with them. This occurred when the British brought their preference for sugar to Australia, and later when new immigrants reduced the national average of sugar intake because they preferred less sugar. Foods often are used to convey cultural values, such as convenience and modernity, urban lifestyle (sweetened beverages in Thailand), hospitality (tea and sweets in Japan), and socialization and moral education for children (Nigeria and Australia). Foods such as sugar and meat also can convey nationalistic or hierarchical cultural values that privilege certain groups of people above others. Sugar may have been the aim of some colonial exploits, and at other times simply the spoils of war, but through slavery and indentured labor, production of sugar has influenced the global movement of people and their cultures. Now sugar (and similarly historically rare foods such as meat) provides a window through which to explore many variations on the theme of food–culture interactions. Cross-cultural comparisons highlight the dangers of reducing foods such as sugar and meat to their biomedical functions and stress the need to understand the complex social roles. These multi-directional influences and nuanced local cultural factors have wide-ranging implications for studies of food and public health.

Implications for Health Professionals

In order to design nutrition education messages and programs that will connect with clients and counteract food beliefs that might negatively impact health, it is important that health professionals be aware of the cultural values underlying food beliefs so that the messages produced will have a greater chance of being effective.[103] Attending to cultural values is particularly important because nutrition education and other interventions carried out to influence traditional beliefs are developed within the biomedical worldview, which tends to overemphasize the biological function of food as a source of nutritional requirements over its non-biological, social functions. Traditional cultures have a broader view of food functions, which often include symbolic reasons underlying food beliefs and practices. This difference in what is emphasized with food, that is, the biomedical versus traditional worldview, often leads to a misunderstanding that impairs communication between the nutrition educator trained in the biomedical worldview model and the recipient with little understanding of the biomedical framework.[92,104,105]

A need has been identified for several decades for health professionals to analyze concepts of health and nutrition within their overall cultural context.[106–109] This need, however, has not been effectively addressed in practice. One reason for this may be that the culture of the clients is often seen as a problem and therefore a barrier to care.[104] Framing culture as problematic may arise from health professionals being trapped in the Western perspective with the erroneous belief that this framework is the only valid way of interpreting the world.[109] Yet to understand the cultural values underlying food belief systems, health professionals need to have a deeper awareness of the worldview encompassing these health beliefs.[110]

Discussion Questions

1. As the Yoruba in Nigeria undergo economic development, will they have the same problems with sugar? Why or why not? How could cultural understandings be used to prevent problems seen in Thailand or Australia, for example?
2. What are the pros and cons of a sugar tax, or meat subsidies for children to achieve healthful eating and growth, particularly for vulnerable sub-populations?
3. For successful public health interventions, is it critical to take "culture" into consideration? Discuss "culture-inclusive" interventions and policies to improve public health in each of the four case studies.

Quiz Questions

Multiple Choice Questions

1. In the Australian case study, which factor influenced the shift from sugar consumption in foods prepared at home to manufactured products?
   a. Rewarding children with candy
   b. Industrialization contributed to cheaper sugar
   c. Women entering the workforce and having less time for baking
   d. Concerns about high-fat diets led to replacement of fat with sugar
   e. Increased availability of ready-to-drink tea with added sugar
2. How does Japanese tea culture contribute to sugar consumption?
   a. Increased sweetened ready-to-drink tea sold from vending machines has replaced traditional brewed tea.
   b. Japanese are drinking more and more tea, thus sugar consumption is increasing.
   c. Sugar is very expensive in Japan, so sugar consumption is low although most people would like to eat more.
   d. Japanese green tea is very bitter, and must be consumed with sweets to be palatable.
   e. Japanese prefer to drink unsweetened tea, and thus sugar consumption is not as high as in other developed countries.
3. In Thailand, which cultural factor contributed to the greatest increase in sugar intake in the latter part of the 20th century?

a. Sweetness (*waan*) is the most important flavor component in Thai cuisine.

b. Ecologically, in a tropical country such as Thailand, there is widespread availability of palm sugar.

c. In a developing country with high poverty, such as Thailand, many poor people were swayed by marketing ploys to buy sweetened beverages.

d. Development of politically strong sugar industry and changing consumption habits in sugary food and drinks

e. Government tariffs on imported sugar supported the domestic sugar industry, so it produced great quantities, leading to high local intake.

4. What is the most important cultural factor influencing malnutrition in children among the Yoruba in Southern Nigeria?

a. British colonial influence taught people that meat should be reserved for upper-class white people.

b. Parents are concerned that feeding children meat is morally and economically indulgent.

c. Their rudimentary understanding of nutrition and physiology lead them to think that meat is not healthful for children.

d. They live in remote villages and have not had the benefit of public health education.

e. Due to the tsetse fly, they cannot raise livestock.

5. Which of the following is the most important cultural factor influencing the difference in sugar consumption between Australia and Japan?

a. Japan was closed to Western influence for many years during the Edo period and did not discover sugar until later; thus, the Japanese are catching up in terms of their preferences.

b. Australian cuisine is influenced by Western taste preferences for sugar, which comes from the United States and is thus more widely available in Australia.

c. Japanese prefer bitter tastes, while Australians prefer sweet tastes in the context of tea drinking.

d. Australians descend from the British, and require more sugar in the hot climate of Australia, to which they are not accustomed.

e. Sugar is more expensive in Japan than in Australia, so the Japanese cannot afford to indulge their innate taste preferences.

Short Answer/Essay Questions

1. What do you think would happen to childhood malnutrition among the Yoruba in Nigeria if meat prices fell? Why?

2. Examine Figure 11.1. Pick two case studies and describe how they highlight different levels of culture and the impacts on food preferences. Compare and contrast them.

3. Based on the case studies presented here, to what extent do you think economic development, as opposed to other cultural factors, plays a role in determining food preferences?

4. For food preferences, what is the appropriate scale for analysis and intervention? For example, which sub-groups should we examine (based on economics, gender, age, religion, etc.)?

5. To what extent has food moved from sustenance to symbol for humans (e.g., of status, modernity, urbanism, convenience)?

References

1. Rozin P. Past, present and future perspectives on the meal and the restaurant. *International Research Symposium 2015: Experimental restaurant of the future;* December 1, 2015; Taylor's University Lakeside Campus in Malaysia.

2. Rozin P. The meaning of food in our lives: a cross-cultural perspective on eating and well-being. *Journal of Nutrition Education and Behavior.* 2005;37:S107–S112.

3. Appadurai A. *Modernity at Large: Cultural Dimensions of Globalization.* Vol 1. Minneapolis: University of Minnesota Press; 1996.

4. Carr S, Unwin N, Pless-Mulloli T. *An Introduction to Public Health and Epidemiology.* Berkshire: McGraw-Hill Education (UK); 2007.

5. Kalofonos IA. "All I Eat Is ARVs." *Medical Anthropology Quarterly.* 2010;24(3):363–380.

6. Allen LH, De Benoist B, Dary O, Hurrell R, Organization WH. *Guidelines on Food Fortification with Micronutrients.* Geneva: World Health Organization and Food and Agricultural Organization of the United Nations; 2006.

7. World Health Organization. *Global Prevalence of Vitamin A Deficiency in Populations at Risk 1995–2005: WHO Global Database on Vitamin A Deficiency.* Geneva: World Health Organization; 2009.

8. Betancourt JR, Green AR, Carrilo JE, Park ER. Cultural competence and health care disparities: key perspectives and trends. *Health Affairs.* 2005;24(2):499–505.

9. Robert Wood Johnson Foundation. 2014 President's Message. 2014; http://www.rwjf.org/en/library/annual-reports/presidents-message-2014.html. Accessed June 17, 2017.

10. Wilk R. The extractive economy: an early phase of the globalization of diet. *Review (Fernand Braudel Center).* 2004:285–306.

11. Van der Veen M. When is food a luxury? *World Archaeology.* 2003;34(3):405–427.

12. Popkin BM. Nutritional patterns and transitions. *Population and Development Review.* 1993:138–157.

13. Monteiro CA, Moubarac JC, Cannon G, Ng SW, Popkin B. Ultra processed products are becoming dominant in the global food system. *Obesity Reviews.* 2013;14(S2):21–28.

14. Symons M. *One Continuous Picnic: A Gastronomic History of Australia.* Melbourne: Melbourne University Press; 2007.

15. Department of Foreign Affars and Trade (DFAT). Agricultural trade.http://dfat. gov.au/trade/organisations/wto/Pages/agricultural-trade.aspx. Accessed April 24, 2018.

16. World Bank. World Bank Country and Lending Groups. 2017; https://datahelp-desk.worldbank.org/knowledgebase/articles/906519-world-bank-country-and-lending-groups. Accessed April 24, 2017.

17. United Nations. Sustainable Development Goals. 2015; https://sustainabledevel-opment.un.org/sdgs. Accessed June 18, 2017.

18. Australian Bureau of Statistics. 4364.0.55.001 National Health Survey: First Results, 2014–15. 2015; http://www.abs.gov.au/ausstats/abs@.nsf/mf/4364.0.55.001. Accessed April 24, 2017.

19. Australian Bureau of Statistics. Australian Health Survey: Consumption of added sugars, 2011–12. 2016; http://www.abs.gov.au/ausstats/abs@.nsf/Lookup/4364.0.55.011main+features12011-12. Accessed June 20, 2017.

20. Griggs P. Sugar plantations in Queensland, 1864–1912: Origins, characteristics, distribution, and decline. *Agricultural History.* 2000;74(3):609–647.

21. Miller I. Sugar slaves. 2010; http://www.qhatlas.com.au/content/sugar-slaves. Accessed May 4, 2017.

22. Australian Sugar Milling Council. Australian sugarcane industry overview. http://asmc.com.au/industry-overview/. Accessed May 24, 2017.

23. United States Department of Agriculture. Sugar: world markets and trades. 2017; https://apps.fas.usda.gov/psdonline/circulars/sugar.pdf. Accessed April 24, 2018.

24. Griggs P. Black poison or beneficial beverage?: Tea consumption in colonial Australia. *Journal of Australian Colonial History.* 2015;17:23–44.

25. Griggs P. "A natural part of life": The Australian sugar industry's campaign to reverse declining Australian sugar consumption, 1980–1995. *Journal of Australian Studies.* 2006;30(87):141–154.

26. Banwell C, Broom D, Davies A, Dixon J. *Weight of Modernity: An Intergenerational Study of the Rise of Obesity.* New York: Springer; 2012.

27. Farrer K. *To Feed a Nation: A History of Australian Food Science and Technology.* Collingwood: CSIRO Publishing; 2005.

28. Australian Bureau of Statistics. 4364.0.55.011-Australian Health Survey: Consumption of added sugars, 2011–12. Canberra: Australian Bureau of Statistics; 2016.

29. Barclay AW, Brand-Miller J. The Australian paradox: a substantial decline in sugars intake over the same timeframe that overweight and obesity have increased. *Nutrients.* 2011;3(4):491–504.

30. Brand-Miller JC, Barclay AW. Declining consumption of added sugars and sugar-sweetened beverages in Australia: a challenge for obesity prevention. *The American Journal of Clinical Nutrition.* 2017;105(4):854–863.

31. Ministry of Agriculture, Forestry, and Fisheries. Heisei 28 sato nendo ni okeru sato oyobi iseikato no jyukyu mitoshi (Outlook of supply and demand of sugar and sweeteners in sugar year 2016). 2017; http://www.maff.go.jp/j/seisan/tokusan/kansho/attach/pdf/satou-4.pdf. Accessed April 24, 2017.

32. Kushner B. Sweetness and empire: sugar consumption in imperial Japan. In: Francks P, Hunter J, eds. *The Historical Consumer: Consumption and Everyday Life in Japan, 1850–2000.* New York: Palgrave Macmillan; 2012:127–150.

33. Morinaga & Co. Ltd. Morinaga museum special exhibition. 2014; https://www.morinaga.co.jp/museum/exhibition/140718/index.html. Accessed June 20, 2017.

34. Yamaura J. Saitama ken nai no satou shiyoujyokyo ni kansuru ichikousatsu (A study on sugar consumption in Saitama area). *Saikatsu kagaku kenkyu.* 1989;11(35):50–58.

35. Mintz SW. Time, sugar, and sweetness. In: Counihan C, Van Esterik P, eds. *Food and Culture: A Reader.* New York: Routledge; 2013:91–103.

36. Ludwig TM. Before Rikyū. Religious and aesthetic influences in the early history of the tea ceremony. *Monumenta Nipponica.* 1981;36(4):367–390.

37. Rath EC. Banquets against boredom: towards understanding (Samurai) cuisine in early modern Japan. *Early Modern Japan 16.* 2008:43–55.

38. Surak K. From selling tea to selling Japaneseness: symbolic power and the nationalization of cultural practices. *European Journal of Sociology.* 2011;52(02):175–208.

39. Agriculture and Livestock Industries Corporation. Sugar price: sugar open-market quotation, yearly and monthly sugar price in Tokyo area. 2017; http://sugar.alic.go.jp/japan/data/jd2-(1).pdf. Accessed April 24, 2017.

40. Organisatopm fpr Economic Co-operation and Development – Food and Agriculture Organization of the United Nations (OECD-FAO). OECD-FAO Agricultural Outlook 2016–2025. OECD Publishing; 2016.

41. Japan Soft Drink Association. *Seiryo inryo no 50 nen (50 years of non-alcoholic beverages).* Chuo, Tokyo: Japan Soft Drink Association; 2005.

42. Japan Soft Drink Association. *Seiryo inryo sui kankei toukei shiryo (Documents related to non-alcoholic beverages).* Chuo, Tokyo: Japan Soft Drink Association; 2016.

43. Statistics Bureau of Japan. Kakei chosa (Household survey: Yearly amount of expenditures, quantities and average prices per household, two or more person household, from 1993 to 2015). Shinjuku, Tokyo: Statistics Bureau of Japan; 2016.

44. Fukuda H, Dyck JH, Stout J. *Sweetener Policies in Japan.* Washington DC: U.S. Department of Agriculture, Economic Research Service; 2002.

45. Ministry of Agriculture, Forestry, Fisheries. Touka chosei seido no anteitekina unei ni muketa torikumi ni tsuite (Regarding an approach to stable management of

sugar price adjustment system). 2010; http://www.maff.go.jp/j/council/seisaku/kanmi/h22_1/pdf/07_siryo5_torikumi_2.pdf. Accessed April 24, 2018.

46. Agriculture and Livestock Industries Corporation. Nihon no satou wo sasaeru shikumi (Structure to support sugar industry in Japan). Minato, Tokyo: Agriculture and Livestock Industries Corporation; 2011.

47. Ministry of Commence. Foreign Trade Statistics of Thailand. 2017; http://www2.ops3.moc.go.th/. Accessed June 22, 2017.

48. Siamwalla A. A history of rice policies in Thailand. *Food Research Institute Studies.* 1975;14(3):233–249.

49. Dixon J, Takeda W, Kelly M, Banwell C, Seubsman S. Two approaches to health promoting food systems: Thailand and Japan. In: Lin V, Fawkes S, Engelhardt K, Mercado S, eds. *Health Promotion Systems and Strategies in Asia: Preparing for the Asia Century.* New York: Springer; In press.

50. Thailand Board of Investment. Thailand Investment Review: Thailand gears up to become the world's food innovation hub. 2016; http://www.boi.go.th/upload/content/TIR_JULY_82855.pdf. Accessed June 22, 2017.

51. Seubsman S, Suttinan P, Dixon J, Banwell C. *Thai Meals.* Cambridge: Woodhead Publishing; 2009.

52. Ramsay A. The political economy of sugar in Thailand. *Pacific Affairs.* 1987;60(2):248–270.

53. Ingram JC. *Economic Change in Thailand, 1850–1970.* Stanford, CA: Stanford University Press; 1971.

54. Vandergeest P. Peasant strategies in a world context: contingencies in the transformation of rice and palm sugar economies in Thailand. *Human Organization.* 1989;48(2):117–125.

55. Food and Agriculture Organization of the United Nations. Food Balance Sheet. Rome: Food and Agriculture Organization of the United Nations; 2017.

56. Department of Health, Ministry of Public Health, School of Public Health, Mahidol University. The third national nutrition survey of Thailand 1986. Nonthaburi: Division of Nutrition; 1995.

57. Department of Public Health, Ministry of Public Health. The fourth national nutrition survey of Thailand 1995. Nonthaburi: Ministry of Public Health; 1996.

58. Bureau of Nutrition. The fifth nutrition survey in 2546 (2003). Nonthaburi: Bureau of Nutrition, Department of Health, Ministry of Public Health; 2005.

59. National Health Examination Survey Office (NHESO). Thai food consumption survey: Thai health survey no. 4 in 2546-2547 (2008–2009). Nonthaburi: National Health Examination Survey Office; 2011.

60. National Bureau of Agricultural Commodity and Food Standards (ACFS). Food consumption data of Thailand. Chatuchak, Bangkok: National Bureau of Agricultural Commodity and Food Standards; 2016.

61. Han E, Powell LM. Consumption patterns of sugar-sweetened beverages in the United States. *Journal of the Academy of Nutrition and Dietetics.* 2013;113(1):43–53.

62. National Statistical Office (NSO). National survey on health and welfare 2013. Nonthaburi: National Statistical Office; 2013.

63. *Ryokucha no puraido wo kaketa tatakai (Fights over the pride of "green tea")*. Minato, Tokyo: TV Tokyo Corporation; 2005.

64. Ichitan Group Public Company Limited. Opportunity day 1H/2016. Ichitan Group Public Company Limited; 2016.

65. Amornpetchkul TB. Ichitan group and the price war in Thailand's ready-to-drink tea market. *Journal of the International Academy for Case Studies*. 2016;22(3):4–21.

66. Ichitan Group Public Company Limited. Annual Report 2014. 2015; http://ichi.listedcompany.com/misc/AR/20150424-ichi-ar2014-en.pdf. Accessed May 6, 2017.

67. The Excise Department. Excise Tax Rate. October 1, 2013; http://interweb.excise.go.th/contents.php?lang=en&m=4. Accessed May 6, 2017.

68. Jou J, Techakehakij W. International application of sugar-sweetened beverage (SSB) taxation in obesity reduction: factors that may influence policy effectiveness in country-specific contexts. *Health Policy*. 2012;107(1):83–90.

69. Sattaburuth A. Sugar tax for public health: soft drinks 20–25% price rise. *Bangkok Post*. April 27, 2016.

70. Global Database on Body Mass Index: An Interactive Surveillance Tool for Monitoring Nutrition Transition. Geneva: World Health Organization; 2017. http://apps.who.int/bmi/index.jsp. Accessed May 6, 2017.

71. International Diabetes Federation. *IDF Diabetes Atlas – 7th edition*. Brussels: International Diabetes Federation; 2015.

72. Pisuthipan A. Sugar tax just a quick fix. *Bangkok Post*. May 30, 2016.

73. Bhadrakom C. A sugar tax is not the answer to obesity. *Bangkok Post*. June 15, 2016.

74. Israngkura A. *Rethink the Tax on Sugar Drinks*. Wangthonglang, Bangkok: Thailand Development Research Institute; 2016.

75. Kelly M, Seubsman S, Banwell C, Dixon J, Sleigh A. Traditional, modern or mixed? Perspectives on social, economic, and health impacts of evolving food retail in Thailand. *Agriculture and Human Values*. 2015;32(3):445–460.

76. Kham Paka. Sugar: the history of the Thai elite and the journey from the 'the sacred' to 'dangers' (in Thai). February 10, 2017; http://themomentum.co/momentum-opinion-history-of-sugar-thai. Accessed May 6, 2017.

77. Carlsen MH, Blomhoff R, Andersen LF. Intakes of culinary herbs and spices from a food frequency questionnaire evaluated against 28-days estimated records. *Nutrition Journal*. 2011;10(1):1–6.

78. Yasmeen G. Not "from scratch": Thai food systems and "public eating." In: Counihan C, Van Esterik P, eds. *Food and Culture: A Reader*. New York: Routledge; 2012:320–329.

79. Wolfson JA, Bleich SN. Is cooking at home associated with better diet quality or weight-loss intention? *Public Health Nutrition*. 2015;18(08):1397–1406.

80. United Nations Economic Commission for Africa. The demographic profile of African countries. 2016; http://repository.uneca.org/handle/10855/23177. Accessed May 22, 2017.

81. Inyang H, Adebayo E, Anyanwu S. Consumption of animal protein in Adamawa State: an empirical analysis. *Journal of Studies in Social Sciences.* 2014;7(1):41–64.

82. Fanzo J. The nutrition challenge in sub-Saharan Africa. 2012; http://www.undp. org/content/dam/rba/docs/Working%20Papers/Nutrition%20Challenge.pdf. Accessed April 24, 2018

83. Guerrant RL, Oriá RB, Moore SR, Oriá MO, Lima AA. Malnutrition as an enteric infectious disease with long-term effects on child development. *Nutrition Reviews.* 2008;66(9):487–505.

84. Neumann C, Harris DM. Contribution of animal source foods in improving diet quality for children in the developing world. 1999; http://www.international-food-safety.com/pdf/diet-quality.pdf. Accessed April 24, 2018.

85. Gittelsohn J, Vastine AE. Sociocultural and household factors impacting on the selection, allocation and consumption of animal source foods: current knowledge and application. *The Journal of Nutrition.* 2003;133(11):4036S-4041S.

86. Leroy JL, Frongillo EA. Can interventions to promote animal production ameliorate undernutrition? *The Journal of Nutrition.* 2007;137(10):2311–2316.

87. United Nations International Children's Emergency Fund (UNICEF). *Improving Child Nutrition: The Achievable Imperative for Global Progress.* New York: UNICEF; 2013.

88. National Population Commission (NPO) and ICF Macro. *Nigeria Demographic and Health Survey 2008.* Abuja: National Population Commission and ICF Macro; 2009.

89. Maziya-Dixon B, Akinyele IO, Oguntona EB, Nokoe S, Sanusi RA, Harris E. *Nigeria Food Consumption and Nutrition Survey 2001–2003: Summary.* Ibadan, Nigeria: International Institute of Tropical Agriculture; 2004.

90. Rowland MG, Rowland SG, Cole TJ. Impact of infection on the growth of children from 0 to 2 years in an urban West African community. *The American Journal of Clinical Nutrition.* 1988;47(1):134–138.

91. Ekwochi U, Osuorah CD, Ndu IK, Ifediora C, Asinobi IN, Eke CB. Food taboos and myths in South Eastern Nigeria: The belief and practice of mothers in the region. *Journal of Ethnobiology and Ethnomedicine.* 2016;12(7).

92. Sanjur D. *Social and Cultural Perspectives in Nutrition.* Englewood Cliffs,NJ: Prentice-Hall; 1982.

93. Ikpe EB. *Food and Society in Nigeria: A History of Food Customs, Food Economy and Cultural Change 1900–1989.* Stuttgart: Franz Steiner Verlag; 1994.

94. United Nations International Children's Emergency Fund (UNICEF). *Strategy for improved nutrition of children and women in developing countries.* New York: UNICEF;1990.

95. Bascom WO. Yoruba Concepts of Soul. Paper presented at: Fifth International Congress of Anthropology and Ethnological Sciences1949/1956; University of Philadelphia.

96. Onuoha GB. The changing scene of food habits and beliefs among the Mbaise people of Nigeria. *Ecology of Food and Nutrition*. 1982;11(4):245–250.

97. Vemury M, Levine H. *Beliefs and Practices that Affect Food Habits in Developing Countries: A Literature Review*. New York: CARE; 1978.

98. Ogbeide O. Nutritional hazards of food taboos and preferences in Mid-West Nigeria. *The American Journal of Clinical Nutrition*. 1974;27(2):213–216.

99. Aina TA. *Beyond Benign Neglect: Early Childhood Care, Development and Nutrition in Metropolitan Lagos, Nigeria*. Lagos, Nigeria: Malthouse Press; 2008.

100. Colecraft E, Marquis GS, Aryeetey R, et al. Constraints on the use of animal source foods for young children in Ghana: a participatory rapid appraisal approach. *Ecology of Food and Nutrition*. 2006;45(5):351–377.

101. Boseley S. Mexico's sugar tax leads to fall in consumption for second year running. The Guardian. February 22, 2017.

102. Sanger-Katz M. Yes, Soda taxes seem to cut soda drinking. The New York Times. October 13, 2015.

103. Launer LJ, Habicht J. Concepts about infant health, growth, and weaning: A comparison between nutritional scientists and Madurese mothers. *Social Science & Medicine*. 1989;29(1):13–22.

104. Tripp-Reimer T, Choi E, Kelley LS, Enslein JC. Cultural barriers to care: inverting the problem. *Diabetes Spectrum*. 2001;14(1):13–22.

105. Ikeda JP. Culture, food and nutrition in increasingly cultural diverse societies. In: Germov J, Williams L, eds. *A Sociology of Food and Nutrition: The Social Appetite*. South Melbourne: Oxford University Press; 2004:288–313.

106. Cassel J. Social and cultural implications of food and food habits. *American Journal of Public Health and the Nation's Health*. 1957;47(6):732–740.

107. Cassidy CM. Benign neglect and toddler malnutrition. In: Green LS, Johnston FE, eds. *Social and Biological Predictors of Nutrition Status, Physical Growth and Neurological Development*. New York: Academic Press; 1987:109–136.

108. Adetunji JA. Preserving the pot and water: a traditional concept of reproductive health in a Yoruba community, Nigeria. *Social Science & Medicine*. 1996;43(11):1561–1567.

109. Hassel CA. Reconsidering nutrition science: critical reflection with a cultural lens. *Nutrition Journal*. 2014;13(1):1–11.

110. Setiloane KT. Beyond the melting pot and salad bowl views of cultural diversity: advancing cultural diversity education of nutrition educators. *Journal of Nutrition Education and Behavior*. 2016;48(9):664–668.

From Soil to Stomach

AGRITOURISM AND PUBLIC HEALTH

Erecia Hepburn and Allison Karpyn

Chapter Highlights

- The concept of agritourism
- Defining agritourism
- Global perspectives on agritourism
- Agritourism and public health
- Agritourism linkages

For those experiencing a daily commute of asphalt and smog only to arrive at a cubicle and screen, the farm holds a special allure. With open space and chirping birds, it represents a throwback to a simpler way of life and for many stimulates desires to go back to life before the cell phone, e-mail era. For tourists, the farm allows the opportunity to unplug and recharge while engaging in hands-on opportunities to learn about a new culture, space, and way of life. And for farmers, the demand for ecologically minded getaways has created an important new source of income.

Indeed, agritourism represents a popular and growing tactic, which addresses challenges in small farm profitability while supporting the recreational interests of travelers eager to explore and better understand their agricultural heritage. Agritourism furthers the goals of public health as the field continues to push beyond traditional definitions and strategies toward recognizing the importance of wellness. Presented with a multidimensional approach that provides people with engaging, hands-on educational activities, as well as nutritious local foods that limit carbon footprints, states across the United States and nations across the globe have begun to invest in agritourism efforts as a way of building local economies and ensuring that agricultural traditions remain for future generations.

Agritourism also offers public health practitioners a novel mechanism to connect agriculture with public health. Those most vulnerable to poor health are also those who struggle most for employment, at the nexus of which is food security and malnutrition. Sustainable enterprises that support the growth of jobs as well as healthy affordable foods for the farmers' "own" consumption and for market sale are critical mechanisms to ensure food security.[2]

The United Nations' 17 Sustainable Development Goals (SDGs) are a good example of the coming together of these approaches for comprehensive global policy and planning. Intended to help frame global agendas over the next 15 years, the SDGs emphasize the ways in which governments can improve the lives of the poor. Recognizing the critical importance of economic development, health, education, equity, safety, justice, conservation, and sustainability, the 17 SDGs are supported by 169 targets, which provide measurable benchmarks toward progress. Goal Two, for example, is to "End hunger, achieve food security and improved nutrition and promote sustainable agriculture" and is backed by targets including Target 2.3, which seeks to, "By 2030 double the agricultural productivity and incomes of small-scale food producers, in particular women . . . "[3]

The Concept of Agritourism

Agritourism has many varying definitions and applications to various industries and countries around the world, but the one commonality is the link between agriculture and tourism. Of course, the merger of agriculture and tourism is not a recent phenomenon; many studies suggest agritourism has been a recognized development strategy worldwide since the early 20th century. Together, the approach represents a way to utilize local resources in a sustainable and often economically beneficial way, which benefits local residents.[4]

Agritourism has taken on various names depending on the region, much like the common names of plants and animals in different countries. For example, agritourism has been referred to as agricultural tourism, farm tourism, vacation farms, farm-based tourism, county hospitality, and on-farm recreation. Although the idea of agritourism is distinctive, this form of tourism can fall under several broader tourism headings, such as rural tourism and

---

BOX 12.1

Fun Fact: AGRI versus AGRO Tourism

The terms agritourism and agrotourism were used interchangeably in the literature until Jolliffe (2014) tried to make a distinction between the two concepts. His research indicated that there was a difference between the terms; namely, that agritourism implies a style of vacation that is normally spent on farms, and that agrotourism denotes the management of the agricultural estate. The literature has not agreed with these distinctions as yet, and both are still used as synonyms.

---

sustainable tourism and now agroeco-tourism (Box 12.1). Agritourism and all of its synonyms are also at times classified under sustainable agriculture and agri-health. Tourists, who can be domestic or international, participate in a variety of activities in forward linkage operations, including "U-picks" of fruits and vegetables, horseback rides, sampling and tasting of items such as honey, classes about wine coupled with wine tasting, shopping at gift shops and farm stands for local and regional produce or handcrafted gifts, and numerous other activities.[5]

Although agritourism has had a long history in the eastern hemisphere, in countries such as England, where approximately 15% of farms have a tourism component, and Germany, where estimates of around 20,000 farm holidays are offered, it is a relatively new concept to the western hemisphere.[6] Wine growing regions such as those in Ireland, Germany, France, and Denmark have had successful agritourism ventures for decades. Since 1991, European Union (EU) countries have spent €2 billion to subsidize agritourism development in rural farming areas.[7] Studies carried out by the European Union, have showcased the value of the economic subsidy, finding that when a tourist stays on a farm, about €70 remains in the region. Other research has shown that agritourism has positive and statistically significant effects on farm profitability and is particularly beneficial to the small- to medium-sized farm, with fewer benefits for large farms.[8] Many European countries, including Austria, Denmark, England, France, Germany, Ireland, and Norway have government policies to encourage agritourism. Most of these countries have ways of categorizing and rating their agritourism operations, which receive aid from central and local governments (Box 12.2 and Figure 12.1).[9]

BOX 12.2

Italian Agritourism: Adding Cycling to the Mix

"Agriturist Qualità"

In Italy a certificate is awarded to agrotourism enterprises that offer a wide variety of activities with particular focus on "holiday accommodation in agrotourism."

The designation is intended to brand the industry and provide tourists with a premium and trustworthy experience while also promoting and protecting the land, culture, and local food customs. http://www.agriturismo.it

A related effort is AgriCycle Venento, which offers farm guest housing to those interested in bicycling across Italy. Founded in December of 2013, the effort currently has 38 guest houses across the provinces of Venetia, which provide cyclists with covered and protected overnight bike storage, along with information about where to rent bikes, how to transport luggage, do laundry, and connect to nearby bicycle maintenance for repairs. A breakfast "suitable for active guests" is also part of the service (www.agricycleveneto.net).

In America, the history of agritourism dates back to the late 1800s when individuals left the city for short visits on family farms to escape city life. Agritourism has now become widespread in the western hemisphere and includes any farm open to the public at least part of the year. The U.S. Census of Agriculture, for example, reports a 30% increase in farms providing agritourism opportunities from just over 10,000 in 2007 to more than 13,000 in

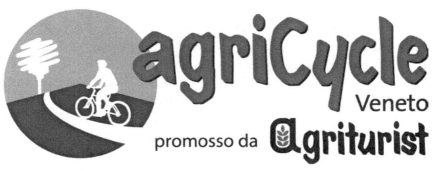

FIGURE 12.1 Agritourism.

2012. Incomes from agritourism sources have shown 23% increase in the same period.[10]

In many ways, Caribbean agritourism is still in its infancy, though more and more island nations have embraced the concept. Countries such as The Bahamas, St. Lucia, Grenada, Guyana, Dominica, Barbados, and Jamaica have welcomed the idea of forging strong linkages among their agriculture, health, and tourism sectors.[4] Researchers and others have argued for the importance of connecting tourism and agriculture in small-island developing states (SIDS), in particular given the critical opportunities to obtain income from foreign exchange and tax dollars, jobs, and improvements to local infrastructure (such as roads and utilities), which benefit locals and tourists alike.

Agritourism Definitions

In its simplest form the word agritourism is derived from the terms "agriculture" and "tourism," representing the intersection of these two industries. Defining what the tourism industry includes and does not include can be a challenge, however, as evidenced by its lack of an industry classification code (NAICS code), for example. When combined with agriculture, the definition becomes even more complex, and together results in a variety of interpretations.[4]

Agritourism has been defined as "an economic activity created when tourists actively seek out farms and farm products during their vacations."[5] Agritourism is a style of vacation in which hospitality is offered on farms, or it can be described as "the act of visiting a working farm or any agricultural, horticultural, or agribusiness operation for the purpose of enjoyment, education or active involvement in the activities of the farm operation."[11] Agritourism also is viewed as "an alternative enterprise that links value-added or nontraditional agricultural production or marketing with travel to a farm or ranch."[12] This may include the opportunity to assist with farming tasks during the visit.[13] Agritourism also has been defined as an enterprise that combines elements of agriculture and tourism, where enterprise refers to the overall agritourism operations and the operation should include at least two attractions; for example, U-pick operations and some form of a maze (corn or sugar cane) or ride (hay or pumpkin), a tasting station, and even accommodations.

"In sum, agritourism is defined as an interactive activity that involves agricultural producers, tourists, and the products and facilities of agricultural producers. Mahoney (1987) particularly indicated that such activity was to "use agriculturally related facilities and activities to draw visitors' attention and attempted to sell agricultural products to tourists."[14] Although there are several definitions in the literature for agritourism, one of the most comprehensive definitions is:

Agritourism is an all-encompassing term, which embraces a wide range of activities and operations, but essential to all of them is an interaction between the agricultural producer, his/her products, and the tourists. Agritourism applies to products and services, which combine agriculture—its natural setting and products—with a tourism experience. It includes providing tourists with opportunities to experience a broad spectrum of products and services, including fruit stands, winery tours, farm-based bed and breakfast accommodation, and farm tours. It implies economic activity between tourists and farm operators, an activity that links travel with agricultural products, services, and experience.

As described, there are numerous forms and definitions surrounding the concept of agritourism, but for the purpose of this chapter, agritourism will be defined in two parts to include the forward and backward linkages that take place within it. Further, we recognize that agritourism is linked with sustainable tourism, a kind of tourism that integrates with regional resources and promotes environmental quality; minimizes adverse economic, ecological, and sociocultural impacts; and promotes the educational and recreational experience that is important to visitors. Agritourism also is connected to sustainable agriculture, which has similar integrated qualities and promotes ecological and social health, and which will be examined in greater detail in the next section.

Forward and Backward Linkages in Agritourism

Defining and measuring the impact of agritourism has been a topic of interest since its emergence. One way that experts in the field have sought to comprehensively understand agritourism is in terms of forward and backward linkages.[5,15] This definition complements a more traditional, and perhaps more straightforward, approach to simply calculating the economic benefits of tourism on the economy of the destination location, a practice that remains quite common.[15] At the crux of the concept lies a distinction between two different types of businesses. The first type, a *forward linkage*, describes businesses whose operations create new local opportunities for tourism-related products and services broadly (e.g., a national marketing campaign). The second type of business, a *backward linkage*, relies on specific products and services provided to the customer (e.g., a retail store that sells souvenirs).

The *forward linkage* definition of agritourism is any form of agricultural activity that takes place at the agricultural enterprise that persuades and encourages visitors to participate and spend discretionary income on any of the activities offered on site. The *backward* linkage is defined as the association and usage of the agriculture sectors in the destination/region/nation so as to encourage the economy as a whole and to formulate interaction between distinctive areas such as tourism and health, which often also have a long history of non-collaboration and lack of integration. In the case of agritourism, a way to enhance the backward linkage is to increase the amount of local foodstuffs utilized in the tourism sector of the economy. This would be done through encouraging the promotion of an agricultural product, such as Neep (featured later in this chapter), to the tourism market. Marketing efforts or partnerships with travel agents or local travel brokers, or ideas such as that featured in Italy to brand cycling as an agritourism industry, would magnify forward linkages.

As a measurement framework, forward and backward linkages recognize both the local impact of the tourism dollar to the larger economy while also valuing the ways in which the tourism sector connects with other industry sectors alongside the economy as a whole.[15]

Agritourism: Sustainable Agriculture and Agri-Health
Sustainable Agriculture

Agriculture throughout the world has changed dramatically as more countries move away from an agrarian society. The United States Department of Agriculture's Sustainable Agriculture Research and Education (SARE) program defines sustainable agriculture as an activity that promotes environmental stewardship, generates an acceptable level of income, and maintains stable farm families and communities. All sustainable agriculture research promotes these three foundational guidelines. In addition, Environmental health, economic profitability, and social/economic equity all can be fostered through the development of agritourism. Agritourism has the ability to incorporate each of these foundational guidelines, which would ensure overall healthier humans. Although agritourism is seen by many as primarily a way to assist family farms financially, this concept actually utilizes numerous other sectors in a myriad of ways.

There are three main pillars of sustainable agriculture: environmental health, economic profitability, and social and economic equity. One of the major tenets of sustainable agriculture is stewardship of human resources, which includes consideration of social responsibilities such as the needs of communities and consumer health and safety. Consumer health is a major factor and agritourism development can play a contributory role in ensuring that consumers, who in this case would be called tourists, have access to healthy food. Agritourism promotes farmers markets and venues where farmers and their consumers have the ability to learn from each other and discuss what is in their food, connect with other customers, and preserve the local farming heritage.

Agritourism can be placed under the umbrella of sustainable agriculture, although neither has a definitive definition. Fazio et al. (2008) define this concept as a method in which resources are kept in balance whether through conservation, recycling, or preservation that prevents environmental damage to the farm while profits remain at acceptable levels. Sustainable agriculture first came to general public awareness in the western hemisphere in the 1980s, with the merging of three different, but related, agricultural concerns.[16] Organic farmers and environmental groups were concerned with the impacts of agricultural chemicals on the natural environment and on human health. Some conventional farmers and agricultural groups were concerned about the impacts of rising costs and falling prices on the agricultural economy. Small farmers and rural advocacy groups were concerned about the impacts of agricultural industrialization on farm families, rural communities, and society as a whole.

The growing trend of the locavore movement also ties into agritourism's forward and backward linkages, as people have become more interested in knowing where their food originates. The term locavore is commonly defined as a person who seeks to consume mainly local foods from within a 100- to 200-mile radius of his or her residence.[17] The physical activity of working or recreating on a farm coupled with consuming healthier products has now become a fast growing trend. By using agritourism as a form of sustainable development in tourism, health and agriculture, land, labor, and other resources could be maximized while minimizing the amount of environmental degradation and competition.

Agri-Health

The marriage of food and agriculture is longstanding; however, connections between agriculture and public health from the perspective of preventive health and wellness have only come about in recent decades. The global rise of non-communicable diseases (NCDs) in the major developed and developing countries, coupled with the high rates of malnutrition, which now encompasses both hunger and obesity, clearly indicates that a shift and review of the food system needs to take place.

Non-communicable diseases, or chronic or lifestyle-related diseases, are the major global causes of morbidity and mortality. Approximately 63% (36 million) of the 57 million global deaths in 2008 were due to NCDs, a figure that has increased to 70% in 2017.[1,2] The four major NCDs, namely, cardiovascular disease (CVD), cancer, chronic respiratory disease, and diabetes, account for about 80% of total NCD deaths and share four common modifiable risk factors: unhealthy diet, physical inactivity, smoking, and alcohol consumption.[3] Although NCDs place an extreme burden on developed and developing countries, it is now evident that the prevalence of NCDs in low- and middle-income countries is increasing. Agritourism is not the answer to eliminating or preventing NCDs, but it is another tool to address the growing problem. Globally, we have witnessed a rapid increase of NCDs, and according to the World Health Organization they are projected to exceed communicable, maternal, perinatal, and nutritional diseases as the most common cause of death by 2030. NCDs will take more lives than all other causes combined if appropriate responses are not undertaken; agritourism properly administered can be one of these responses.

Example in Practice

Abaco Neem Farm: An Agritourism Operation in Abaco

Nicholas Miaoulis, a Greek Bahamian, has been living on Abaco in The Bahamas for 30 years after moving from Florida. At age 61, Miaoulis has owned and operated a tree farm named The Abaco Neem Farm for 26 years (Figure 12.2). It is a certified organic farm and has 110 acres cultivated with certified organic aloe, citronella, coconuts, and Neem trees. These are ingredients used in the production of the Abaco Neem products

---

1. World Health Organization. Global status report on noncommunicable diseases 2010, available online: World Health Organization. Global status report on noncommunicable diseases 2010.

2. World Health Organization. 2017. Non communicable disease progress monitor 2017. ISBN 978 92 4 151302 9, pp 231. Available online: http://www.who.int/nmh/publications/ncd-progress-monitor-2017/en/.

3. World Health Organization. The Global strategy for prevention and control of noncommunicable diseases, a report by the Director-General, 22 March 2000.A53/14. Available online: http://www.afro.who.int/sites/default/files/2017-06/NCD-Global_Strategy_for_the_Prevention_and_Control_of_NCD_2000.pdf

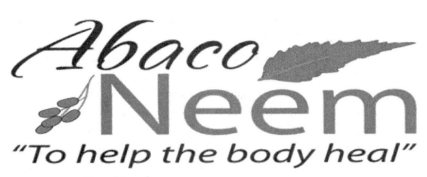

FIGURE 12.2   Abaco Neem logo.

sold locally at most major stores throughout the country and at their farm (Figure 12.3).

The farm is located in South Abaco near the settlement of Cassurina. Although the primary focus of the farm is to produce the ingredients that go into its Neem production, it also is developing the *forward linkages* of agri-tourism by incorporating a wide variety of tropical floral and fruit-bearing trees for U-pick operations (Figure 12.4). They have constructed a small, solar paneled, visitor cottage, which requires no electricity and is considered to be

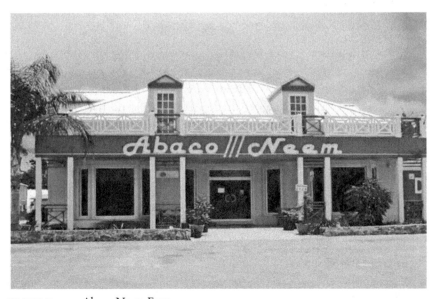

FIGURE 12.3   Abaco Neem Farm.

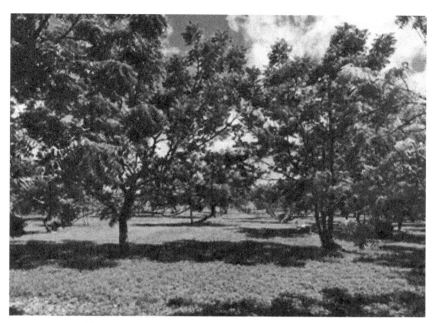

FIGURE 12.4 Neem trees.

totally off the grid. The company, Abaco Neem Limited, has a separate off-site production center where they manufacture over 23 different Neem products from the raw commodities grown on the farm.

In the case of the Neem farm, the goal was always to support both health and agricultural production and, in the words of the owner, "The more I researched the Neem tree and the value of Neem; I came to appreciate its medicinal value and focused on how preventable diseases hypertension and diabetes both prevalent throughout The Bahamas."

The farm today makes a variety of medicinal products including creams for the body and items for pets, as well as agricultural products (Figure 12.5). "We make soaps, creams, lotions, balms and a salve for treating extreme dry skin issues as well as a tooth powder and Neem leaf extract for dental hygiene, and an insect repellent. A key ingredient in the products is neem oil pressed from the seeds (Figure 12.5). A valuable agricultural byproduct derived from pressing the seed to extract the oil is Neem Cake, a natural pesticide and fertilizer for organic crop cultivation. On The Neem Farm, in addition to the cottage, they have constructed bathrooms and an open-plan kitchen with plans for future expansion to include an on-site restaurant where residents and tourists alike can learn and gather (Figure 12.6).

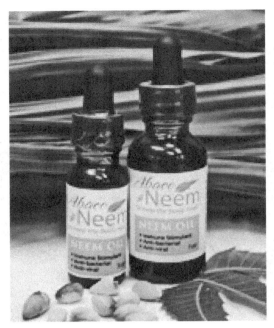

FIGURE 12.5 Neem oil.

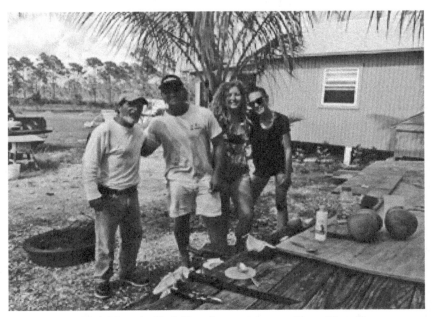

FIGURE 12.6 Nick Miaoulis (far left) and some visitors to Abaco Neem Farm.
Photo Credit Abaco Neem.

Agritourism Worldwide

The previously accepted notion that large numbers of tourists are not interested in participating, absorbing, or sampling the local culture or food is no longer the case today. The popularity of *Travel Channel* programs such as *Anthony Bourdain No Reservations* or *Bizarre Foods with Andrew Zimmern,* have contributed to the heightened interest on the part of tourists to explore local food cultures in new ways. Tourists are now looking for more than just a typical "tourist experience" of "sun, sand, and sea."[18]

With the local food movement becoming quite popular in America and in Europe, there is a great opportunity to see local food producers growing and producing various foodstuffs. And as more and more of the world's population is based in cities, rural and agritourism has an increasing appeal.[19]

Agritourism is now a global phenomenon. As countries that primarily focus on tourism or agriculture look for ways to provide a kaleidoscope of attractions to build their economic base in rural areas, agritourism has become a primary focus. "In 2004, approximately 52,000 U.S. farms—2.5% of all farms—received income from farm-based recreation, totaling about $955 million."[4] Hosts of websites now can assist with the planning of an agritourism adventure in places like Africa, Australia, North America, the Middle East, and Latin America.

Europe

In European countries, agritourism, or as more commonly cited there, *farm-tourism*, has a long history, perhaps dating back one hundred years. In the European Union, "Agritourism is the subject of social, agricultural and economic policy, known as multifunctional economic development of the agricultural farms and multifunctional development of rural areas."[11]

Over two decades, these countries have spent approximately $2 billion to subsidize agritourism development in rural farming areas.[20] Several European countries (Austria, Denmark, England, France, Germany, Ireland, and Norway) have governmental policies to encourage agritourism. In France, for example, according to figures from the agricultural statistics of 2010,

---

4. Brown D. and Reeder R. Agrotourism Offers Opportunities for Farm Operators, Amber Waves Newsletter, United States Department of Agriculture Economic Research Service. Feb 1, 2008.

about 100,000 farms (37%) are engaged in some type of agritourism initiative. European organizations and governments have supported farm-tourism through direct and indirect means, such as reducing taxes and providing financing for farms. The Ministry of Agriculture, Food and Fisheries of France, for example, has implemented several rural tourism development polices, including (1) Measure 311: Diversification into non-agricultural activities for farmers and (2) The Development of Rural Areas, including several provisions adopted in the law 2005-157 of February 23, 2005.

Most of these countries have ways of categorizing and rating their agritourism operations, which receive aid from central and local governments.[9] One of the top-rated agritourism operations in France is Bienvenue à la Ferme, a trademark of Chambers of Agriculture. It is the largest network of farm producers and entrepreneurs offering tourist accommodation in farms. There are more than 6,500 members on French territory (http://www.bienvenue-a-la-ferme.com/en/).

The way that rating systems score sites varies from nation to nation. In Great Britain, the National Board of Tourism, using the same criterion for the rural and urban areas, assesses the quality of agricultural farms and their accommodations for overnight stays. In France, assessment is undertaken in strict accordance with a series of benchmarks, designating quality and symbolized by the image of an ear of corn, awarded to high-ranking operations.[21]

In Austria, a daisy is the symbol of quality, and the best quality farms get four daisies. Agritourism has become a way of life for Europeans; both Frater (1983) and Lack (1997) have found that a large percentage of them take farm holidays. In Italy, for example, 73% of persons are in the agritourist sector. Additionally, "according to the latest studies the annual turnover in agrotourism sector is around €1,17 billion."[21]

Canada

Agritourism in the western hemisphere has made tremendous strides. In Canada, places like Alberta, British Columbia, and Saskatchewan have seen significant growth in agritourism. In Alberta alone, there are approximately 200 agritourism operations, 120 farmers markets, and 160 gardeners and fruit growers. Saskatchewan has 60,000 farms and ranches with a wide range of agritourism attractions from museums to fairs to tour operations. The Ministry of Agriculture and Food in Saskatchewan offers one-day workshops to producers in the area to assist with their agritourism program development.[22]

The Ontario Ministry of Tourism, Culture and Recreation developed a strategy to implement a Rural Visitation Program in 1993. Although there is some governmental involvement in the development of agritourism in Canada, it has not reached the scale of involvement in Europe. With agencies such as the Canadian Rural Adaptation and Rural Development, Manitoba Agri-Ventures Initiatives, Country Roads Agritourism Product Club, and Niagara Agritourism, Canada has made significant inroads in its investment in agritourism.

United States of America

In the United States, a five-year census of farms found that over 33,000 U.S. farms benefitted from agritourism activities in 2012, up from 23,000 farms in 2007. As a result, the income from agritourism activities also has expanded in recent decades. Between 2007 and 2012, annual farm income from agritourism increased by more than $137 million.

In 1998, the U.S. Department of Agriculture's (USDA) Agricultural Marketing Service (AMS) developed a Direct Marketing Action Plan designed to support the operation of small farms by providing support to market their products. In 2004, the USDA printed a comprehensive guide to agritourism via the Natural Resources Conservation Service and has issued a resource manual to help support farm profitability. The guide is extensive, with some 20 chapters and 2,300 pages.[23]

In Vermont, for example, agritourism is well established. Between the years 2000 and 2002, agritourism in the state experienced a growth of 86% ($19.5 million). A 2006 report found that about 30% of the state's farms were engaged in agritourism, amounting to 2,300 farms—on average benefitting from $8,900 in agritourism income per small farm (Evan et al., 2006).

California is second only to Texas as the state with the largest amount of income generated from agritourism in the United States. With 1,700 agritourism operations in 2012, California more than doubled the 685 enterprises recorded in 2007. In 2012, the state grossed more than 64,520,000 in agritourism income (Figure 12.7).

Policy also has helped to support the growth in agritourism in the United States. A summary of *States' Agritourism Statutes*[24] for example, reveals an array of state mechanisms in place to regulate safety concerns and ensure farm marketing efforts are supported.

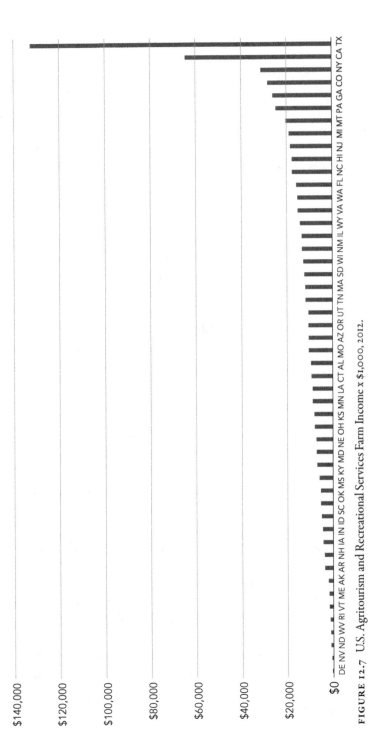

FIGURE 12.7 U.S. Agritourism and Recreational Services Farm Income x $1,000, 2012.

Source: 2012 Census of Agriculture—State Data.

Latin American and the Caribbean

Caribbean agritourism is not often studied, though reports indicate that investment in this area is worthwhile. Organizations such as Inter-American Institute for Cooperation on Agriculture (IICA) also have worked to support the promotion and development of agritourism in the region.[25-27] A few examples of efforts regionally illustrates the diversity of opportunities available in the region.

Places such as Costa Rica have coffee plantations where tourists play an interactive role in the agritourism process or have the option of just touring the estates. Among projects taking place in Barbados are workshops for the encouragement of agritourism. In the Dominican Republic, visitors plant crops and are encouraged to return to reap the crop as a part of their tourism package. St. Lucia has mastered the forward and backward linkage—visitors are invited to come onto farms in the area and farmers sell their produce to Sandals resorts. The Inter-American Institute for Cooperation on Agriculture (IICA) is in the process of developing a strategy for several islands in the Caribbean to advance agritourism in one way or another. The Bahamas has several vibrant agritourism destinations including Abaco Neem, Goodfellow Farms, and Down to Earth Farm, in addition to highly innovative efforts such as the One Eleuthera Foundation's Center for Training and Innovation Hotel (Box 12.3).

Among Jamaica's agritourism operations, several promote the health and wellness aspects in their model. Woodford Market Garden is a small organic farm in Jamaica that originated over 20 years ago. Its primary products are packaged salads—the most popular brand is called "Super Greens Salad Blend"—that are sold in local supermarkets; it is the only farm that sells certified organic produce in Jamaica.[28] Visitors to the farm are given free samples of organic produce, along with product information and recipes for the farm's clients, which include hotels, restaurants, and supermarkets.

Linkages: Tourism, Health, Agriculture, and a Sustainable Way Forward

Although growth of the agricultural sector has suffered in terms of investment and research, in a lot of developing and least developed countries, the public health need for them to "catch up" is evident. There are clear differences between agriculture in developed and less developed countries, but both face

BOX 12.3

One Eleuthera Foundation: Bringing Jobs and Sustainable Development to the Forefront

Another innovative example of the ways in which nations are integrating agritourism and health to promote sustainable development is the *Centre For Training and Innovation* (CTI), a tertiary-level institution created by the One Eleuthera Foundation, a nonprofit organization in Eleuthera, in The Bahamas.

The 110-mile-long island is home to more than 11,000 residents, many of whom are under- or unemployed and struggle with low incomes in a place where the cost of living is exceptionally high. CTI helps to create jobs while at the same time offering the opportunity to complete vocational education training, all while promoting sustainable agriculture. In 2017, CTI opened its doors to a newly renovated training hotel and farm. In The Bahamas, where the tourism industry is the largest economic driver in the nation, industry training is highly relevant yet until CTI opened its doors, there was no training hotel or teaching farm in the area. Although this component of the work is of critical importance, what is even more notable is how the hotel and farm were constructed.

About two years earlier, the land and the run-down, vine-covered remnants of an old dilapidated hotel were acquired. After a short training program in general maintenance with a local institution, participants were asked if they would be interested in working on the site earning minimum wage to repair the hotel and start a farm—all while receiving training from expert carpenters, electricians, plumbers, and local farmers. In the end, participants would earn a certificate in their area of study. Over 50 people enrolled in the *Learn and Earn* program, with an equal mix of men and women. Twenty-two students graduated, sixteen received employment prior to graduation, and three became instructors.

nutritional issues, even if these issues are not identical. The rise of agritourism with its forward and backward linkages has the ability to assist with combatting some of these nutritional challenges. The promotion of functional foods, foods that promise consumers improvements in targeted physiological functions, such as lowering cholesterol or hypertension, can take place with agritourism.

The term "linkages" for most studies is synonymous with investigation of the proportion of imported food to domestic food utilized by the tourism industry.[27] "The aim of creating linkages is to reduce the high import content in the tourism sector, which is achieved by substituting foreign imports with local suppliers."[26]

This chapter has broken linkages into two different components, the forward linkage and the backward linkage. Both forward and the backward linkages have the ability to stimulate agricultural production while also enhancing the tourism product. The forward linkage is defined as any variety of agricultural activity or service that takes place at the agricultural enterprise that convinces and promotes visitors to participate and spend a portion of their discretionary income on any of the activities offered on site.

The backward linkage related to agritourism as used in this research is generally defined as the collaboration and usage of other economic sectors so as to stimulate the economy as a whole and to create synergy between distinctive sectors. These sectors often have a long history of non-collaboration and lack of integration. Several studies have advanced the need to establish linkages with particular focus on "backward linkages" with the agriculture sector.[4,26,29,30] These linkages promote a variety of activities, such as agri-health, agricultural production, food security, and diversification of the tourism product, thus making agriculture a viable option.

Several elements are thought to pervade both the characteristics and strength of linkages (see figure 12.8). These factors are categorized as demand-related, supply- or production-related, and marketing/intermediary factors. One principal demand-related factor influencing linkages is the environment

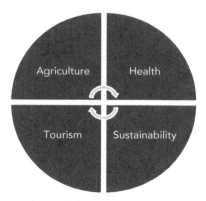

FIGURE 12.8 An Integrated Model of Agritourism: Addressing Linkages in Agriculture, Health, Tourism and Sustainability.

of tourism development. Studies note a trend for foreign-owned or managed enterprises to rely mainly on imports, thus creating only weak links to local production. Others have suggested that the opportunity to advance agritourism lies in a more niche audience of adventure seekers and those committed to spending their tourism dollars to do good, as opposed to attracting the masses. Others have suggested that greater emphasis on the promotion of regional foods should be undertaken to build the sector.[31,4,8,19,32,33]

The need for collaboration between the agricultural sector and the tourism sector is not a new concept. Critical review of current activities, where and how agritourism could be implemented, and what systems and supports are in place at the national and local levels to do so is needed. As the forward and backward linkage model exemplifies, there are a number of facets to defining and measuring the impacts of agritourism efforts. Suggested linkages include agriculture, tourism, health, and sustainability, given that they enhance local revenue for industry and reinvest in the environment, as well as promote equitable distribution of economic benefits to local communities.

Model of the Intersectoral Linkages

Although a change in consumers' tastes is another issue that is thought to constrain the development of backward linkages, this can be rectified by introducing visitors to the local produce at farmers markets (a forward linkage) or through import substitution. While local food purchases by the tourism industry can strengthen the linkages within the traditional market sector, a series of natural and human barriers also can exist, which can prevent a potentially symbiotic relationship between the two sectors from evolving. The lack of communication and understanding that often exists between the industries needs to be remedied.[35] In the case of agritourism, the call for clear communication among all parties can be achieved through a variety of mechanisms.

One way is to ensure that education and information are gathered on the benefits of consuming local produce, coupled with information on the positive health, environmental, social, and cultural impacts that agritourism provides. Second, opening lines of communication through the formation of linkages within the sectors of agriculture, health, sustainability, and tourism creates a reciprocal relationship among the sectors. This evolution of agritourism also has the ability to educate tourists about the significance of conserving natural and cultural heritage, while promoting ethical behavior and responsibility toward the natural and cultural environment.

Agritourists have the ability to get to know on a personal level where their food comes from.

Linkage creation is not only possible but also necessary for a myriad of reasons, perhaps above all to ensure food safety, access to good nutrition, and food security. Ensuring food security would take a long time for a nation to achieve. Although it is acknowledged that the development of forward and backward linkages are important, it should be noted that "not all linkages are the same, nor are they likely to have a similar effect on local agricultural producers and hotel purchasers. Redefining linkages as relations, including such characteristics as information flows between demand and supply as well as access to agricultural inputs, a more informed understanding of the effects that hotel demand has on agricultural production can be gained."[35]

Agritourism Classifications

The complementary phases (CP) listed here depict the integrated system that agritourism capitalists utilize in the Caribbean.

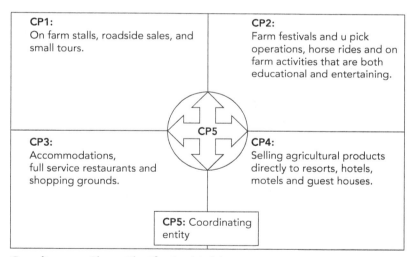

Complimentary Phases Classification Model.

CP1: is a business enterprise that is in the initial stage of agritourism development on its farm. These agritourism operators attract tourists to purchase produce or their agricultural commodity either on their premises or through stalls located near the premises. Many of these entrepreneurs also utilize a coordinating agency to assist with marketing and continued development of their agritourism firms. Some of these enterprises are focused on creating and/or continuing backward linkages.

CP2: businesses often start out as CP1 and mature into CP2 enterprises that still have at least one component of the CP1 venture but have expanded their production to include festivals and training with more interaction with tourists at the forward linkage level. These enterprises are normally also working on increased production to enter into the backward linkage area. Some of these undertakings utilize the CP5 portion of the model, but this varies depending on the national commitment of the country and the number of organizations playing a role in coordination.

CP3: The agritourism endeavors classified mainly in this CP3 segment are permanent elements of the farming operations. These enterprises continually and actively seek tourists to participate in their farming/tourism activities. These businesses utilize aspects of CP5 to expand their market share through on-site visits.

CP4: This agritourism activity is classified as a backward linkage toward the tourism sector. Blair (1995,1997) describes a backward linkage that involves buyers attracting suppliers. Agritourism operators of the other three segments, CP1–3, all strive to participate in this segment. The backward linkage in this model is the collaboration and usage of the agricultural sector to stimulate the country's economy as a whole and to create synergy between agriculture and tourism. In this model, the agricultural producers are trying to increase the amount of local foodstuffs utilized in the tourism sector of the economy, through fresh and value-added products.

CP5: This component of the model could be a governmental agency, a non-governmental agency, an international agency, or a financial agency that assists the producers with the development of their agritourism venture. Several countries around the world have some form of coordinating entity that assists with agritourism development either directly or indirectly. Frater (1983) provides an extensive list of European agencies, governmental and non-governmental, that assist farmers with development, marketing, and resources. This agency also has to ensure that it keeps consumer health in perspective when assisting the agricultural operations.

The model depicts different complementary phases of agritourism development. "The advancement of agritourism is commonly attributed to the repercussions of agricultural restructuring and to the forces driving this structural adjustment."[36] At the same time as tourists with more adventurous spirits and palates set foot in new lands, successful local agritourism efforts are also recognizing that tourist tastes are changing and require native dishes to soothe their exploratory palate. Other factors, such as individuals' interest in where their food comes from, along with health and well-being, accentuate the rationale for a country to look into developing an agritourism program. Several studies have examined tourist interest in health and where their food comes from with growing recognition for the importance of local and sustainable food.[21] Globally, it's clear that with assistance from global governments and other agencies, such as Inter-American Institute for Cooperation of Agriculture (IICA) and the Food and Agriculture Organization (FAO), more farmers can advance from CP1 to other segments of the classification system.

Conclusion

For many countries, including rural and island nations, tourism is critical as a mechanism for developing the economy. Yet there often can be a tug-of-war between local development and development efforts that originate from external forces acting on the region. For many nations, political and financial realities create challenges to achieving a double bottom line with tourism: to both build local capacity while at the same time supporting economic and business growth. Challenges are magnified when it comes to rural tourism, where new communications, outreach, and internal supports are needed to cultivate this niche market. Nations such as Italy and the United States have created certification programs and online resources to help farmers and tourists alike. For farmers, agritourism is an important source of alternative income for farm households. In the case of the One Eleuthera Foundation, the integration of hospitality management, farming, and tourism can create new opportunities for job development and economic growth for local communities, which, in turn, supports public health. These examples and others reveal how agritourism functions as an important mechanism for creating new opportunities in lower income areas, both by providing an economic boost and creating more local leisure spaces for both tourists and residents to enjoy. Ultimately, agritourism can boost local job creation, provide additional income sources for residents, and create opportunities for cooperative development, empowerment, and local control at the community level. It also may provide women, in particular, with new skills and experience that offers them qualifications for additional growth.

Agritourism has the benefit of advancing local products and dishes and explaining the benefits of conscientious consumption. McElroy (2002) lists three directives to sustain vacation quality: (1) restoring environmental damage; (2) managing visitors; and (3) developing smaller-scale specialty alternatives to mass tourism.[37] Agritourism embodies all of these, making it a "win-win" for development in any country. Creating tourism and agriculture linkages calls for entrepreneurial skills within the agricultural sector to be able to respond and meet the demands of the most frequently encountered tourist nationalities.

With current global conditions such as food shortages and increased population growth, citizens are now looking for a new sustainable direction. And although there is no definitive model for the transition from one economic sector to another, support for agritourism may have far-reaching benefits. The utilization of local foods not only alleviates or minimizes the consumer's carbon foot print, it also reduces the import balance, while promoting a local industry—connecting sustainability, economic development, health, and community development in new ways.

Quiz Questions

1. Agritourism addresses challenges in small farm profitability while supporting the interests of travelers eager to explore and better understand their agricultural heritage. True or false?
2. Agritourism furthers the goals of public health. True or false?
3. The United Nations has published how many Sustainable Development Goals (SDGs)?
   a. 9
   b. 12
   c. 15
   d. 17
   e. 21
4. Although not an explicit goal, the UN SDGs incorporate hunger and food security as embedded priorities. True or false?
5. Which of the following countries *has not* had a long-established agritourism industry supported in part by government resources?

a. The Bahamas
b. Ireland
c. Germany
d. France
e. Italy

6. Agritourism in America dates back to the late 1800s when families left farms to visit family in the city. True or false?

7. Agritourism can be understood in terms of:
   a. Forward linkages
   b. Backward linkages
   c. Lateral linkages
   d. All of the above
   e. a and b only

8. Sustainable agriculture's main pillars are:
   a. Environmental health, economic profitability, and social and economic equity
   b. Environmental health, economic profitability, and social and economic innovation
   c. Environmental health, economic innovation, and social and economic equity
   d. Environmental modernization, economic innovation, and social and economic equity
   e. None of the above

9. In part due to the popularity of travel-related television shows, tourists are increasingly interested in agritourism. True or false?

10. Ministries of Agriculture have played a role in developing local agritourism efforts by:
    a. Sponsoring workshops
    b. Marketing
    c. Subsidizing experiences
    d. Documenting impacts of growth
    e. All of the above

References

1. One Eleuthera Foundation. One Eleuthera Foundation's Center for Training and Innovation CTI.
2. Dorward A, Dangour AD. Agriculture and health. *BMJ*. 2012;344.
3. United Nations General Assembly. Transforming our world: the 2030 Agenda for Sustainable Development. New York: United Nations; 2015:35.

4. Karampela S, Kizos T, Spilanis I. Evaluating the impact of agritourism on local development in small islands. *Island Studies Journal.* 2016;11:161+.

5. Hepburn EST. *Agritourism as a Diversification Strategy for The Bahamas.* Agriculture, University of the Bahamas; 2008.

6. Lack JK. Agritourism Development in British Columbia. *Master's thesis in Natural Resource Management. Simon Fraser University.* 1997.

7. Hackett CN. *Vines, Wines and Visitors: A Case Study of Agricultural Diversification into Winery Tourism.* Master's thesis. Simon Fraser University; 1998.

8. Schilling BJ, Attavanich W, Jin Y. Does agritourism enhance farm profitability? *Journal of Agricultural and Resource Economics.* 2014;39(1):69–87.

9. Frater JM. Farm tourism in England—planning, funding, promotion and some lessons from Europe. *Tourism Management.* 1983;4:167–179.

10. United States Department of Agriculture: National Agriculture Statistics Service. Census of Agriculture Highlights: Farmers Marketing; 2012.

11. Lobo RE, Goldman GE, Jolly DA, Wallace BD, Schrader WL, Parker SA. Agrotourism Benefits Agriculture in Sand Diego County, UC Small Farm Program; Nov-Dec 1999, http://sfp.ucdavis.edu/agritourism/Case_Studies/agritourSD/.

12. Maetzold J. Nature-based tourism & agritourism trends. Unlimited Opportunities; 2002.

13. Che D, Veeck A, Veeck G. Sustaining production and strengthening the agritourism product: linkages among Michigan agritourism destinations. In: Values AaH, ed. Vol 222005:225–234.

14. Hsu C-C. *Identification of Intangible Resources Essential to Agritourism Enterprises in Taiwan: A Delphi Study*: Agriculture, Ohio State University; 2005.

15. Cai J, Leung P, Mak J. Tourism's forward and backward linkages. *Journal of Travel Research.* 2006;45:36–52.

16. Fazio RA, et al. Barriers to the Adoption of Sustainable Agricultural Practices: Working Farmer and Change Agent Perspectives. Sustainable Agriculture Research & Education Final Report, November 2008. Available online https://projects.sare.org/sare_project/ls03-183/.

17. The Local Foods Wheel. Are you a locavore? Vol 2017.

18. Hepburn E. *Agritourism as a Viable Strategy for Economic Diversification: A Case Study Analysis of Policy Options for The Bahamas.* Clemson University; 2008.

19. Rogerson CM, Rogerson JM. Agritourism and local economic development in South Africa. *Bulletin of Geography. Socio-Economic Series.* 2014;26:93–106.

20. Tagliabue J. Preserving a heritage via beg and barns; European governments subsidize agritourism. *New York Times.* Aug 13, 1998.

21. Black Sea Economic Centre. Research of Good Practices in Agrotourism in Italy (Tuscany), France (Provence) and Germany (Bavaria); 2014.

22. Williams P. The evolving images of wine tourism destinations. *Tourism Recreation Research.* 2001;26:3–10.

23. United States Department of Agriculture National Resources Conservation Service. *Alternative Enterprises and Agritourism: Farming For Profit and Sustainability Resource Manual.* Washington DC; 2004.

24. Alexander A, Rumley E. States' Agritourism Statutes. National Agricultural Law Center; 2017.

25. African, Caribbean and Pacific Group of States deepen ties with FAO/Agreement. Will enhance 79 countries' pursuit of upcoming Sustainable Development Goals. *M2 Presswire.* Coventry; 2015.

26. Meyer D. Caribbean Tourism, Local Sourcing and Enterprise Development: Review of the Literature; Pro-Poor Tourism Partnership Working Paper 18: January 2006, available online https://www.odi.org/sites/odi.org.uk/files/odi-assets/publications-opinion-files/4038.pdf 2006.

27. Pattullo P. Last Resorts: The Cost of Tourism in the Caribbean. Ian Randle Publishers; 1996.

28. Rhiney K. Geographies of vulnerability in a changing climate: lessons from the Caribbean. *Geography Compass.* 2015;9(3):97–114.

29. Ramsaran R. The Commonwealth Caribbean in the World Economy. New York: Macmillan Publishers Ltd; 1989.

30. Taylor BE, Morison JB, Fleming EM. The economic impact of food import substitution in the Bahamas. *Social and Economic Studies.* 1991;40:45–62.

31. Gooding E. Food Production in Barbados with Particular Reference to Tourism. *Tourism Marketing and Management in the Caribbean.* London: Routledge; 1971.

32. Momsen J. Linkages between Tourism and Agriculture: Problems for the Smaller Caribbean Economies. *University of Newcastle Upon Tyne Seminar Paper*: University of Newcastle Upon Tyne; 1984.

33. Momsen JH. Caribbean tourism and agriculture: new linkages in the global era? *Globalization and Neoliberalism: The Caribbean Context.* 1998:115–134.

34. Milne S. Tourism and development in South Pacific microstates. *Annals of Tourism Research.* 1992;19:191–212.

35. Timms B. Caribbean agriculture—tourism linkages in a neoliberal world. Problems and prospects for St. Lucia. *IDPR.* 2006;28(1):35–56.

36. Hackett C. Vines, Wines and Visitors: A Case Study of Agricultural Diversification into Winery Tourism. In: University MSF, ed1998.

37. McElroy JL. The impact of tourism on small islands: A global comparison. *Tourism, Biodiversity and Information.* 2002:151–167.

Appendix: Answers to Quiz Questions

Chapter 1

1. D
2. C
3. E
4. B
5. A
6. E
7. C
8. A
9. E
10. C

Chapter 2

1. E
2. False
3. E
4. A
5. True
6. False
7. True
8. D
9. D
10. True

Chapter 3

1. D
2. True
3. True
4. D
5. True
6. B
7. E
8. True
9. False
10. C

Chapter 4

1. False
2. C
3. False
4. B
5. True
6. C
7. D
8. C
9. D
10. True

Chapter 5

1. C
2. C
3. False
4. A
5. True

Chapter 6

1. True
2. False
3. B
4. B
5. False
6. C

7. False
8. False
9. B
10. True

Chapter 7

The open ended questions in this chapter are meant to stimulation discussion of its themes and, as such, have no set answers.

Chapter 8

1. True
2. C
3. D
4. E
5. False
6. False
7. E
8. False
9. D
10. False

Chapter 9

1. B
2. B
3. A
4. A
5. A
6. B
7. B
8. C
9. A
10. A

Chapter 10

1. B
2. C
3. A

4. C
5. B
6. A
7. D
8. B

Chapter 11

1. C
2. E
3. D
4. B
5. C

Chapter 12

1. True
2. True
3. D
4. False
5. A
6. False
7. E
8. A
9. True
10. E

About the Editor

Allison Karpyn, PhD, is Associate Professor of Human Development and Family Sciences; Behavioral Health and Nutrition; Education and Public Policy & Administration at the University of Delaware; she is also Senior Associate Director of the Center for Research in Education and Social Policy at the University of Delaware and Associate Fellow for the Center for Public Health Initiatives at the University of Pennsylvania. Karpyn previously served as the Director of Research and Evaluation at The Food Trust, a pioneering nonprofit in Philadelphia. Her research focuses on understanding how to increase access to affordable nutritious foods, healthy food purchasing and consumption behavior, especially among children.

Index

Tables, figures, and boxes are indicated by an italic *t, f,* and *b* following the page/paragraph number.

AAA (Agricultural Adjustment
    Administration), 3–4
Abaco Neem Farm, 325–27, 328, 333
Aboriginal peoples, 108–9
ABS (Australian Bureau of
    Statistics), 290–91
ACA (Affordable Care Act) of 2010, 108,
    185–86, 190
Academy of Nutrition and Dietetics
    (formerly American Dietetic
    Association), 16
acculturation
    health disparities, 87–88, 93
    immigrants, 93
    Satia-Abouta model of dietary
        acculturation, 93–95, 106–7
Active Design Verified initiative, 135
Adams, John, 227
advertising and marketing, 18–19, 125–38
    to children, 125–29, 161–62
    4 Ps of marketing, C5.P19–C5.P24
    government policy and regulation,
        142–43, 161–62
    industry standards, 161–62
    in-store marketing, 130–32
    multicultural marketing, 89, 107
    new media, 127–29
    priming and, 54–55
    school food environments and, 133–37
    Smarter School Lunchroom
        movement, 136–37

social marketing, 18
sugary products in Japan, 293, 294
affect
    avenue through which mental models
        operate, 55–56
    behavior influenced by, 54–55
Affordable Care Act (ACA) of 2010, 108,
    185–86, 190
affordance, 52–53
African Americans
    advertising and multicultural
        marketing, 107
    chronic stress from discrimination, 104–5
    cultural influences, 95–96
    employment status, 103
    food insecurity, 106, 179–80
    food marketing to children, 125–26
    gender, 97
    health disparities, 88–89, 95–96, 97,
        101–3, 104–5, 106, 107, 108
    healthcare access, 108
    historical contexts, 101
    incarceration rates, 178–79
    as racial category, 84–85
    sharecropping, 2, 3
    socioeconomic status and class, 101–3
After-School Snacks and Suppers
    program, 155
age. *See* elderly and seniors
Agricultural Act of 2014, 145, 146–50.
    See also farm bill

Agricultural Adjustment Administration
    (AAA), 3–4
agricultural production, 1–6
    Great Depression and Dust Bowl, 3
    New Deal-era, 3–4
    post-World War I, 2–3
    post-World War II, 4–6
    St. Kitts-Nevis "farm to fork project,"
        264, 268
    transformation in farming in 20th
        century, 2
    World War I-era, 2
    World War II-era, 4
Agriculture Adjustment Act of 1933, 145. *See
    also* farm bill
AgriCycle Venento, 320
agritourism, 317–40
    Abaco Neem Farm example, 325–27
    agri-health, 324–25
    agrotourism vs., 319
    in Canada, 330–31
    Complimentary Phases Classification
        Model, 320, 337–39
    concept of, 318–21
    defined, 321–22
    in Europe, 329–30
    as global phenomenon, 329
    in Italy, 320
    in Latin American and Caribbean, 333
    linkages in, 322–23, 333–37
    sustainable agriculture, 322–24
    in United States, 331, 332
Alaskan Natives. *See* Native Americans
Alliance for a Healthier Generation, 161–62
allostatic load, 105
Amazon, 127, 132
American Academy of Pediatrics,
    154–55, 193
American Beverage Association, 159, 161–62
American Cookery (Simmon), 16, 17
American Heart Association, 241
American Indians. *See* Native Americans
American Medical Association, 34
American Red Cross, 15

Amornpetchkul, T. B., 299–301
Anthony Bourdain No Reservations
    (TV program), 329
Antigua and Barbuda, 263
antiretrovirals (ARVs), 283–84
architectural depth, 52
Asian Americans
    advertising and multicultural
        marketing, 107
    cultural influences, 95
    health disparities, 92, 93–95, 101–3, 107
    immigration, 93–95
    socioeconomic status and class, 101–3
Atkins Diet, 11, 241–42
Atwater, Helen Woodard, 11–12
Atwater, Wilbur O., 11, 16–18
Aunt Sammy (fictional radio character), 19
Australia, 285–92, 305–6
    health disparities, 108–9
    overview of, 285–87
    prevalence of non-communicable
        diseases, 287
    sugar consumption, 287, 289–90, 292
    sugar industry, 287–89, 291–92
    sweetened tea consumption, 289–90
Australian Bureau of Statistics
    (ABS), 290–91
Australian Sugar Milling Council, 289
Austria, 319, 329–30
Avery, Alex, 228
azodicarbonamide, 243

backfire effect, 246–47
backward linkages, 322–23, 333, 335, 336
Bahamas
    Abaco Neem Farm, 325–27, 328, 333
    One Eleuthera Foundation, 333, 334
Balance Calorie Initiative, 161–62
Banwell, C., 290
Barbados, 333
Barker, Roger, 53
Bascom, W. O., 304–5
"Basic Four" food guide, 13–14
"Basic Seven" food guide, 12, 13, 14

Bayer corporation, 233
Beard, James, 19
behavior change theory, 48
behavior settings, 53
behavioral design, 47–72
  descriptive geography of
    experience, 56–57
  disciplines contributing to, 48, 49
  dual-system model of cognition, 53–55
  environmental psychology, 51–53
  ethics of modifying exposure, 62–65
  experience and agent-exposure interface,
    47–48, 49, 56–67
  food and beverage environment, 61–62,
    69, 71, 72
  physical activity environment, 65–67
  roots of, 50
behavioral economics, 48, 50, 137
behavioral insight teams, 50–51
Benach, J., 103–4
Berry, John, 93
Bienvenue à la Ferme, 329–30
Bill and Melinda Gates Foundation, 233–34
biotechnology
  genetically modified organisms, 6, 159–61,
    225–26, 232–34, 240
  hybrid seeds, 3
Bizarre Foods with Andrew Zimmern
    (TV program), 329
Blacks. *See* African Americans
Blair, P. D., 338
blogs, 19–20
Bloomberg, Michael, 236–37
body mass index (BMI), 256
Bon Appétit, 19
Borges, J. L., 47
bounded rationality, 58, 64
bovine spongiform encephalopathy ("mad
    cow" disease), 242
Bracero Program, 4–6
Brazil
  health disparities, 108–9
  school feeding programs, 261, 274
breakfast cereals, 126–27

Bronfenbrenner, U., 142
built environment, 48–49, 50. *See also*
    behavioral design; obesogenic
    environments
  ethics of modifying exposure, 62–65
  food and beverage environment, 61–62
  physical activity environment, 65–67
  restaurant food environment, 72
  retail food environment, 71
  school food environment, 69
  strategies to facilitate integration of, 61
  strategies to support better choices, 62
Burton, Robert, 247

CACFP (Child and Adult Care Food
    Program), 155, 187–89
cake mixes, 10
calorie content, mandatory posting of, 236
Canada
  agritourism, 330–31
  framework for disease prevention, 33
cancer
  agricultural workers, 6
  agri-health, 325
  food insecurity, 183
  obesity and, 210, 256
  race and ethnicity, 92–93
carbohydrates
  Atkins Diet, 241–42
  dietary guidelines, 11, 14, 32
cardiovascular disease (CVD), 112, 325
  in Australia, 287
  changing defaults, 211
  chronic stress from discrimination, 105
  employment status, 103–4
  food insecurity, 177
  gender, 96–97
  obesity, 256
  race and ethnicity, 87, 88–89, 92–95,
    97, 177
  sexual orientation, 97–98
Caribbean. *See also names of specific countries*
  agritourism, 321, 333
  Farm-to-School programs, 264–75

Caribbean Commission on Health and
    Development, 263–64
Caribbean Community and Common
    Market (CARICOM), 262–75
    St. Kitts-Nevis, 264–75
Caribbean Food and Nutrition Institute
    (CFNI), 263
Carson, Rachel, 6
CCC (Commodity Credit Corporation),
    3–6, 20
CDC (Centers for Disease Control and
    Prevention), 67, 83–84, 92–93, 210,
    219, 229
CDCs (Community Development
    Corporations), 214
CDFIs (Community Development
    Financial Institutions), 214
celebrity chefs, 19
Center for Food Safety, 160–61
Center for Global Food Issues (CGFI), 228
Centers for Disease Control and Prevention
    (CDC), 67, 83–84, 92–93, 210, 219, 229
Centre for Training and Innovation (CTI),
    333, 334
cerebrovascular disease and stroke
    gender, 89, 96–97, 109
    race and ethnicity, 87, 89, 90, 92–93, 109
CFBAI (Children's Food and Beverage
    Advertising Initiative), 161–62
CFNI (Caribbean Food and Nutrition
    Institute), 263
CFP (Community Food Projects), 148–49
CGFI (Center for Global Food Issues), 228
Chick-fil-A, 218
Child, Julia, 19
Child and Adult Care Food Program
    (CACFP), 155, 187–89
Child Nutrition Act of 1966, 21, 144–45,
    155, 187–88
Child Nutrition and WIC Reauthorization
    Act of 2004, 154–55, 185–86, 187–88
Children's Food and Beverage Advertising
    Initiative (CFBAI), 161–62
Children's HealthWatch, 192–93
Children's Hospital of Philadelphia, 193

choice architecture, 48, 72, 144
cholesterol, 14, 32, 34
chronic respiratory disease, 256, 325
Civil Rights Act of 1964, 101
climate change, 6–7, 239–40
Coca-Cola, 126, 237, 299
Color of Wealth in Boston, The, 102
commodification
    creation of new products, 9
    federal commodity programs, 148
    food as fungible commodity, 7–8
    homogenization and standardization, 8–9
Commodity Credit Corporation (CCC),
    3–6, 20
Commodity Supplemental Food Program
    (CSFP), 148–49
Communities Putting Prevention to Work
    grants, 211
Community Development Corporations
    (CDCs), 214
Community Development Financial
    Institutions (CDFIs), 214
Community Food Projects (CFP), 148–49
"community food security" initiatives, 191
Community Servings food delivery
    program, 193–94
Community Supported Agriculture (CSA),
    6–7, 215, 238
Complimentary Phases Classification
    Model, 320, 337–39
Comprehensive Africa Agriculture
    Development Programme, 261–62
consumer culture, 1–2, 16–20. *See also*
    advertising and marketing
    advertising, 18
    cookbooks, 16
    mass media, 19
cookbooks, 16, 19, 290
Cornell Food and Brand Lab, 136–37
corner stores, 214–15
Costa Rica, 333
Council of Better Business Bureaus, 126
countercuisine movement, 11
CPS (Current Population Survey), 93,
    175–76, 184–85

critical nutrition studies, 16
Crocker, Betty (fictional advertising character), 19
crop insurance, 148
Cruz, Joanna, 171–73, 182, 184, 187, 192, 194, 196
CSA (Community Supported Agriculture), 6–7, 215, 238
CSFP (Commodity Supplemental Food Program), 148–49
CTI (Centre for Training and Innovation), 333, 334
cultural influences and contexts, 281–307
    in Australia, 285–92
    health disparities, 95–96
    implications for health professionals, 307
    influence on food preferences, 282, 283
    in Japan, 285–87, 292–97
    in Nigeria, 285–87, 302–5
    in Thailand, 285–87, 298–302
    traditional public health interventions and, 283–84
cultural niche construction, 96
Current Population Survey (CPS), 93, 175–76, 184–85
CVD. *See* cardiovascular disease

Davis, William, 240–42
Dawson, Shane, 128
depression, 175–76, 181, 182–83, 184
DGA. *See Dietary Guidelines for Americans*
DGAC (Dietary Guidelines Advisory Committee), 14–15, 34, 39, 150
diabetes, 112, 325
    in Australia, 287
    food insecurity, 177, 183
    gender, 96–97
    race and ethnicity, 87, 88–89, 90, 91, 92–93, 104, 177
    socioeconomic status, 98
diet cultures and fads, 11
Dietary Goals for the American People, 14, 32, 150
Dietary Guidelines Advisory Committee (DGAC), 14–15, 34, 39, 150

Dietary Guidelines for Americans (DGA), 14–15, 16, 31–43, 154–55
    1980, 14–15, 33 C2.P15–C2.P18, 150
    1985, 35 C2.P19–C2.P21
    1990, 35–36
    1995, 36–37
    2000, 38–39
    2005, 39, 40
    2010, 39, 41
    2015, 42 C2.P27–C2.P31
    critiques and attacks against, 15, 34, 43, 150
    process for creating, 150–51
    school lunches and meal programs, 145
Dinour, L. M., 183
Dione Lucas Show, The (TV program), 19
direct lobbying, 157
disabilities, people with
    food insecurity, 179, 193–94
    Supplemental Nutrition Assistance Program, 152, 186–87
discrimination and racism
    food insecurity and, 179–80, 195
    health disparities and, 83–84, 101, 104–5
Dominican Republic, 333
"double burden of disease," 110
"double burden of malnutrition," 256–57, 263
"Double-Up Food Bucks" approach, 153
Down to Earth Farm, 333
downstream policies, 258–59, 260
Drèze, Jean, 173
drip irrigation, 268
dual-system model of cognition, 53–55
    automatic thought processes, 54–55
    mental models, 55–56
    social thought processes, 55
Dust Bowl, 3

ecological framework and approaches, 51, 174, 176–77, 195
Ecological Systems Theory, 142, 143
ego
    avenue through which mental models operate, 55–56
    behavior influenced by, 55
    ego depletion, 58

elderly and seniors
    food assistance programs, 148–49,
        188–89, 193–94, 217
    food insecurity, 183–84
    socioeconomic status and class, 98–99
Elderly Nutrition Program, 188–89
Emergency Food Assistance Program
    (TEFAP), 148–49
employment status
    food assistance program eligibility, 186
    food insecurity, 184–85
    during Great Recession, 186
    health disparities, 103–4
environmental determinism, 52–53
environmental psychology, 51–53
    affordance, 52–53
    behavior settings, 53
    focus of, 51
    layout of interior spaces, 52
    origins of, 51
    sustainable behavior, 51–52
EPA (U.S. Environmental Protection
    Agency), 160–61, 228
ethnicity. *See names of specific races and
    ethnicities*; race and ethnicity
European Union (EU). *See also names of
    specific countries*
    agritourism, 319, 329–30
    growth hormones, 242–43
Evans, Dwight, 214
"ever-normal granaries," 3–4

family-operated farms
    collapse of, 6
    decrease in, 2, 148
FAO (Food and Agricultural
    Organization), 299
FAO (Food and Agriculture
    Organization), 339
farm bill, 145–49
    changing priorities of, 146–47
    commodity programs, 148
    drafting and passing, 146
    effects on food supply and dietary
        patterns, 147–48, 149

food insecurity, 185–86
    funding, 146, 147
    future of, 149–50
    nutrition assistance, 148–49, 186–87
Farm to Fork online course, 225
Farmer's Bulletin, 11
Farmers Market Nutrition Program
    (FMNP), 187–88, 217
farmers markets, 215–17
    economic and community impact
        of, 216–17
    number of, 215
    research studies about, 217
Farm-to-School programs, 134–35, 138,
    259, 261
    in Brazil, 261
    in St. Kitts-Nevis, 264–75
    in sub-Saharan Africa, 261–62
fast food, 21, 217–19
    food swamps, 106
    marketing to children, 126
    multicultural marketing, 89
    revenues, 218
    top companies, 218
    zoning, 219
fats
    dietary guidelines, 11–12, 15, 32
    shifts in scientific opinions of,
        43–44, 241–42
Fazio, R. A., 324
FCC (Federal Communications
    Commission), 128
FDA. *See* U.S. Food and Drug
    Administration
Fed Up (documentary), 230, 236–37
federal agricultural aid and subsidies. *See also*
    farm bill
    commodity programs, 148
    New Deal-era, 3–4, 9
    obesity and, 230
    post-World War II, 4–6
    World War I-era loans, 2
Federal Communications Commission
    (FCC), 128
federal dietary guidelines, 1–2, 11

"Basic Seven" and "Basic Four," 12–14
  for children, 11–12
  combating chronic disease, 14
  critiques and attacks against, 15–16
  Dietary Guidelines for Americans, 14–15,
    16, 31–43
  early years of, 11–12
  food groups, 11–14, 15
  graphic devices for nutrition education, 15
Federal Reserve, 101–3
Federal Trade Commission (FTC), 126, 128
fertilizer
  algae blooms, 6
  synthetic, 3, 4–6
FFQ (Food Frequency
    Questionnaire), 301–2
FFVP (Fresh Fruit and Vegetable Program),
    135, 148–49, 155
FINI (Food Insecurity Nutrition Incentive)
    Grant Program, 153
Fischler, Claude, 282
floorplan openness, 52
fluoride, 211
FMNP (Farmers Market Nutrition
    Program), 187–88, 217
FNV (Fruits & Veggies) marketing
    campaign, 135
Food & Wine, 19
Food and Agricultural Organization
    (FAO), 299
Food and Agriculture Organization
    (FAO), 339
food and beverage environment. *See also*
    obesogenic environments; school food
    environment
  behavioral design, 61–62, 69, 71, 72
  restaurant food environment, 72
  retail food environment, 71
Food and Drug Administration (FDA), 7–8
Food and Nutrition Board, 12
Food and Water Watch, 247
food beliefs and taboos, 304
  in Nigeria, 303, 305
food controversies, 225–49
  causes of obesity, 229–30

chasm between facts and
    conclusions, 226–27
  conflating specific policies and social
    movements, 235–39
  debating science and policy
    simultaneously, 239–40
  each person as a lifeworld, 247
  gluten sensitivity, 231–32
  interacting in, 248
  lack of sufficient facts, 227–32
  local foods movement, 238–39
  motivations for argument, 226, 227, 240
  movement against soda, 236–37
  neural networks, 243–45
  pesticides and organic foods, 228–29
  as positive, 248–49
  power of intuition, 240–43
  as proxy wars, 232–34
"Food: Cookbook Boom" (Owen), 19
food deserts, 106, 212, 213, 214, 238
Food for Fitness-A Daily Food Guide, 13–14
Food for Young Children (Hunt), 11–12
Food Frequency Questionnaire
    (FFQ), 301–2
Food Guide Pyramid, 15, 36–37
food insecurity, 106, 171–96
  in Caribbean, 263
  cultural and regional contexts, 257–58
  defined, 174–77
  disabilities, people with, 179
  discrimination and, 179–80
  economic circumstances of, 184–85
  first-hand experiences with, 171–73, 182,
    187, 192, 194
  food deserts, 106, 238
  food swamps, 106
  formerly incarcerated and their
    families, 178–79
  gender, 176
  getting involved, 190–92, 193–94
  global trends in, 257
  government policy and regulation,
    144, 185–90
  immigrants, 176, 177
  LGBTQ youth and adults, 178

food insecurity (*cont.*)
  obesity and, 257
  prevalence of, 174, 175–76
  public health impact of, 180–84
  race and ethnicity, 174, 176, 177
  rights-based approach, 195–96
Food Insecurity Nutrition Incentive (FINI)
    Grant Program, 153
Food Marketing Institute, 130
food markets, groceries,
    and supermarkets
  behavioral design and retail food
    environment, 71–72
  corner stores, 214–15
  as economic anchors, 213–14
  expenditure trends, 131, 132
  food deserts, 106, 212, 213, 214
  historical changes to, 211, 212–13
  in-store marketing, 130–32
  national chains, 8, 10
  Progress Plaza, 211
food media, 19
Food Network, 19–20
food policy councils, 190–91
Food Politics (Nestle), 15
"food porn," 19–20
food sovereignty, 233–34
food stamps. *See* Supplemental Nutrition
    Assistance Program
food swamps, 106
food systems response, 258, 259, 261
Food Trust, 214
Ford, Henry, 3
foreclosures, 2
forward linkages, 322–23, 326–27, 333, 335, 336
Fourth National Survey of Ethnic
    Minorities, 104
Fragile Families and Child Well-Being
    Study, 178–79
Fram, M. S., 181
"A Framework for Public Health Action"
    (Frieden), 210
France
  agritourism, 329–30
  "mad cow" disease, 242
Frater, J. M., 330, 338

French Chef, The (TV program), 19
Fresh Food Financing Initiative, 214
Fresh Fruit and Vegetable Program (FFVP),
    135, 148–49, 155
Frieden, Tom, 143–44, 210, 211
frozen foods, 9–10
Fruits & Veggies (FNV) marketing
    campaign, 135
fruits and vegetables. *See also* Farm-to-
    School programs
  dietary guidelines, 13–14, 38–39, 261
  farmers markets, 216–17
  federal subsidies, 230–31
  genetically modified organisms, 160
  obesity and cost of, 257
  pesticides, 228–29
  school food environment, 144–45,
    148–49, 155
FTC (Federal Trade Commission),
    126, 128

gender
  advertising and multicultural
    marketing, 107
  cultural influences, 96
  defined, 85
  employment status, 103
  food insecurity, 176
  health disparities, 85, 87, 89, 96–97, 98–99,
    103, 107, 110, 112
  incarceration rates, 178–79
  race and ethnicity, 87, 89, 97
  socioeconomic status and class, 98–99
gene-culture interactions, 96
General Mills, 127
genetically modified organisms
    (GMOs), 6, 240
  controversy over, 225–26, 232–34
  labeling, 159–61
Germany, 319
Ghana, 110
Glenn, John, 10
globalization
  evolution of culture and food
    preferences, 282
  food insecurity, 186, 256

health disparities, 110
nutrition transition, 256
gluten sensitivity, 231–32
GMOs. *See* genetically modified organisms
God's Love We Deliver food delivery
program, 193–94
"Golden Rice," 6
Goodfellow Farms, 333
Google, 128–29
Gourmet, 19
government policy and regulation, 142–62. *See
also names of specific policies, regulations,
and programs*
advertising and marketing,
142–43, 161–62
altering choice architecture, 144
dietary guidelines, 150–51
farm bill, 145–49
food assistance programs, 152–56
food insecurity, 144, 185–90
getting involved in, 156–57
importance of in shaping food
environments, 143–44
industrialization and, 7–8
innovative approaches to, 158–62
lobbying, 157–58
marketing to children, 125
obesity, 143–44, 146, 258, 260
preemption, 144
Grassley, Chuck, 159–60
grassroots lobbying, 157, 158
Great Depression, 3, 12, 20, 146–47
Great Migration, 3, 101
Great Recession, 186
Green Revolution, 259–61
Griggs, P., 290
groceries. *See* food markets, groceries, and
supermarkets
Guiding Stars nutritional scoring system,
131–32, 133
Guyana, 263

Haber process, 3
Hager, E. R., 193
Haiti, 263
Hannaford Supermarkets, 131–32

Harvard School of Public Health, 15
Hassle-Free Daily Food Guide, 14
Health Belief Model, 53
health disparities, 83–113
advertising and multicultural
marketing, 107
cultural influences, 95–96
discrimination and chronic stress, 104–5
employment status, 103–4
environmental factors, 106
gender, 85, 89, 96–97
global, 108
health inequities vs., 83–84
healthcare access, 108
historical contexts, 101
immigrants, 87–88, 93
race and ethnicity, 84–92, 93–96
sexual orientation, 97
social determinants of health, 99, 100
socioeconomic status and class,
98–99, 101–4
Health Impact Pyramid, 143–44, 210
"Health in All Policies" approach, 108
health inequities, 83–84
health insurance coverage, 108
healthcare access, 108
Healthy, Hunger-Free Kids Act
of 2010 (HHKA), 21, 134, 136, 144–45,
146, 155, 261
Healthy Eating Pyramid and Healthy Eating
Plate (Harvard), 15
Healthy Food Financing Initiative, 214
"healthy immigrant effect," 87–88
Healthy People 2020, 185–86
Healthy Weight Commitment
Foundation, 161–62
HGSFPs ("home grown school feeding
programs"), 261–62
HHKA (Healthy, Hunger-Free Kids Act
of 2010), 21, 134, 136, 144–45, 146,
155, 261
HHS (U.S. Department of Health and
Human Services), 214
high-fructose corn syrup
(HFCS), 297
Hilaire, Belloc, 235

Hispanics and Latinos
advertising and multicultural
marketing, 107
cultural influences, 95
as ethnic category, 84–85
food insecurity, 106
food marketing to children, 125–26
health disparities, 85–87, 93–95, 101–3,
106, 107, 108
healthcare access, 108
immigration, 93–95
incarceration rates, 178–79
socioeconomic status, 101–3
HIV/AIDS, 97–98, 183, 283–84
home economics texts, 16–18
"home grown school feeding programs"
(HGSFPs), 261–62
hormones, 4–6, 242–43
House Committee on Appropriations, 34
Housing Choice Voucher Program (Section
8), 189
How to Select Foods (Hunt), 11–12
HUD (U.S. Department of Housing and
Urban Development), 189
Hulu, 127
Hunger and Public Action (Drèze and
Sen), 173
"Hunger Vital Sign" screening, 193
Hunt, Caroline, 11–12
hybrid seeds, 3
hypertension
in Australia, 287
chronic stress from discrimination, 104–5
employment status, 103–4
food insecurity, 177
gender, 89, 96–97
race and ethnicity, 87, 88–89, 90, 92,
104–5, 109, 177
sugar-sweetened beverages, 159

I Love to Eat (TV program), 19
IDRC (International Development Research
Centre), 264
"If Monsanto Loses Its Name, What
Will Opponents Oppose?" (*WSJ*
article), 233

IICA (Inter-American Institute for
Cooperation on Agriculture), 333, 339
Illuminati (Wise Intelligent), 233
immigration and migration
acculturation, 93
food insecurity, 176, 177
health disparities, 87–88, 93
"healthy immigrant effect," 87–88
labor, 4–7
incarceration, 179
industrialization, 1–2, 7–11
commodification, 7–9
consolidation of agribusiness, 6
critiques and attacks against, 6, 11
government policy and regulation, 7–8
homogenization and standardization, 7–9
invention of new foodstuffs, 9, 10
processing, 7, 9–11
purity and sanitation, 7, 8–9
socioeconomic status and, 101
20th century increase in, 2
industry standards, 161–62
Inhofe, Jim, 239
Institute of Medicine, 161–62, 186–87
Inter-American Institute for Cooperation on
Agriculture (IICA), 333, 339
Internal Revenue Service (IRS), 157, 185, 189
International Development Research Centre
(IDRC), 264
Internet, 16
marketing to children, 127–29
online food purchases, 132
Iowa State University, 233–34
IRS (Internal Revenue Service), 157, 185, 189
Italy, 289, 320, 323, 330

"Jagdeo Initiative," 263–64
Jamaica, 333
James, William, 56
Japan, 286, 292–97
beverage exports to Thailand, 299–301
high-fructose corn syrup, 297
overview of, 285–87, 292–93
ready-to-drink beverage consumption,
295, 296
sugar consumption, 293–95

as sugar deficit country, 292–93
sugar production and importation,
    292–93, 295, 297
tea consumption, 293, 297, 306
Jell-O, 9
Jim Crow racial segregation laws,
    101, 179–80
Johnson, Lyndon B., 187–88
Jolliffe, L., 319
Jones, Susannah Mushatt, 242
Jungle, The (Sinclair), 7–8

Kellogg's, 127
Kham Paka, 301–2
Kimmel, Jimmy, 231
Kraus, B., 247
Krieger, Nancy, 104–5
Kushner, B., 293

Lack, J. K., 330
Ladies' Home Journal, 19
"Latino/Hispanic paradox," 87–88
Latinos. *See* Hispanics and Latinos
Lavizzo-Mourey, Risa, 284
Lawrence, M., 258
layout of interior spaces, 52
Lend-Lease Act of 1941, 4
Let's Move! initiative, 135
LGBTQ community. *See* sexual orientation
Library of Economics and Liberty, 238
life course perspective, 182
lifeworld, 247
LIHEAP (Low-Income Heating and Energy
    Assistance Program), 189
LIHTC (Low Income Housing Tax
    Credit), 189
liver disease, 90
lobbying, 3–4, 157–58
local foods movement, 6–7, 238–39, 243,
    324, 329
locavore movement, 324
Lockton, Dan, 62–63
Low Income Housing Tax Credit
    (LIHTC), 189
Low-Income Heating and Energy Assistance
    Program (LIHEAP), 189

Lu, Chensheng, 228
Lucas, Dione, 19

"mad cow" disease (bovine spongiform
    encephalopathy), 242
magazines, 16–18, 19, 107
Mahoney, E., 321–22
Manna food delivery program, 193–94
marketing. *See* advertising and marketing
McDonald's, 107, 126, 218
McElroy, J. L., 340
McGill University, 264
MCNs (multi-channel networks), 127–28
Meals on Wheels, 193–94
Meatless Mondays, 18
Medicaid, 108, 158–59, 190
Medicare, 158–59, 190, 193–94
Miaoulis, Nicholas, 325, 327
midstream policies, 258–59, 260
Migration Policy Institute, 93
Mintz, S. W., 293–94
Missouri Sharecroppers Roadside
    Demonstration, 3
Modern Farmer, 233
Monsanto, 233, 234
Monsanto Years, The (Young), 233
Mozambique, 283–84
multi-channel networks (MCNs), 127–28
MyPlate, 15
MyPyramid Food Guidance System, 15

National Academy of Sciences (NAS),
    12, 247
National Aeronautics and Space
    Administration (NASA), 10
National Agricultural Worker survey, 6–7
National Association of Convenience
    Stores, 215
National Collaborative on
    Childhood Obesity Research
    (NCCOR), 48–49
National Commission on Hunger, 196
National Food Guide, The, 12
National Health and Nutrition Examination
    Survey (NHANES), 98, 105
National Livestock and Meat Board, 34

National Nutrition Monitoring and Related
    Research Act of 1990, 34–35, 36–37
National School Lunch Act of 1946, 20–21,
    155, 259–61
National School Lunch Program (NSLP),
    20, 21, 98–99, 135, 144–45, 151–52,
    155–56, 187–88
National War Garden Commission, 2
National Wartime Nutrition Guide, 12
Native Americans
    chronic stress from discrimination, 104
    food insecurity, 176, 177, 179–80
    health disparities, 89–90, 101, 104
    historical contexts, 101
    Navajo Indians, 101, 177
    Pima Indians, 90, 91, 101
    as racial category, 84–85
Native Hawaiians and other Pacific
    Islanders, 92
"natural" foods, 6
Natural Resources Conservation Service, 331
Navajo Indians, 101, 177
NCCOR (National Collaborative on
    Childhood Obesity Research), 48–49
Neem, 323, 325–27, 328
NEL (Nutrition Evidence Library), 39
Nestle, Marion, 15
Netflix, 127
neural networks, 243–45
New Deal, 3–4, 9, 20
*New Perspective on the Health of
    Canadians, A*, 33
New York Times, 19, 43, 247
NHANES (National Health and Nutrition
    Examination Survey), 98, 105
Nielsen, 126, 127
Nigeria, 286, 302–6
    animal source foods, 303–4, 305
    food taboos and beliefs, 303, 305
    nutritional status of children, 303
    overview of, 285–87, 302–3
    vegetation zones, 304–5
non-food uses for crops, 6
norms, behavior influenced by, 55

NSLP (National School Lunch Program),
    20, 21, 98–99, 135, 144–45, 151–52,
    155–56, 187–88
Nutrition and Your Health: DGAs, 32
Nutrition Evidence Library (NEL), 39
Nutrition Facts labeling, 36–37, 42–43, 161
nutrition transition, 256
nutritional scoring systems, 131–32, 133

Obama, Barack, 160–61
Obama, Michelle, 21, 135
obesogenic environments, 209–20
    in Australia, 292
    changing defaults, 210–11
    corner stores, 214–15
    defined, 210
    farmers markets, 215–17
    fast food, 217–19
    food deserts, 212, 213, 214
Office of Experiment Stations, 11
Older Americans Act of 1965, 188–89
On Being Certain (Burton), 247
"On Food" (Hilaire), 235
One Eleuthera Foundation, 333, 334
organic farming and food, 6, 240
    controversy over, 228–29
    industrialization of, 6–7
    pesticides, 228–29
Organisation for Economic Co-operation
    and Development, 112
overstaffed behavior settings, 53
overweight and obesity, 255–56
    in Australia, 287, 292
    in Caribbean, 262–75
    controversy over causes of, 229–30
    costs of, 158–59, 210
    cultural and regional contexts, 257–58
    "double burden of malnutrition,"
        256–57, 263
    Farm-to-School programs, 259, 261
    food insecurity, 177, 181
    gender, 89, 99
    global health disparities, 110–12, 113
    global trends in, 255–57

government policy and regulation, 143–44, 146, 258, 260
measurement of, 256
nutrition transition, 256
prevalence of, 256
race and ethnicity, 87, 89, 90, 92–93, 177
socioeconomic status, 99
sugar-sweetened beverages, 158–59
Owen, June, 19
Oz, Mehmet (Dr. Oz), 236–37

Pacific Islanders and Native Hawaiians, 92
Parks and Recreation (TV program), 236–37
Partnership for a Healthier America (PHA), 135, 138, 161–62
"A Pattern for Daily Food Choices," 15
Peapod, 132
Pedestrian Question-What is Gluten? (video), 231
pesticides
contamination from, 6
controversy over, 228–29
organic farming and food, 228–29
rise of, 4–6
Pew Research center, 101–3, 240–41
PHA (Partnership for a Healthier America), 135, 138, 161–62
Photovoice methodology, 191–92
physical activity, 38–39
environmental impediments to, 66
nutrition transition, 256
relationship of behavioral design to, 65–67
PICO (population, intervention, comparator, outcome) approach, 39
Pima Indians, 90, 91, 101
Plank, Max, 241
Population Research for Identity and Disparities for Equality (PRIDE) case study, 97–98
"Port of Spain Declaration," 263–64
PRIDE (Population Research for Identity and Disparities for Equality) case study, 97–98

priming, 54–55
processed and prepared foods, 7, 9–11, 42–43, 101, 243
in Australia, 290–91, 292
Cold War-era, 10
critiques and attacks against, 11
multicultural marketing, 89
in schools, 259–61
World War II-era, 9–10
Progress Plaza, 211
Progressive Era, 18
Project for Public Spaces, 66
protein
animal protein consumption in Nigeria, 285–87, 303, 304–5
dietary guidelines, 12, 14, 42–43
public policy. *See* government policy and regulation
Pure Food and Drug Act of 1906, 7–8

race and ethnicity. *See also names of specific races and ethnicities*
advertising and multicultural marketing, 107
in Brazil, 108–9
census questions, 84–85, 86
chronic stress from discrimination, 104–5
cultural influences, 95–96
defining, 84–85
employment status, 103
food deserts, 213
food insecurity, 106, 174, 176, 177, 179–80
food marketing to children, 125–26
gender, 87, 89, 97
global, 108–9
health disparities, 85–92, 93–96, 97, 99–101, 103, 104–5, 106–9
health insurance coverage, 108
healthcare access, 108
historical contexts, 101
immigration and migration, 93–95
incarceration rates, 178–79
social determinants of health, 99
radio, 19

Ramsay, A., 298–99
rational actor model, 53, 55
Rausa, Alfio, 212
Recommended Dietary Allowances
    (RDAs), 12
red meat, 42–43
redlining, 101
reflective system, 54, 63
Reinvestment and Recovery Act of 2010, 211
renal disease, 87, 89, 90, 92
Research Training Institute for the National
    Commission on Hunger, 190
Richard R. Russell National School Lunch
    Act. *See* National School Lunch Act
    of 1946
Richmond, Julius, 33
Rodale, J. I., 6
Rolling Stone, 233
Roosevelt, Franklin Delano, 3–4, 9, 20
Round Up Ready Soybeans, 232–33
Rozin, Paul, 281–82, 284, 305–6
Rudd Center for Food Policy & Obesity, 107

Sacks, G., 258
salience, 54–55
"salmon bias" theory, 87–88
Satia-Abouta model of dietary acculturation,
    93–95, 106–7
School Breakfast Program (SBP), 135, 155,
    156, 187–88
School Feeding Law of 2009 (Brazil), 261
school food environment, 136, 259–61
    behavioral design, 69
    birthdays and special occasions, 133, 136
    Farm-to-School programs, 134–35, 138,
        259, 261
    food allergies, 134
    food marketing to children, 126
    local school wellness and nutrition
        policies, 133, 135–36
    school gardens, 238
school lunches and meal programs,
        20–21. *See also* National School Lunch
        Program; School Breakfast Program
    food assistance programs, 144–45, 148–49

New Deal-era, 20
    World War II-era, 20–21
School Meals Centre (SMC), 264, 265–66
School Nutrition Councils, 261
SCRI (Specialty Crop Research
    Initiative), 147–48
SDGs (United Nations Sustainable
    Development Goals), 285–87, 318
Section 8 (Housing Choice Voucher
    Program), 189
Sen, Amartya, 173
Senate Select Committee on Nutrition and
    Human Needs, 14, 150
Senior Farmers Market Nutrition Program
    (SFMNP), 148–49
seniors. *See* elderly and seniors
sexual orientation, 85. *See also* gender
    food insecurity, 178, 179–80
    health disparities, 97–98, 108
SFMNP (Senior Farmers Market Nutrition
    Program), 148–49
SFSP (Summer Food Service Program), 135,
    155, 187–88
sharecropping, 2, 3, 4–6
Shiva, Vandana, 249
Silent Spring (Carson), 6
Simmon, Amelia, 16
Sinclair, Upton, 7–8, 226
slavery, 2, 84
Smart Snacks in School Nutrition
    Standards, 136
SMC (School Meals Centre), 264, 265–66
SMP (Special Milk Program), 135
SNAP. *See* Supplemental Nutrition
    Assistance Program
social determinants of health, 99, 100
social ecological (socioecological) model,
    48, 53, 99, 100, 108, 142–43
social media
    blogs, 19–20
    social marketing, 18
socioeconomic status and class
    employment status, 103–4
    fast food, 218–19
    food accessibility, 106

food insecurity, 184–85
health disparities, 98–99, 101–4, 110
obesity, 210
sociofugal seating arrangements, 52
sociopetal seating arrangements, 52
soda. *See* sugar-sweetened beverages
space syntax theory, 52
Spam, 9–10
Special Milk Program (SMP), 135
Special Supplemental Nutrition Program for
    Women, Infants, and Children (WIC),
    14–15, 98–99, 135, 151–52, 154–55, 174,
    187–88, 217
Specialty Crop Research Initiative
    (SCRI), 147–48
SSBs. *See* sugar-sweetened beverages
St. Kitts-Nevis "farm to fork
    project," 264–75
    agricultural production and diversity,
        264, 268
    children's food consumption and
        nutrition intake, 264, 266, 270, 271, 272
    comparison of menus, 266, 267
    costs of, 272–73
    existing school feeding program, 264
    food insecurity issue, 271
    overweight and obesity issue, 270–71
    pillars of project, 264–66
    produce procurement, 264, 265–66, 269
St. Lucia, 333
States' Agritourism Statutes (Alexander and
    Rumley), 331
status quo bias, 54
Stiebeling, Hazel, 12
Storey, Maureen, 159
stroke. *See* cerebrovascular disease and stroke
Subway, 243
Sugar Busters Diet, 11
Sugar Coated (documentary), 230
sugar production and consumption. *See also*
    sugar-sweetened beverages
    in Australia, 287–90, 291–92
    Dietary Guidelines for Americans
        2015, 42–43
    in Japan, 292–95, 297

marketing to children, 125–26, 127
Pima Indians, 91
in Thailand, 298–302
sugar-sweetened beverages (SSBs)
    acculturation, and consumption of, 93–95
    in Australia, 292
    benefits vs. costs, 64–65
    controversy over, 230, 236–37
    corner stores, 215
    Dietary Guidelines for Americans
        2015, 42–43
    food marketing to children, 126
    in Japan, 293–94
    movement against soda, 236–37
    nutrition transition, 256
    St. Kitts-Nevis "farm to fork project," 264,
        266, 273
    Supplemental Nutrition Assistance
        Program, 152–53
    taxes on (soda taxes), 11, 62–63, 158–59,
        230, 236, 237, 301, 306
    in Thailand, 299–302, 306
Sullivan, Leon, 211–12
Summer Food Service Program (SFSP), 135,
    155, 187–88
Sunstein, Cass, 64
supermarket scorecard, 130–31
supermarkets. *See* food markets, groceries,
    and supermarkets
Supplemental Nutrition Assistance Program
    (SNAP), 14–15, 98–99, 152–53,
    154, 174
    block grants, 153
    coverage and benefits by, 149, 152,
        186–87, 188–89
    effect of dietary guidelines on, 151–52
    effect on food supply, 149
    eligibility, 148–49, 152
    employment status and, 186
    first-hand experiences with, 187
    funding, 146, 148–49, 153, 186–87
    future of, 149–50
    incentive-based approach, 153
    online food purchases, 132
    participation by college students, 194

Supplemental Nutrition Assistance
Program (*cont.*)
participation by formerly
incarcerated, 178–79
participation by immigrants, 177
participation by LGBTQ community, 178
proposed restrictions, 152–53
Surgeon General's Report on
Health Promotion and Disease
Prevention, 32–33
Survey of Consumer Finances, 101–3
sustainable agriculture, 322–24
sustainable behavior, 51–52
Swinburn, Boyd, 210, 258
systems model, 48

TANF (Temporary Assistance for Needy
Families), 153–54
Tang, 10
Taubes, Gary, 241
TEFAP (Emergency Food Assistance
Program), 148–49
Teicholz, Nina, 241
television, 16, 19, 107
Temporary Assistance for Needy Families
(TANF), 153–54
Thailand, 286, 298–302
cultural view of sweetness, 298, 301–2
food industry, 298
overview of, 285–87, 298
sugar consumption, 299–302
sugar production, 298–99
taxes on beverages, 301, 306
tea consumption, 299–301, 306
Theory of Planned Behavior, 53
Theory of Reasoned Action, 53
This is the End (film), 231
Thrifty Food Plan, 186–87
tobacco, 142–43, 235
Toy Freaks (video program), 128–29
transgender, 178, 179–80
transgenic seeds and crops, 232–33, 234–35.
See also genetically modified organisms
Travel Channel, 329

unboxing, 127–28
understaffed behavior settings, 53
UNICEF (United Nations International
Children's Emergency Fund),
109–10, 304
United Kingdom
agritourism, 319, 330
census questions, 84–85, 86
"mad cow" disease, 242
sugar consumption, 293–94
United Nations Economic and Social
Council, 195
United Nations International Children's
Emergency Fund (UNICEF),
109–10, 304
United Nations Sustainable Development
Goals (SDGs), 285–87, 318
University of West Indies (UWI), 264
upstream policies, 258–59, 260
urban agriculture, 6–7
U.S. Census of Agriculture, 320–21
U.S. Department of Agriculture (USDA).
*See also Dietary Guidelines for
Americans*; National School Lunch
Program; Supplemental Nutrition
Assistance Program
Administration for Children and
Families, 189
Agricultural Marketing Service, 331
agritourism, 331
Aunt Sammy radio show, 19
"Basic Four" food guide, 13–14
"Basic Seven" food guide, 12, 14
bulk foods purchased and distributed
by, 149
dietary guidelines, 11, 12–15, 16,
31–43, 150–51
Economic Research Service, 175–76
farm bill, 146
Farmer's Bulletin, 11
farmers markets, 215, 217
Food and Nutrition Service, 136
food deserts, 106
Food for Young Children, 11–12

food insecurity definition, 174–75
Healthy Food Financing Initiative, 214
Household Food Security Survey Module, 175–76, 266
mixed messages on nutrition, 43
MyPlate, 15
National Agricultural Worker survey, 6–7
National Commission on Hunger, 190
Nutrition Evidence Library, 39
Office of Experiment Stations, 11
online food purchases, 132
post-World War I, 2–3
pyramid guidelines, 15
safety of GMOs, 160–61
school lunches and meal programs, 21, 259–61
Smarter School Lunchroom movement, 136–37
Sustainable Agriculture Research and Education (SARE) program, 323
Thrifty Food Plan, 151–52
U.S. Department of Health and Human Services (HHS), 214
U.S. Department of Health, Education and Welfare, 32
U.S. Department of Housing and Urban Development (HUD), 189
U.S. Department of the Treasury, 214
U.S. Environmental Protection Agency (EPA), 160–61, 228
U.S. Food and Drug Administration (FDA), 7–8, 237
  "Generally Recognized as Safe" category of ingredients, 243
  nutrition labeling, 161
  safety of GMOs, 160–61
U.S. National Health Interview Survey, 98
U.S. Office of Management and Budget, 84–85
USDA. *See* National School Lunch Program; Supplemental Nutrition Assistance Program; U.S. Department of Agriculture
UWI (University of West Indies), 264

Value-Added Agricultural Product Market Development Grants program, 147–48
vegetables. *See* fruits and vegetables
vegetarianism, 6
Vermont Genetically Engineered Food Labeling Act, 161
Victory Gardens, 4, 5, 18, 20–21
vitamins and minerals
  dietary guidelines, 11, 12
  "double burden of malnutrition," 256–57
  invention of new foodstuffs, 9
  "vitamania," 12

Wall Street Journal, 228, 233
War Food Administration, 20–21
War on Poverty, 187–88
WFP (World Food Program), 261–62
Wheat Belly (Davis), 241–42
Wheatless Wednesdays, 18
WHO (World Health Organization), 108–9, 110, 256, 271–72, 287, 325
whole foods, 6, 14, 38–39, 42, 231
"Why Does Everyone Hate Monsanto?" (*Modern Farmer* article), 233
WIC (Special Supplemental Nutrition Program for Women, Infants, and Children), 14–15, 98–99, 135, 151–52, 154–55, 174, 187–88, 217
William F. Goodling Child Nutrition Reauthorization Act of 1998, 154–55
Williams Institute, 178
Winfrey, Oprah, 236–37
Wise Intelligent, 233
Witnesses to Hunger program, 171–73, 191–92, 196
women. *See* gender
Wonderbread, 11
Woodford Market Garden, 333
World Bank, 55–56
World Food Program (WFP), 261–62
World Health Organization (WHO), 108–9, 110, 256, 271–72, 287, 325
World Trade Organization (WTO), 256

World War I
    advertising, 18
    agricultural production during, 2
    federal agricultural aid, 2
    nationalized food systems, 9
World War II
    advertising, 18
    agricultural production during, 4
    food processing and distribution, 9–10

nutrition levels and dietary habits, 4
processed and prepared foods, 9–10
school lunches and meal programs, 20–21
WTO (World Trade Organization), 256

Yoruba people, 285–87, 302–3, 304–5
Young, Neil, 233
YouTube, 127–29
YouTube Kids app, 128–29